THE COMPLETE BOOK OF

NATURAL PAIN RELIEF

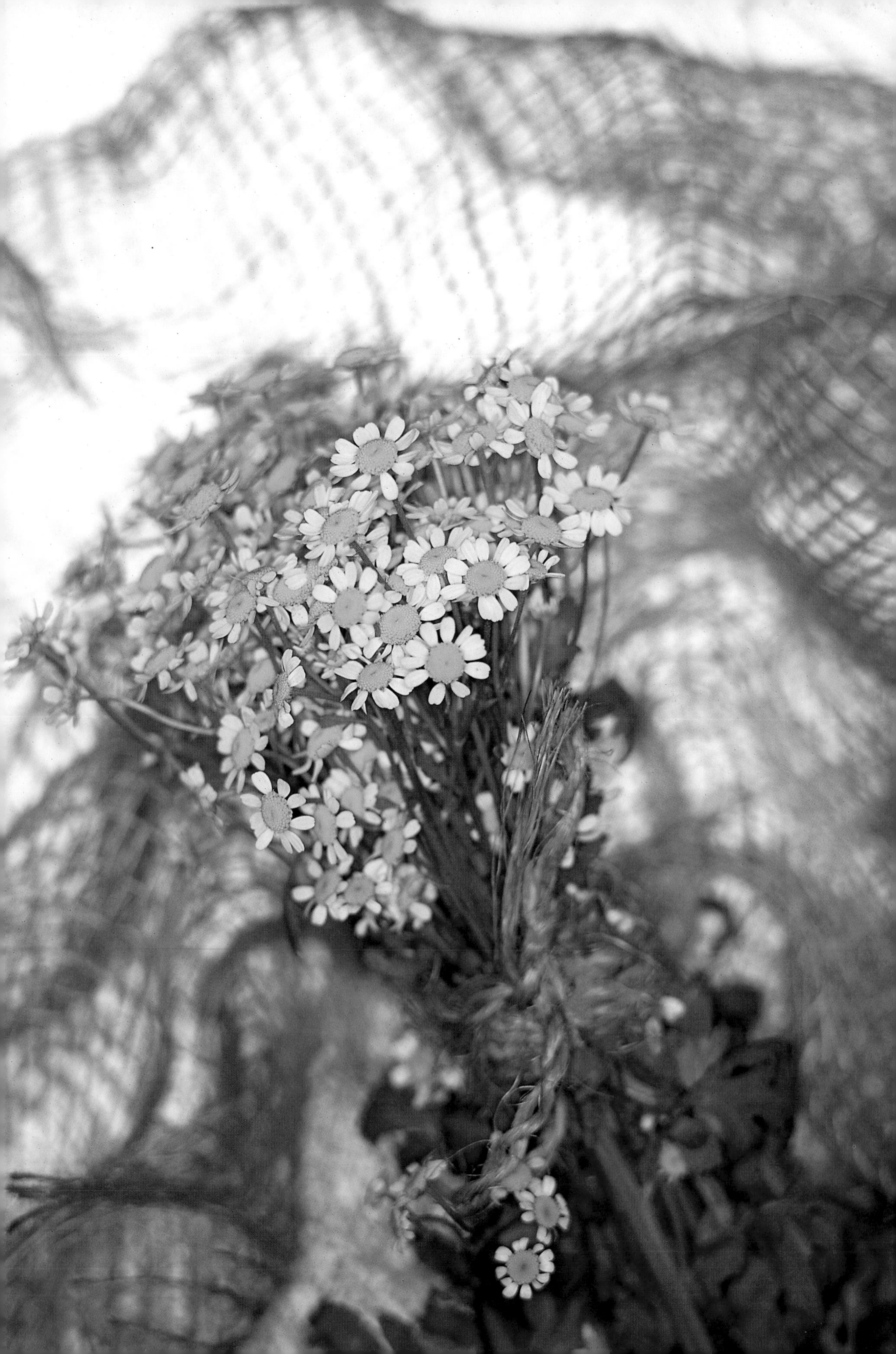

THE COMPLETE BOOK OF

NATURAL PAIN RELIEF

SAFE AND EFFECTIVE
SELF-HELP FOR
COMMON AILMENTS

RICHARD THOMAS

CONSULTANT: PETER ALBRIGHT M.D.

APPLE

A QUARTO BOOK

Published by the Apple Press
6 Blundell Street
London N7 9BH

ISBN 1-85076-983-4

This book was designed and produced by
Quarto Publishing plc
The Old Brewery
6 Blundell Street
London N7 9BH

Senior editor *Michelle Pickering*
Senior art editor *Anne Fisher*
Text editor *Mary Senechal*
Designer *Sheila Volpe*
Illustrators *Vana Haggerty, John Woodcock*
Photographers *Bruce Mackie, Colin Bowling, Paul Forrester*
Picture researcher *Henny Letailleur*
Art director *Moira Clinch*
Assistant art director *Penny Cobb*
Editorial director *Pippa Rubinstein*

Typeset in Great Britain by Central Southern Typesetters, Eastbourne
Manufactured in Singapore by Bright Arts Pte Ltd
Printed in China by Leefung-Asco Printers Ltd

This book is not intended as a substitute for the advice of a health care professional. The reader should regularly consult a health practitioner in matters relating to health, particularly with respect to symptoms that may require diagnosis or medical attention. It is recommended that readers consult qualified practitioners before embarking on a course of self-treatment.

FOREWORD

The management of pain has been a serious consideration in the fields of medicine and healing for as long as people have been feeling pain. In the past few decades, however, the issues around controlling pain have come into sharper focus, spawning a great deal of research into, and understanding of, the nature and mechanisms of pain. There are several reasons for this—the violence of the 20th century, the rising concern over the effects of pollution, the increasing longevity of the population, and the growing stresses of life in the 20th century. Partly as a result of this and the increasing sophistication of scientific methods of research, there has been considerable development of pharmacologic agents for the suppression of pain; this has in turn produced a new set of problems to be dealt with, including toxicity and addiction.

An important part of the concept of holistic medicine is that in the human individual there is unity of body, mind, and emotions. All of these aspects are inextricably interwoven, so that what affects one aspect affects all the others as well. It follows then that if pain is experienced because of a physical injury, for example, such experience reverberates throughout the mind and emotions, as well as the body itself. It also means that the healing of the physical wound does not necessarily produce an immediate cessation of the echoes extending into the other aspects of our being. These interactions have only been partially studied with the methods that are presently available; we are only beginning to understand the full meaning of such connections.

The ambitious book you are now reading takes on the formidable task of presenting this complex subject in a readable form. Further, it aims to provide the reader with the means to take effective action in the face of all of the various guises in which pain appears, from toothache through the anguish of arthritis to that of deep emotional distress. A wide variety of helpful therapies are discussed in relation to specific ailments, and in a special section focusing on each of the therapies in turn. Having read this book very carefully while assisting in a small way in its production, I feel that Richard Thomas and the publisher have had considerable success in producing a very clear and accurate book. It is a book that achieves the breadth as well as the depth of detail required to encompass virtually all that is "out there" to assist the person in pain. At the same time, the material is made so accessible through its very good organization that a great proportion of the reading public will be able to realize its benefits easily. It is a resource that I hope will be readily available in medical offices and pain clinics as well as in the homes of pain sufferers. If so, the book will have made a significant contribution to the current literature of health and healing.

Peter Albright M.D.

CONTENTS

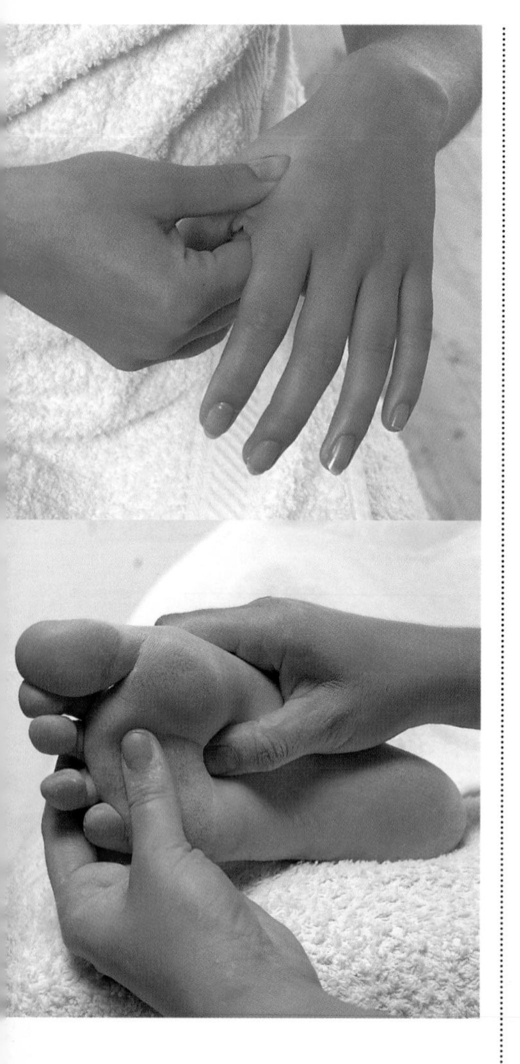

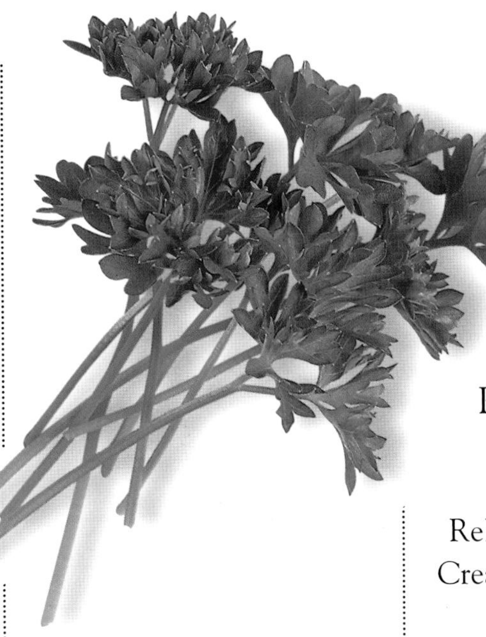

THE THERAPIES

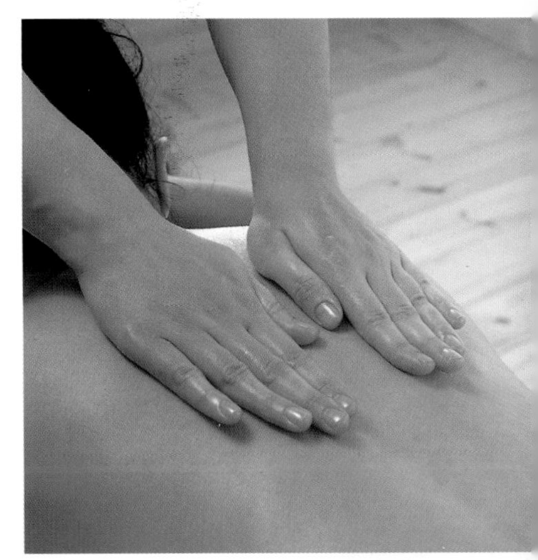

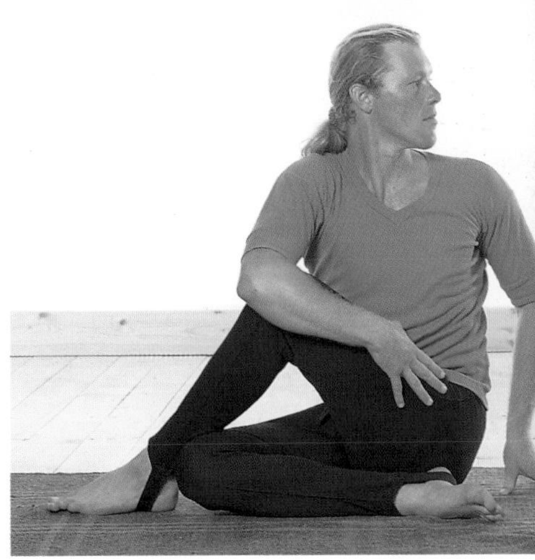

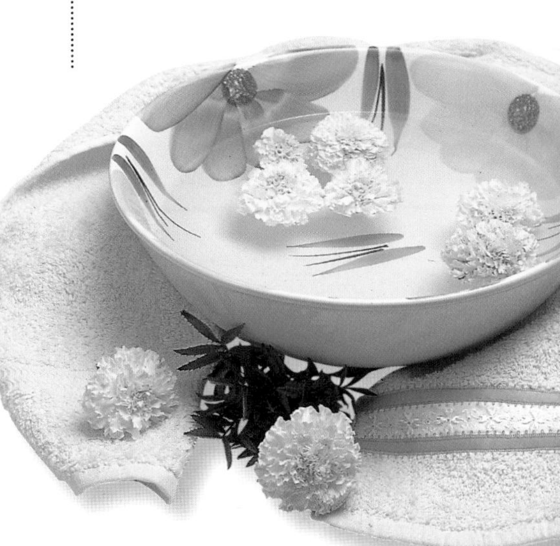

INTRODUCTION

Everyone has suffered pain at one time or another. This is not just because pain is an almost inevitable result of injuring yourself—which virtually everyone does at some stage—but also because aches and pains are a normal part of the great majority of illnesses. And most people get sick at some point in their lives. So whether the pain is a mild ache or an agony, we all know what it is and what it feels like. Or do we?

The truth is that most people only know what pain feels like for them. Because one of the most curious things about pain is that although everyone has felt pain at some time in their lives, pain is elusive and individual. No two people feel it in quite the same way: it is often very hard to describe, it varies in intensity, and it can come and go. Sometimes an action that we have performed for years without any trouble at all can become painful, while another that used to cause a problem no longer does.

So the real mystery about pain is not what it is—we all know it hurts, and we all wish it would go away!—but why it is so individual, indeterminate, and unpredictable. Few of us realize, for example, that pain is not felt in the same way by everyone, even when it comes from the same cause. A bee sting can cause slight discomfort to one person but be excruciatingly painful, and even life-threatening, to another. The reason for this variable quality is the unique mosaic of each person's life. We respond differently to the same stimulii—and what one person can withstand for long periods, another will succumb to almost at once. One thing is clear, however: pain has a purpose. Unpleasant and unwelcome though it may be, it is there for a reason. Pain is a message from the body to the conscious mind that something is wrong.

Accidents are the most obvious and common cause of acute physical pain, but are usually the easiest to treat.

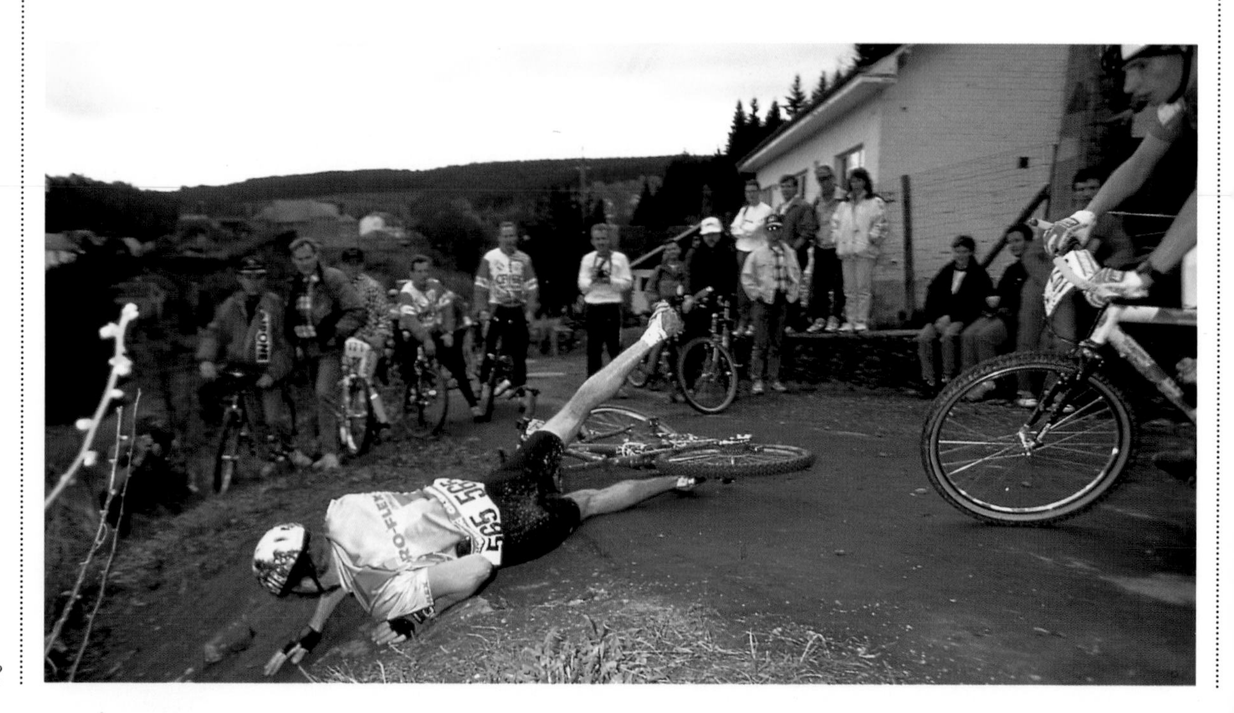

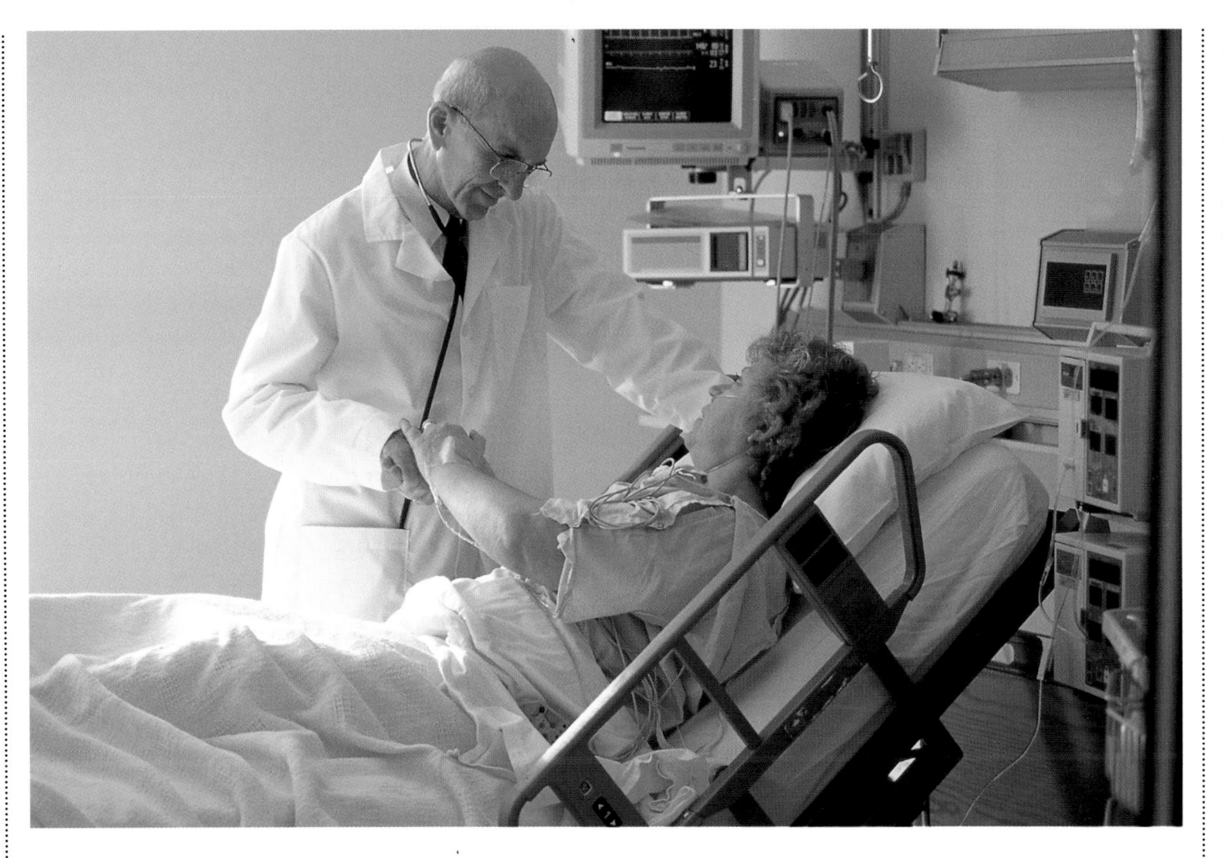

Long-term pain is known as "chronic" pain by doctors and is much harder to treat effectively than short-term, "acute" pain.

Medically, pain is categorized in two fundamental ways. It is either acute pain or chronic pain. Acute pain is immediate, "here-and-now" pain. It is the sort of pain we experience from a fall or bang, from a sprain or break, from inflammation and infection. It is emergency pain. In other words, it warns us quickly and directly that there is a problem and we should do something about it. Chronic pain, by contrast, is long-term pain. Unlike acute pain, which normally eases off and disappears in time, chronic pain has been described as "pain without a purpose." This is not really true, because all pain is a signal that something in the body is not right. But chronic pain is less a sign of threat requiring speedy action than a symptom that simply will not go away. Worse, it can often be inexplicable: there is no obvious reason for it. It is there, constant and nagging, and remains despite everything you do to make it go. Severe chronic pain, as its unfortunate victims know only too well, is its own special kind of hell.

Both acute and chronic pain usually refer to physical pain of one kind or another. But there is another sort of pain, not nearly so well recognized but just as real to many people and now much better understood by doctors and scientists. It is psychological pain. That is the pain and anguish we can feel through our mind and emotions. It is the sort of pain that we can experience, for example, from bereavement or the ending of a relationship (we call it "heartache"), from

Coping with chronic pain

The following advice will not only help victims cope with chronic (long-term) pain but "make life worth living again," according to Dr. Chris Wells, founder and former director of Britain's pioneering and world-famous Pain Research Institute in Liverpool.

- *Never give in to pain, and never allow your pain to become an excuse.*
- *Cultivate positive thinking and actions, by setting goals and getting out and about.*
- *Take regular, gentle exercise.*
- *Learn techniques for deep relaxation, such as meditation, yoga, and biofeedback.*
- *Seek the support of other sufferers doing positive things for their pain.*
- *Aim to come off pain-blocking drugs eventually—pain-blocking drugs can stop the release of natural painkilling chemicals in the body and also stop improvements being felt.*

CAUTION *Do not stop taking pain-blocking drugs without talking first with your doctor.*

redundancy, homelessness, or other apparent forms of rejection and loss of love or of feeling "wanted."

Psychological pain can lead to depression, an all-encompassing description that can extend from feeling a little "down" to such extreme mental and emotional agony that its victims want to end their lives. In depression, mental and emotional pain are usually closely interlinked, but mental pain has its own pain "subset" that can involve yet another type of pain. Nightmares, fears, and phobias are common examples of mainly mental pain, while at the extreme end of the spectrum are obsessions and addictions (to food, drink, drugs, or sex, for example).

Of course, physical pain and psychological pain are closely linked. Physical pain can be mentally and emotionally painful just as psychological pain can lead, we now know, to physical pain. This knowledge grew out of the burgeoning science of mind–body medicine, or what specialists call *psychoneuroimmunology* (PNI), that originated in the United States in the 1980s. PNI is the science of how the mind can help the body heal (and, equally, how the body can affect the mind). It is now known that "mind power"—using the power of the imagination and of thought—promotes the release of chemicals in the brain that actually influence the way the body responds, whether for good or ill. So, for example, positive thought—thinking positively about yourself and your surroundings—has been shown to promote chemicals that assist the healing process, while negative thinking hinders or reduces that process.

REFERRED PAIN

This book offers practical and effective ways of dealing with both physical and psychological causes of pain, but one of the most important features of pain is the phenomenon of "referred pain." This is the term used by doctors and other experts for pain that is felt some way from where it actually originates. In other words, the site of the pain is not necessarily the actual source of the pain. A headache, for instance, can be caused by an infection in the lungs, by digestive or circulatory problems, and by prescription drugs, as well as by a blow to the skull or by depression.

Clearly, it is important to identify the cause of the pain in order to be able to treat it effectively, and that means being able to locate the source. But if the

Pain in the back is not only one of the most severe and disabling forms of pain commonly experienced, but also one of the hardest to recover from quickly.

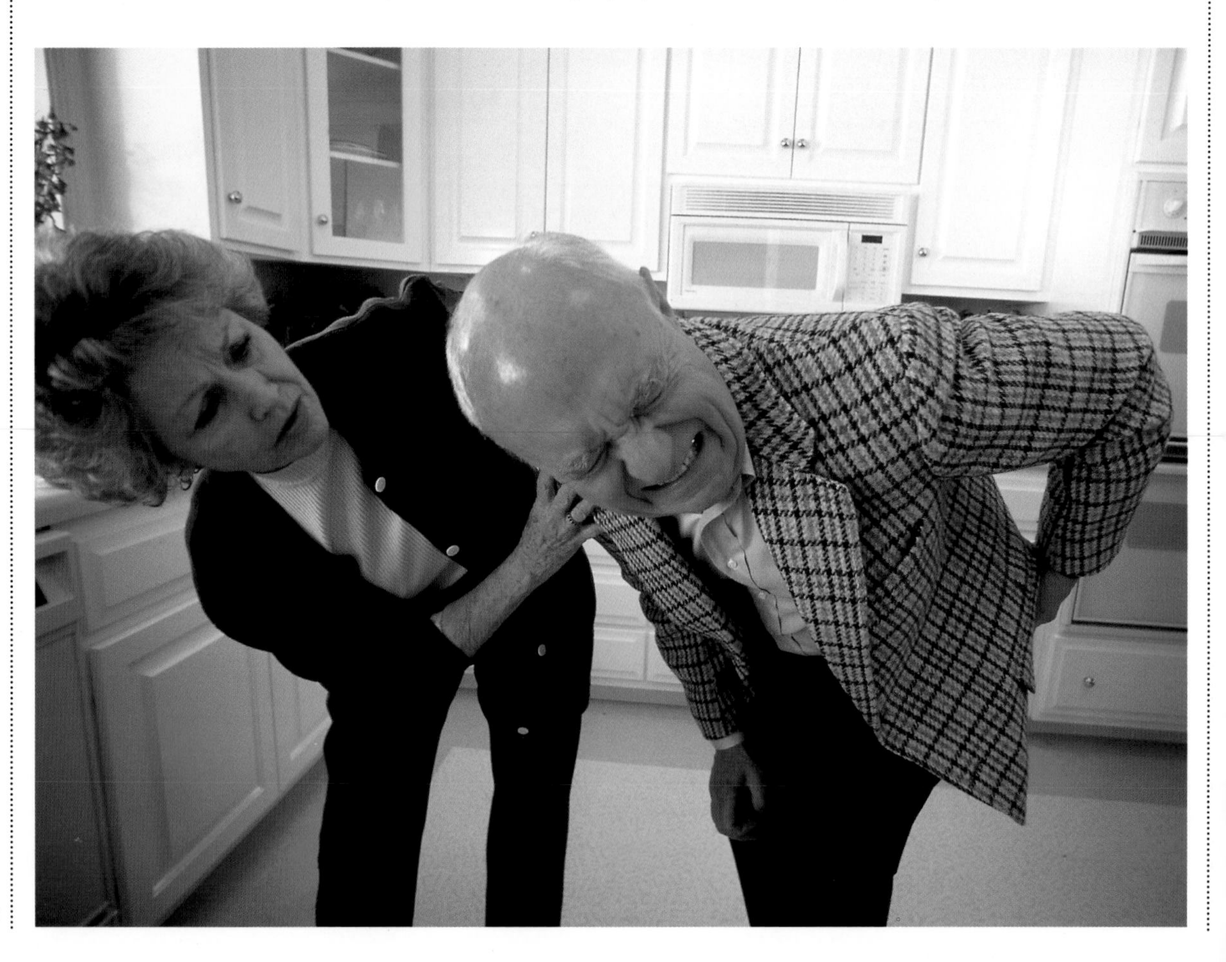

source is not where the pain is actually being felt, identification becomes difficult. This key phenomenon is little understood by nonspecialists, and is the main reason for mistakes in people's treatment of their own pain. Such mistakes could even be fatal—pain in the right shoulder, for example, is one symptom of abdominal cancer—so an important aspect of this book is to indicate very clearly when pain could be referred pain, and when to seek professional, usually medical, advice if this phenomenon is suspected.

HOW AND WHY WE FEEL PAIN

How and why we feel pain, and what the body does when it feels pain, have only recently been understood in any detail. One of the most important breakthroughs came in 1965, when US psychologist Ronald Melzack and British doctor Patrick Wall came up with what became known as the "gate theory."

Before Melzack and Wall's gate theory, pain was even more of a mystery than it is now. No one really knew the mechanism by which it was felt (despite a great deal of scientific research into the subject), it could not be measured, and it meant so many different things to different people at different times that treatment was an almost desperate hit-and-miss affair, sometimes depending as much on luck as on the judgment of an individual doctor.

What was clear was that nerves and the nerve receptors at nerve endings, designed to sense and feel, were involved, but that pain was not a sense (like touch, taste, smell, sight, and hearing) in the strict meaning of the word. Even though pain is relayed to the brain (via the spinal cord) by the nerves, it seems to be more of an emotion than a sense. For example, if you hit your thumb with a hammer hard enough to damage the skin, bones, and tissue, the nerve receptors in the thumb flash a message to your brain that triggers the brain within a split second not only to make you drop the hammer and suck your damaged thumb but also, in most cases, to leap around, yell, and cuss, all at the same time! Stranger still, you may cry, feel angry, or even laugh as a result. And that reaction may well be different every time it happens.

This succession of almost miraculous tricks happens on a mechanical level because of a special "switching station" or "gate," in the spinal cord near where it enters the skull. This gate controls messages going in and out of the brain. The brain reacts to pain signals not only by making the body take action—to run, jump, yell, rub, or cry—but also by releasing certain chemicals into the bloodstream known as hormones, principally endorphins and enkephalins.

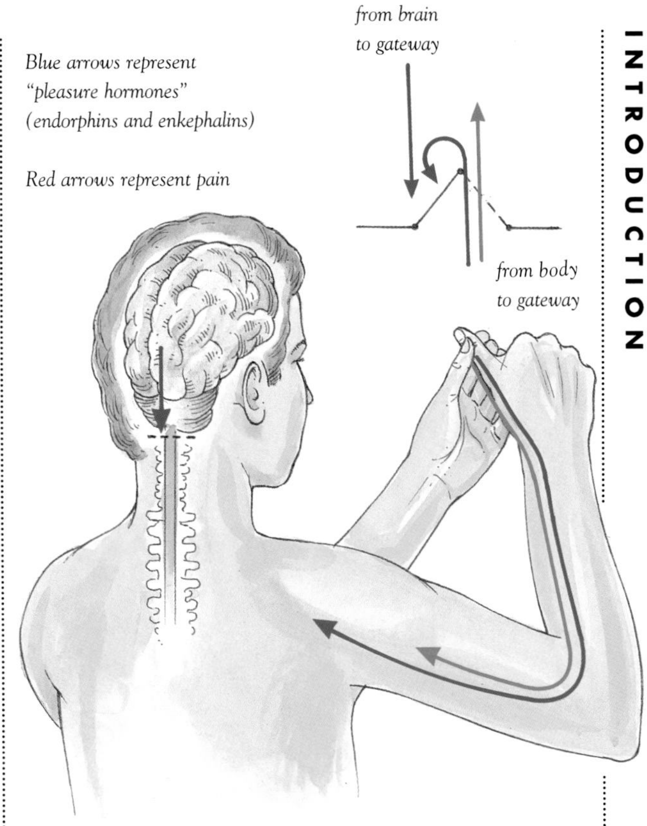

The Melzack–Wall gate theory argues that "pleasure hormones" produced by a positive mental attitude and by the physical reaction to pain (such as "rubbing it better") help to reduce that pain by reaching the "gateway" into the brain first and partially closing it.

Endorphins and enkephalins are especially important because they are the body's natural painkillers, sometimes also known as "pleasure hormones." They partially (not usually completely) block the "pain pathway," so that pain messages do not get through to the brain. The amount of pain that is felt depends on how many endorphins and enkephalins are produced: a lot of endorphins and enkephalins usually means only a little pain is experienced, while fewer of these hormones mean much more pain.

The crucial factor is the amount of pain that gets through the gate. The same degree of damage can cause different measures of pain in different people depending entirely on how much "pain message" passes the gate. This, in turn, varies from person to person according to how many pleasure hormones they produce. Positive feelings, such as love and warmth, can produce pleasure hormones in the brain, just as pleasure hormones produce feelings of love and warmth. Melzack and Wall's key discovery was that pleasurable feelings, such as love and warmth, travel to the brain faster than unpleasant feelings, such as pain. This is because the two types of

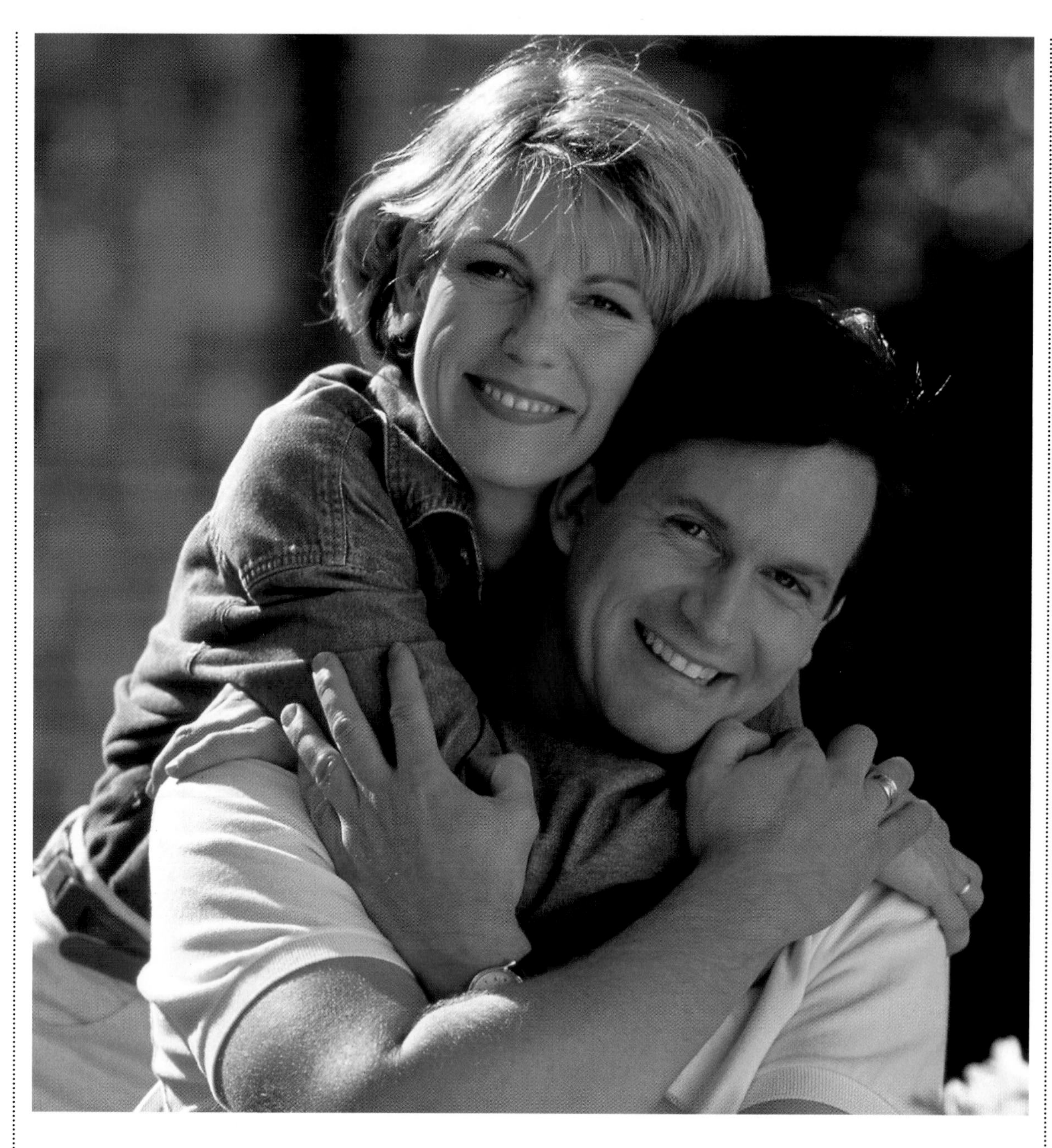

Feeling happy and positive can help overcome pain by producing chemicals in the brain that counter the effects of pain.

feeling travel along different nerve pathways: pleasant feelings travel along "wider" pathways than unpleasant ones, and so move quicker. Pleasure, in other words, seems to be able to reduce pain by getting through the pain gate first and partially closing it, so helping to keep pain out. Thus, in simple terms, Pain=Emotion= Hormone release=Pain control.

This information not only signified the greatest advance in our understanding of pain but, of course, in its treatment also. And it posed a mighty challenge to conventional treatment of pain. Before 1965, the standard medical treatment for pain was drugs, drugs, and more drugs. To a large extent, drugs are still the conventional treatment of choice for pain—and especially for the treatment of severe chronic pain—but the gate theory opened another gate: the gate to pain treatment based on gentler, safer, and often more effective approaches than strong synthetic drugs with powerful, and sometimes dangerous, side-effects. In particular, it opened the way for the so-called "natural" approaches that form the basis of this book.

NATURAL THERAPIES AND PAIN

Research during the last 30 years has confirmed the fundamentally important fact that our mental and emotional state affects the way we feel pain. Depression and

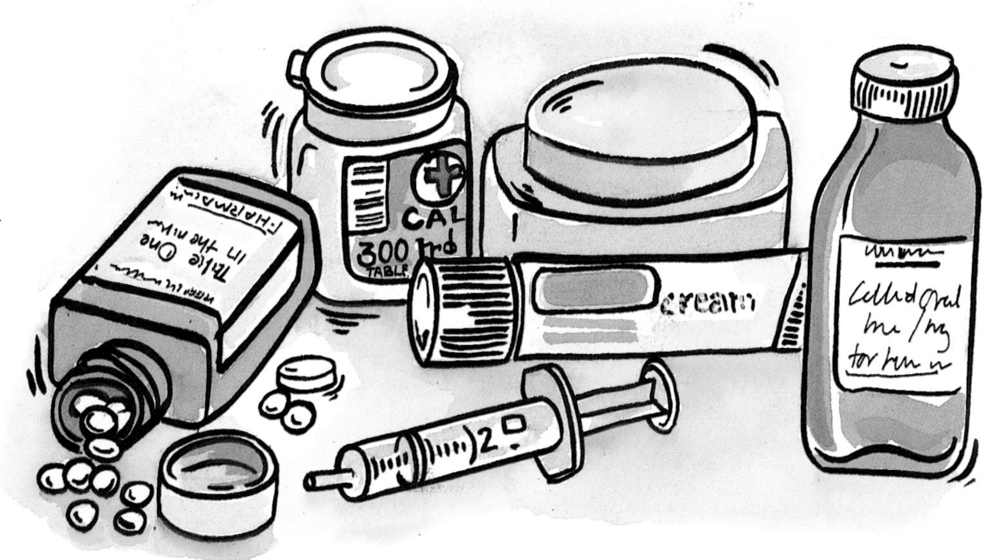

Drugs are still the most common conventional treatment for pain but they can cause additional problems.

simply *expecting* to feel pain opens the pain gate more, while thinking (and acting) positively closes it. So if you are "blue" and depressed, you are likely to feel pain more than if you remain upbeat.

Drugs, of course, also help close the pain gate, and this is the basis of conventional drug therapy in the treatment of pain. But drugs neither cure nor, usually, remove all the pain. Worse, they have the twin disadvantages that they can reduce the body's ability to counteract pain by diminishing its ability to produce endorphins and enkephalins, and they can also be addictive. This means that victims, particularly of severe chronic pain, can become habituated to pain as well as suffering from such unpleasant side-effects as weakness and dizziness. It is almost as if they become so preoccupied with their pain that it controls their lives. The result is obvious, and tragic: a downward spiral of pain, drugs, more pain, and more drugs. Instead of getting better, or feeling better, the patient just gets helplessly worse and worse. The tragedy is that it need not be this way. There are gentler and safer approaches that can help. Such approaches are those known loosely as "natural therapies." (Other terms you will hear are "alternative," "complementary," and "holistic," all covering the same ideas.)

Treatment of pain is one area where natural therapies are coming particularly strongly into their own. As well as thinking positively, other factors that close the pain gate are exercise and deep relaxation. All three are part of such classic mind–body techniques as yoga, tai chi, and meditation, along with the more modern methods of visualization and biofeedback. There are some two dozen natural approaches for pain treatment. They include acupuncture, acupressure, hydrotherapy, aromatherapy, massage, reflexology, hypnotherapy, herbal medicine, homeopathy, psychotherapy and counseling, sound and color therapy, creative arts therapy, and healing. What all these approaches have in common is that, unlike conventional drug therapy, they aim to work *with* the body, mind, and emotions rather than against them. Though research into the effectiveness of many of these therapies is still in its infancy, all those described in this book have shown evidence that they work to reduce, alleviate, and in some cases remove pain completely. They can all be used safely by following the instructions outlined in this book. There are a few cautions, however.

Massaging yourself, or better still being massaged by someone else, is one of the best and quickest ways of alleviating pain.

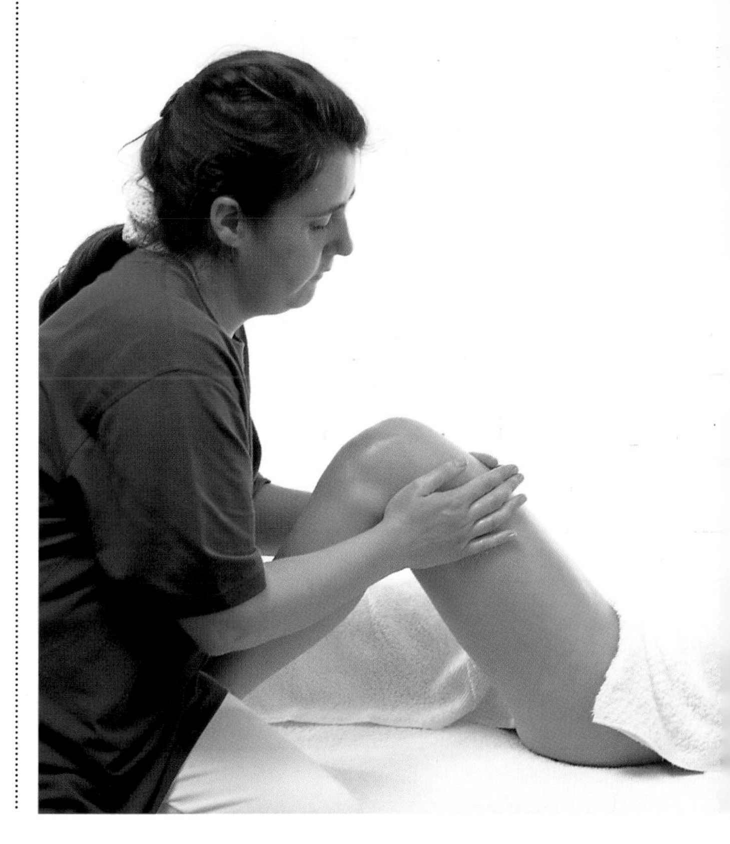

First, you must remember that your pain is individual and specific to you. Therefore what works for others may, unluckily, not work for you (of course it may work even better!). But tailoring treatment to you as an individual is the most important of the principles behind effective natural pain relief. That may mean seeking out the help of a pain clinic or a specialist in natural medicine, such as a qualified natural therapist or naturopath, to get you started on the right track.

Second, it often takes time for many therapies to work fully. This is especially true for chronic (long-term) pain, and it may take perseverance to reverse the trends and habits of years of pain, not least in how you see yourself in relation to the pain (does the pain control you, or do you control the pain?).

Third, it is important to be sure that you have correctly identified the cause of the pain. Accurate self-diagnosis is vital. In most acute cases, the cause is obvious—a cut, bang, scald, or sprain, for example—but

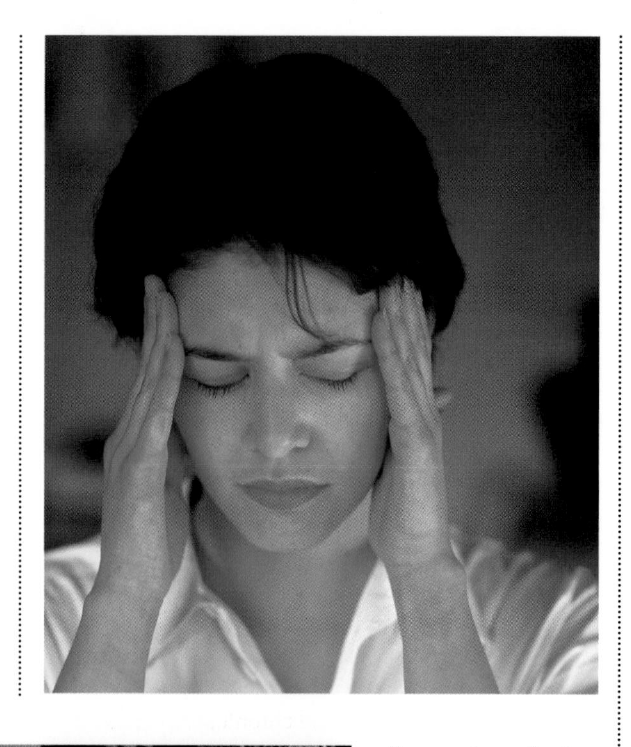

Everyone has suffered pain at one time or another, the most common being headache. However, the cause of the headache can vary, from a bang on the head to an infection in the lungs, and it is important to be sure of this cause before beginning treatment.

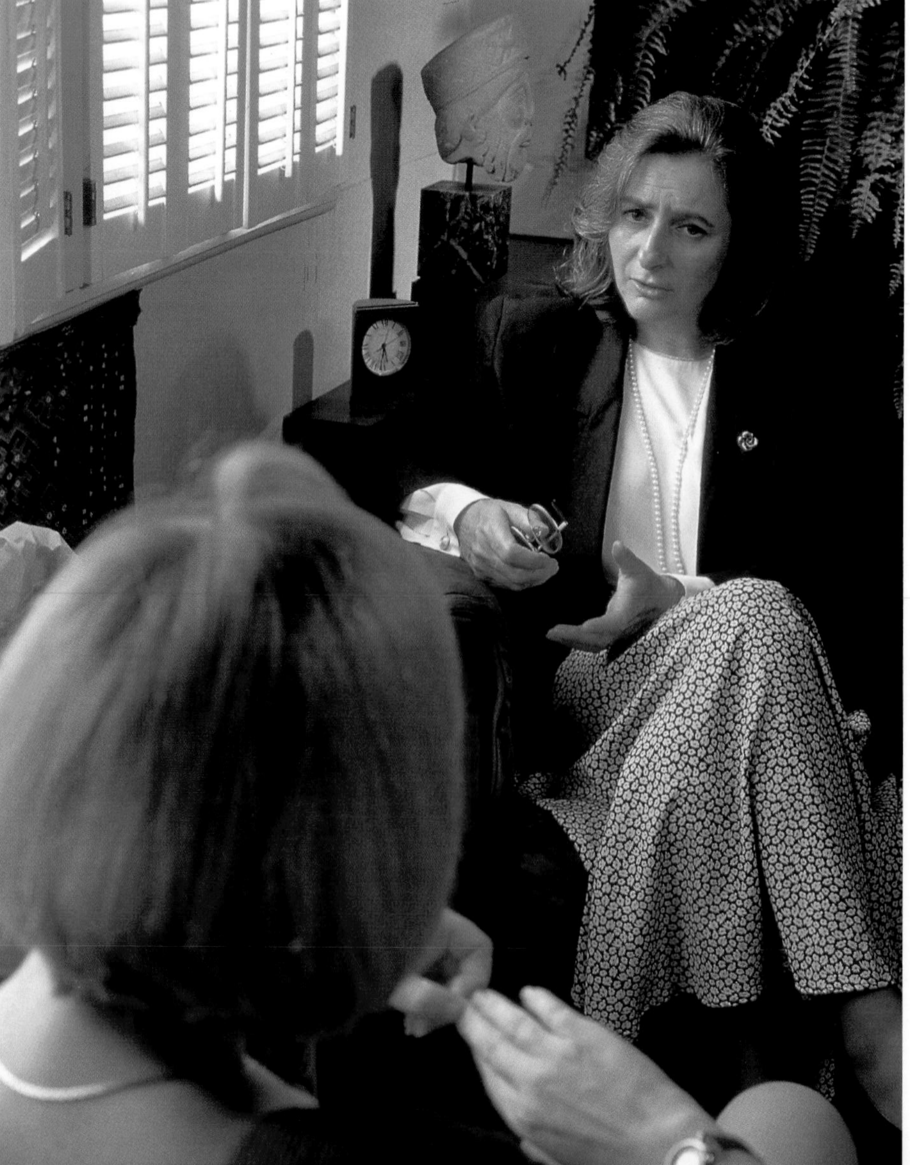

Talking to a trained listener, such as a psychotherapist or counselor, can be a most effective way to overcome mental and emotional pain.

sometimes it is not, and wrong diagnosis can result in wrong treatment. At best, mistaken treatment may do no harm, but it is unlikely to help either. At worst, it may not only do damage but also delay correct treatment. In rare cases, such delay can be fatal. So if in doubt, consult a qualified practitioner, such as your family doctor, before starting.

Remember also that therapies effective for acute pain are not necessarily suitable for chronic pain, and vice versa. A herbal remedy or a massage with an essential oil may help ease an acute headache but do little for chronic arthritis. Equally, emotional pain—whether immediate or long-term—is more likely to be helped by psychological therapies, such as relaxation and meditation, than by acupressure or TENS (transcutaneous electrical nerve stimulation).

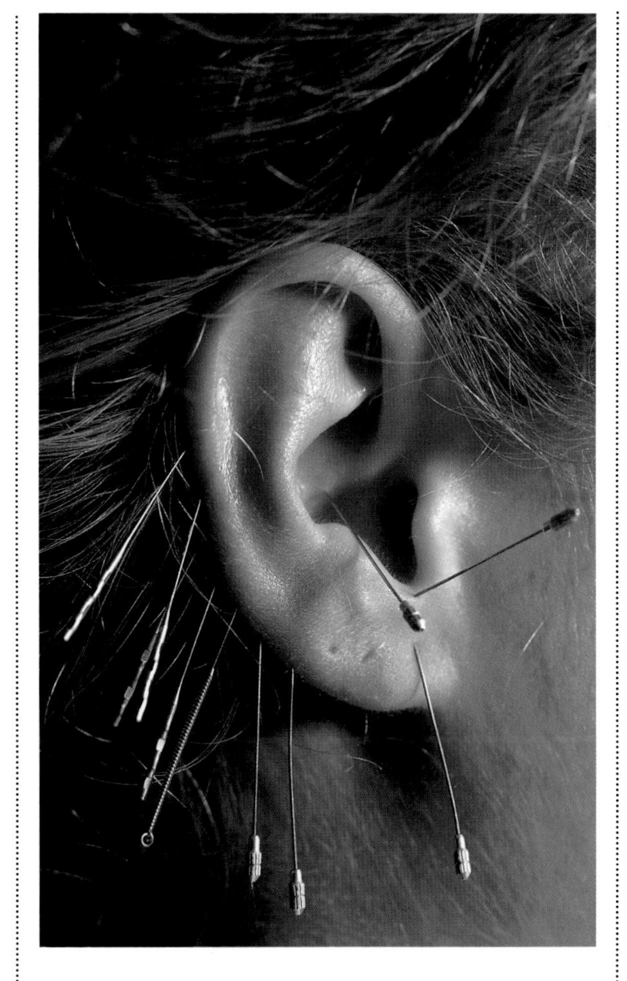

Acupuncture—here shown applied to special points in the ear—is a highly effective oriental form of pain relief now in increasing use in western hospitals and clinics.

ATTITUDES TO PAIN

This book helps you to help yourself—and for most forms of pain, both acute and chronic, physical and psychological, there is usually a great deal you can do for yourself. Helping you to realize that you can do things for yourself and take control of your life again is one of the most significant things this book seeks to achieve. But having the right attitude to pain is important.

Reject outright any idea that your pain is your "fault" or somehow a "punishment" for something. Any notion that the pain (or the disease it represents) is the result of karma, for example, or the act of a vengeful God, or equivalent, should be dismissed out-of-hand. It is not only an unjustified idea but, much more seriously, it could produce negative feelings of guilt or anger that will seriously interfere with the healing process.

Again, some people with chronic pain can become so addicted to their pain that they come to accept it as a sort of support, and even miss it if it goes: in other words, they

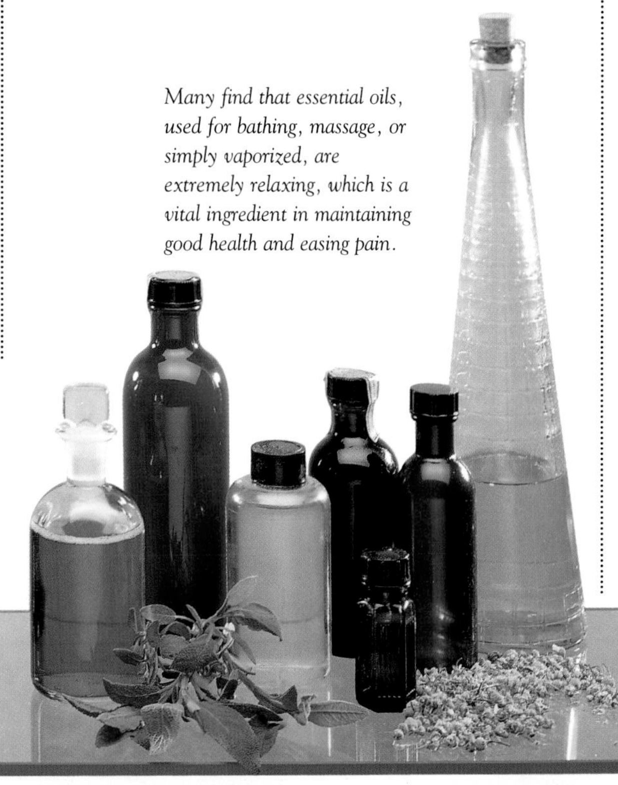

Many find that essential oils, used for bathing, massage, or simply vaporized, are extremely relaxing, which is a vital ingredient in maintaining good health and easing pain.

develop a need for it. Equally, there are people who will do anything to suppress and deny their pain. Pain, in these situations, has become either a "friend" or an "enemy." But it is neither. It is a natural process that is no more nor less than a sign to alert us that something is wrong. Working with and through pain is not only possible, particularly using the natural therapies described in this book, but can be strengthening and life-enhancing if approached with the right attitude.

Using the therapies in this book not only offers you a wealth of choices for effective action in combating pain—action that may enable you to overcome your particular pain—but, most importantly of all, it allows you to reclaim your life and start living again.

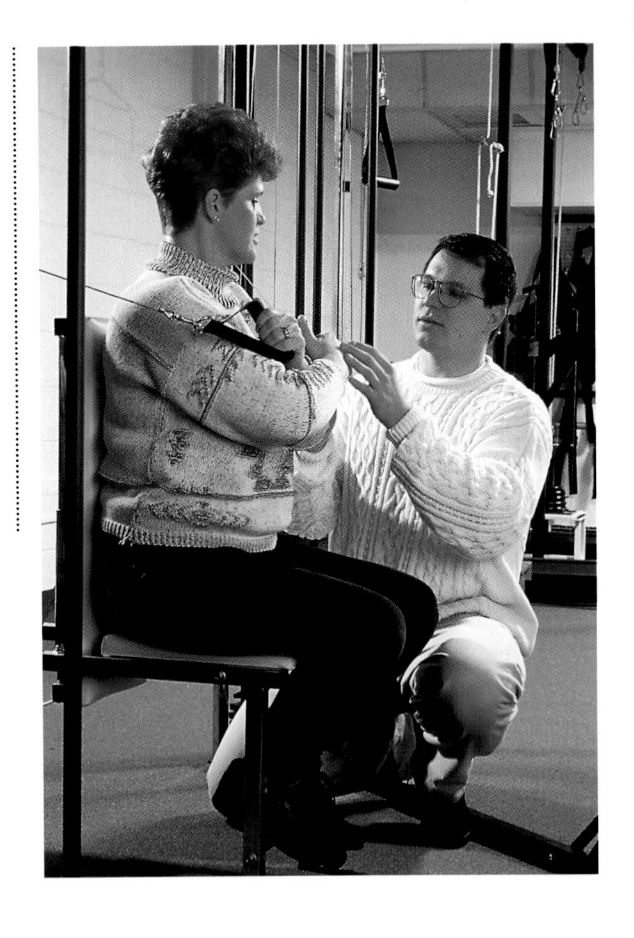

Physical aids applied by trained therapists have a role in helping people with certain types of pain-causing disability.

Regular exercise, particularly in older age, helps prevent aches and pains and aids recovery from them as well.

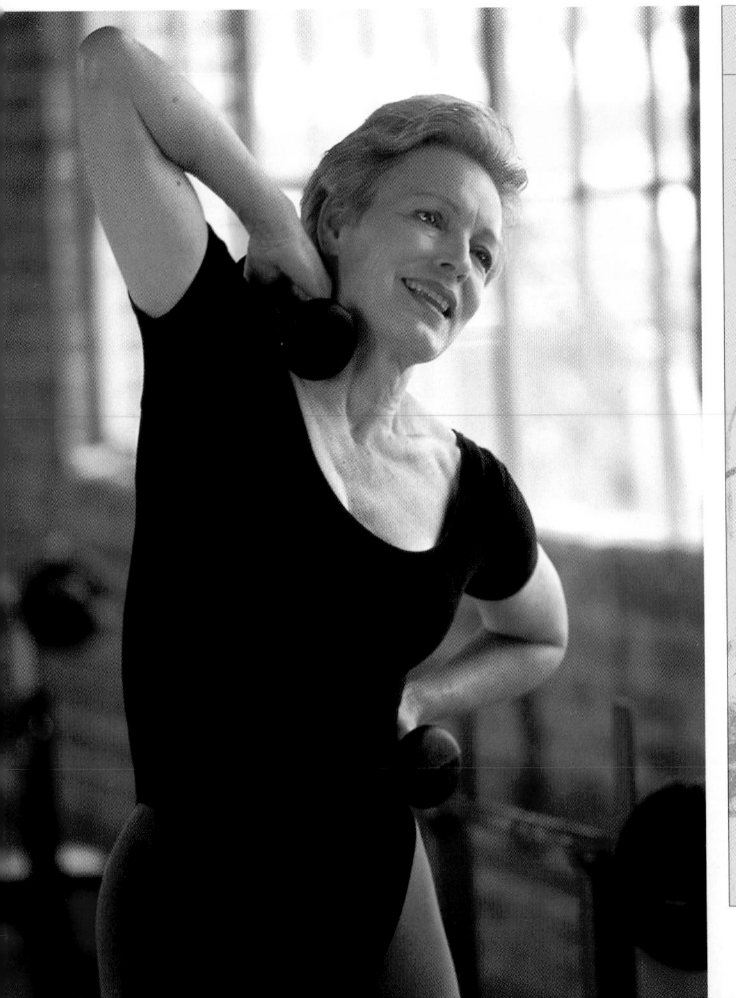

Caution: limits to self-help

Though there is a wide range of effective natural therapies for pain, some natural approaches are beyond the scope of self-help.

- *It is positively NOT recommended that you treat yourself with acupuncture or get a friend to do it. Acupuncture is now widely accepted as a powerful form of pain control, but it must be done by a qualified practitioner.*
- *Do not attempt the severe physical manipulation of the spine that can help back, leg, and neck pain. In untrained hands, techniques such as "high velocity thrusting" and neck "cracking," carried out by chiropractors and some osteopaths, can cause permanent and disabling damage—even paralysis.*
- *The same caution applies to the therapeutic use of most forms of hypnosis or psychotherapy for the treatment of mental and emotional pain.*

In each of the above cases, seek treatment always and only from a fully qualified specialist. These cautions are, of course, mostly common sense and should not discourage you from finding ways to help yourself.

HOW TO USE THIS BOOK

The book is divided into two sections: the "Ailments" and the "Therapies." The Ailments is subdivided into categories according to the site of the pain; for example, pain in the chest and lung area, the back and neck region, the skin, and so on. There is also a special section on first aid for cases of emergency. Within each of these subdivisions you will find a brief overview of the types of problems that may be encountered in that region, a description of the symptoms of each of those ailments, and information on the various natural remedies that may bring relief. Recipes, dosages, and methods of application are outlined as appropriate, together with warnings and cautions for when you should seek medical attention.

The Therapies section concentrates on each of the therapies in turn, giving a description of each one together with any basic techniques or other information that will be necessary in order to use that therapy. For example, in massage, some basic massage strokes are illustrated; in nutritional therapy, a helpful chart outlines the recommended daily supplements.

Both sections also feature an "at-a-glance" chart, for quick reference, so that you can find the appropriate ailments and therapies easily.

The Ailments

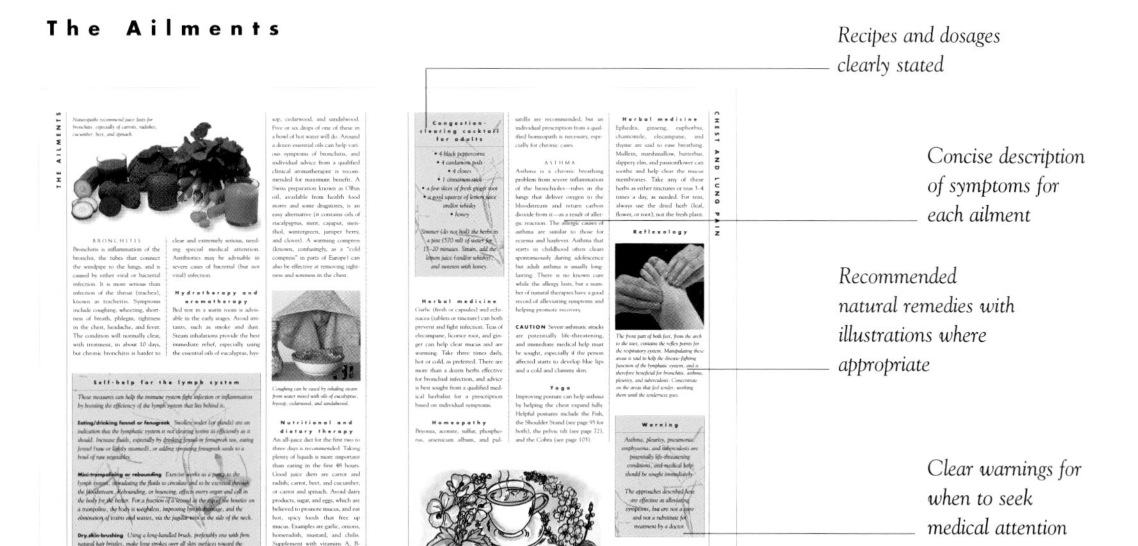

The Therapies

Detailed description of each therapy

Cross-references to the ailments for which each therapy is most appropriate

Basic techniques described and illustrated

Useful charts for quick reference

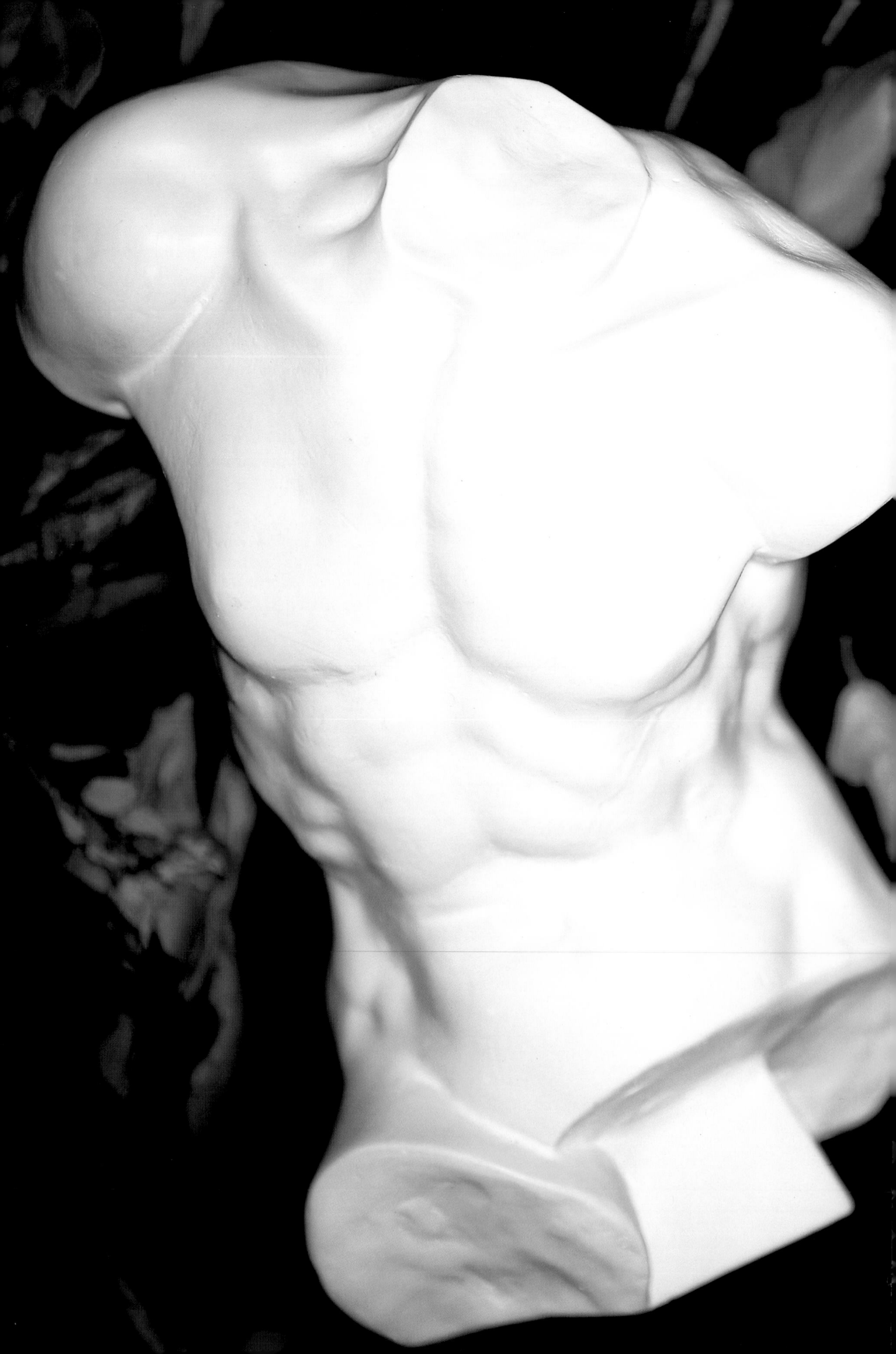

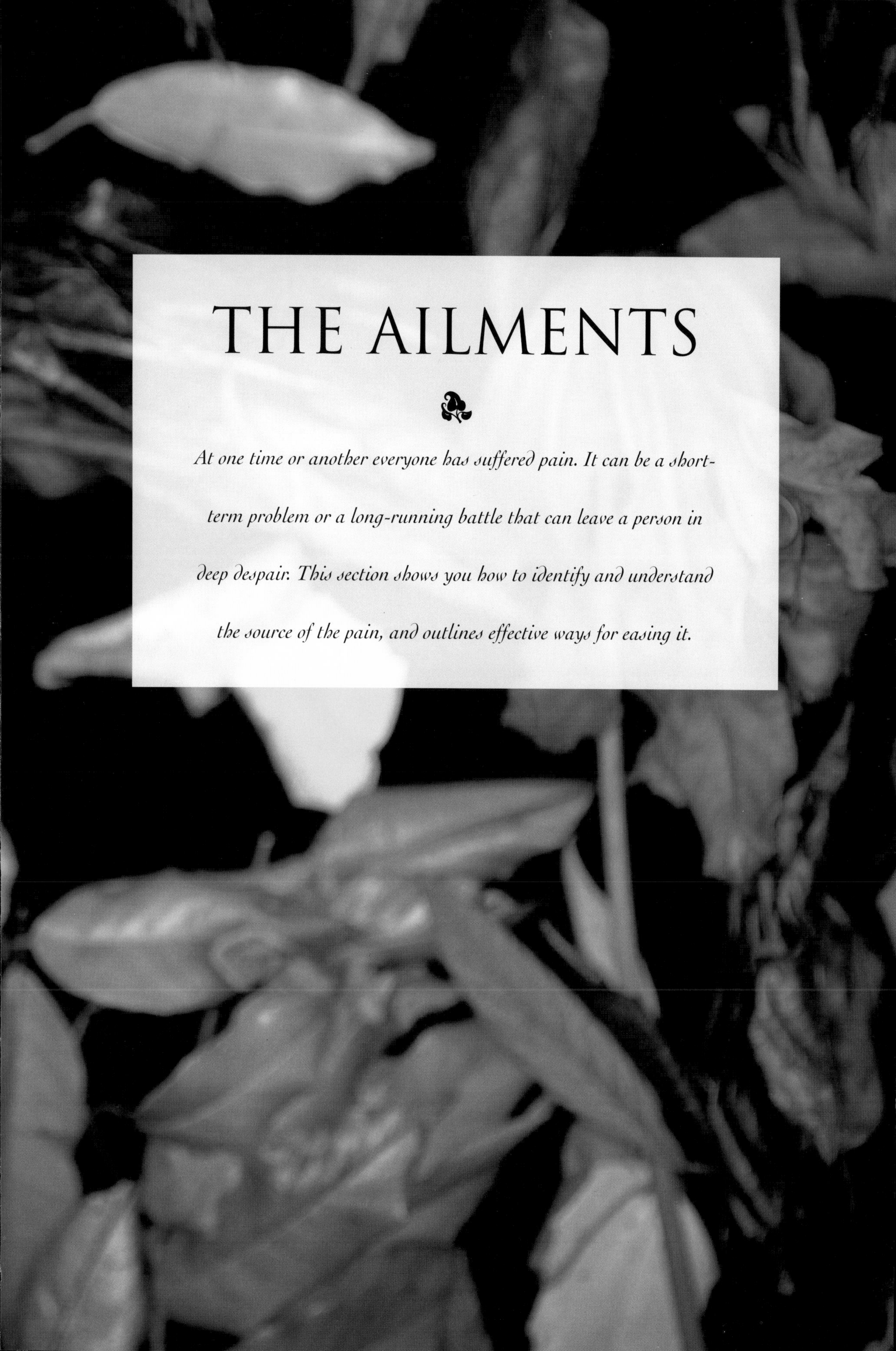

THE AILMENTS

At one time or another everyone has suffered pain. It can be a short-term problem or a long-running battle that can leave a person in deep despair. This section shows you how to identify and understand the source of the pain, and outlines effective ways for easing it.

AT-A-GLANCE GUIDE TO AILMENTS

Site and/or type of pain	Ailment	Page number
First aid	*Bruises*	22
	Sprains	23
	Cuts	23
	Bites	23
	Stings	23
	Burns and scalds	24
	Sunburn	24
	Sunstroke	24
	Chilblains	24
	Frostbite	24
	Nausea and vomiting	25
	Toothache	25
	Hangover	25
	Cramp	25
Mental and emotional pain	*Depression*	28–35
Skin pain	*Heat rash and sunburn*	36–37
	Boils	37
	Blisters	37
	Chapping	37
	Chilblains	37
	Whitelow (felon)	37
	Tinea (ringworm/athlete's foot)	38
	Hives (nettle rash/urticaria)	38
	Eczema/dermatitis	38–39
	Psoriasis	40–41
	Shingles	41
Cancer pain	*Cancer pain*	42–43
Head pain	*Headaches*	45–47
	Migraines	48–49
Eyes, ears, mouth, nose, and throat pain	*Colds and flu*	51
	Eyestrain	52
	Conjunctivitis	52
	Earache (otitis)	52–53
	Tinnitus	53
	Sinusitis	53–54
	Hayfever	54
	Toothache	54
	Gingivitis	55
	Tooth abcess	55
	Face and jaw pain	55
	Cold sores	56
	Mouth ulcers	56
	Sore throat	56
	Tonsillitis	57
Chest and lung pain	*Coughs*	58–59
	Bronchitis	60–61
	Asthma	61–63
	Pleurisy	63
	Pneumonia	63–64
	Emphysema	64–65
	Tuberculosis	65
Neck and back pain	*Kyphosis*	67–68
	Lordosis	68
	Flat back	68
	Sway back	68
	Scoliosis	68–69
	Neckache	69–70
	Whiplash	70–71
	Torticollis	71
	Backache	71–73
	Slipped disk	73

Site and/or type of pain	Ailment	Page number
Nerve, muscle, and joint pain	*Nerve pain (neuralgia/sciatica/neuritis)*	*75–76*
	Carpal tunnel syndrome	*76–77*
	Multiple sclerosis	*77–78*
	Muscle and tendon pain (fibromyalgia)	*78–79*
	Gout	*79*
	Rheumatism and arthritis	*80–81*
	Ankylosing spondylitis	*81*
Digestive and urinary tract pain	*Stomachache*	*83*
	Nausea	*84*
	Indigestion	*84*
	Hiatus hernia	*84–85*
	Ulcers/gastritis	*85*
	Gallstones	*86*
	Constipation	*86–87*
	Diarrhea	*87*
	Gastroenteritis	*88*
	Irritable bowel syndrome	*88*
	Diverticulitis	*88*
	Inflammatory bowel disease	*88–89*
	Cystitis	*89–90*
	Urethritis	*91*
	Kidney stones	*91*
Heart and circulation pain	*Palpitations*	*93*
	Angina	*93–94*
	Circulation pain	*94–96*
	Raynaud's syndrome	*96*
	Varicose veins	*96*
	Hemmorhoids (piles)	*97*
	Phlebitis	*97*
Genital and sexual pain	*Hernia*	*98–99*
	Prostatitis	*99*
	Impotence	*100*
	Vaginismus	*101*
	Vaginitis	*101*
	Thrush	*101*
	Premenstrual syndrome	*102*
	Menstrual cramps	*102–103*
	Prolapse	*103*
	Pelvic inflammatory disease	*103*
	Genital herpes	*104*
	Nonspecific urethritis	*104*
	Chlamydia	*104*
Pregnancy pain	*Morning sickness*	*105*
	Sore breasts	*105*
	Heartburn	*105*
	Childbirth pain	*106–107*
Babies and children in pain	*Diaper (nappy) rash*	*108*
	Colic and stomachache	*108–109*
	Teething	*109*
	Oral thrush	*109*
	Croup	*110*
	Fever	*110*
	Bruising and injuries	*110*
	Earache	*110*
	Whooping cough	*111*
	Cough	*111*
	Sore throat	*111*
	Mumps	*111*
	Skin irritation	*111*

FIRST AID FOR PAIN

Many of the treatments and remedies in this section are to be found later in this book but are summarized here for quick reference in an emergency. The treatments and remedies covered are for adults but may be safely used (unless stated otherwise) for babies and children also. Where medicines are concerned, use half the adult quantity or less, according to the instructions on the bottle or package.

Everyone experiences unexpected injuries and illnesses at one time or another, and quick treatment may be essential both to alleviate pain and to prevent the problem from escalating.

BRUISES

Place anything cold on the affected part as soon as possible, and leave for about 10–15 minutes. An ice pack, a bag of frozen peas from the freezer, or simply a washcloth soaked in cold water will do.

Arnica is the best remedy for mild to moderate bruising, and hypericum for severe bruising. Apply either as a cream over the entire area after icing and drying the bruise. The homeopathic remedy arnica 6c will also help, or if the bones under the bruise feel sore, symphytum 6c (alternatives are ruta and bellis per). For a black eye, lachesis 6c is best. In all cases, take one tablet every hour for four hours.

Alternatives to arnica are comfrey cream and aloe vera gel. A cold compress soaked in tincture of comfrey can also be beneficial.

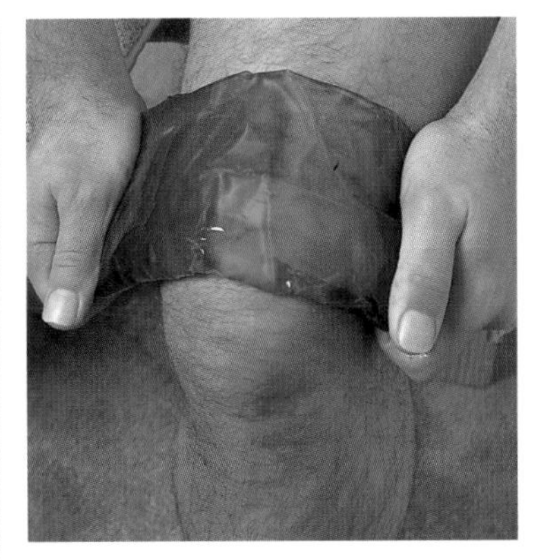

A purpose-made gelatin cold pack is a quick and effective remedy for both bruises and sprains.

SPRAINS

As for bruises, place an ice pack or similar on the affected part, and keep it there for as long as possible.

Immerse the sprain for about 15 minutes in a bowl of cold water containing four drops of the essential oils of rosemary and sweet marjoram. Make a cold compress using the same liquid, wrap it around the sprain, and keep it in place (using a waterproof bandage or similar) for several hours.

Take the homeopathic remedies arnica 6c (every half hour for two hours) and ruta 6c (three times a day for a week).

CUTS

Clean the cut with warm water and flush with calendula tincture (or apply calendula ointment). If the cut is deep, apply firm pressure for several minutes after cleaning to help stop the bleeding, preferably using a lint or cotton pad. Check that there is no loss of sensation or impeded function. Protect with a sterile pad, clean handkerchief, adhesive tape, or bandage.

Hypericum 6c helps to promote healing and overcome shock. Take a pill every hour for four hours.

BITES

Bites from any creature, animal or human, can be serious if deep enough, and infection is always a risk. So, in addition to washing and cleaning the wound, and applying an antiseptic (tea tree oil is excellent), always seek medical help as soon as possible. This step is essential if the bite is from a wild animal, snake, or dog. For minor bites, the homeopathic remedies hypericum, apis, and staphysagria may help reduce any swelling and pain.

STINGS

Calamine lotion is a good general remedy for minor stings, but not for stings from bees and wasps.

Insect stings The homeopathic remedy ledum 6c is good for all stings but particularly those where the skin has been punctured, relieving pain and swelling. Calendula cream and witch hazel tincture can also reduce swelling and soothe pain. The homeopathic tincture pyrethrum, and Bach Rescue Remedy may also help.

Bee stings Sodium bicarbonate will neutralize the poison. Dissolve two teaspoonfuls in a cup of warm water and apply with a cotton ball. Apis 12c (one tablet every half hour until the pain stops) is effective for both bee and wasp stings.

Wasp stings Vinegar or lemon juice, applied to the skin undiluted, will neutralize the poison.

Jellyfish stings A hot bath is the best way to neutralize the poison in jellyfish stings. The temperature should be 100–102°F (38–39°C). For severe stings, take the homeopathic remedy apis 30c (take one tablet every hour until the stinging stops). Ledum and calendula can also be beneficial.

Nettle stings Rubbing a dock leaf onto the affected area is very effective (docks are usually found where nettles grow). The leaf should be rubbed on vigorously, so that the juice from the leaf goes into the skin to neutralize the poison.

Poison ivy stings Cut an onion in half and rub it on the affected area. Wash the area with soap and water to remove the plant's oil, and apply a paste of sodium bicarbonate and water as for bee stings.

CAUTION Reactions to some stings, notably from insects (especially bees and wasps) and jellyfish, can sometimes be so severe as to be life-threatening. This kind of allergic reaction is known as anaphylaxis. Signs are cold, clammy skin with an itchy rash, rapid, shallow breathing, and weak pulse. Seek immediate medical help.

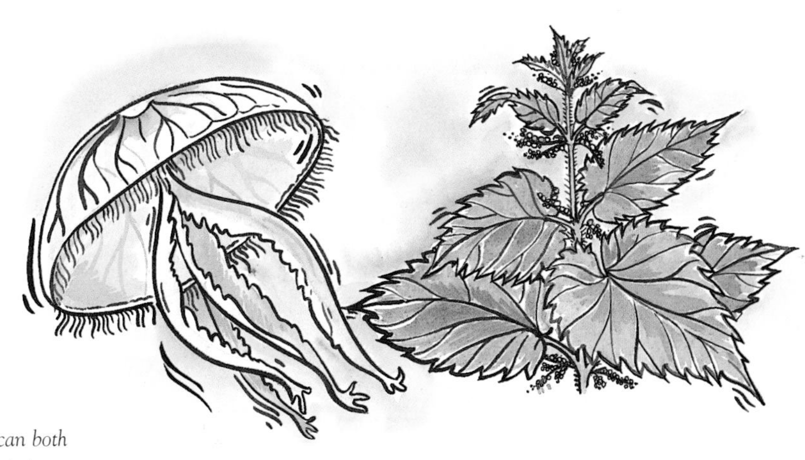

Jellyfish and nettles can both cause severe stinging pain.

BURNS AND SCALDS

For minor burns and scalds, place the affected part under cool running water for at least 10 minutes. Mix 10 drops of hypericum tincture in a glass of cold water and pour over. Dry and cover with a clean, sterile dressing. Bach Rescue Remedy may help any after-effects. For severe pain, one tablet of the homeopathic remedy aconite 12c may bring relief.

Alternatively, place an ice pack on the burn or scald for 10 minutes, then apply aloe vera tincture or calendula ointment. Or, soak some gauze in witch hazel and bandage it carefully onto the affected area.

CAUTION Severe burns or scalds, especially those covering large areas, can produce life-threatening traumatic shock, and require immediate medical attention.

SUNBURN

Soak for 15–20 minutes in a tub of cold water mixed with one of the following: several drops of lavender oil or vinegar, or a sprinkling of sodium bicarbonate or oatmeal. Dry and gently rub in either aloe vera gel, vitamin E cream, or calendula ointment. A cold compress of calendula tincture, held in place, can help soothe badly affected areas. Sunburned eyelids benefit from a slice of fresh cucumber left on them for at least 15 minutes.

SUNSTROKE

Sunstroke (or heatstroke) is characterized by a splitting headache, neck pain, feverishness, dizziness, nausea, and a rapid pulse. The immediate aim is to bring down the body temperature, so sit in a cold bath or wrap the body in a sheet soaked in cold water. Seek *immediate* medical help if body temperature has not dropped after about an hour.

These homeopathic remedies may help: belladonna 6c (for a high temperature), glonoin 6c (for dizziness), and cuprum 6c (for cramp).

CAUTION Too much sun can be extremely dangerous, especially for children and light-skinned people. Severe sunburn and sunstroke can be life-threatening. If in doubt, seek immediate medical help.

CHILBLAINS

Twice a day put the affected hands or feet into hot water for two minutes, then cold water for one minute. Repeat five times. If the affected parts are bleeding, apply calendula cream after the bathing. If they are not bleeding, apply arnica tincture diluted in cold water (six drops to a pint/570 ml). Soak a washcloth in the mixture, wring out, and leave on overnight.

FROSTBITE

Remove anything covering the affected area and warm it slowly between the hands. Do not rub the skin. Dab on Friar's balsam or tincture of myrrh and loosely cover with a dry dressing. Wrap in a blanket to keep warm, and wear gloves and socks. Take agaricus 12c immediately, apis 6c if there is swelling, and pulsatilla 6c if heat makes the condition worse. Take a high-potency vitamin B-complex capsule and 400 iu of vitamin E daily.

CAUTION Frostbite is a serious condition, and immediate medical help is necessary.

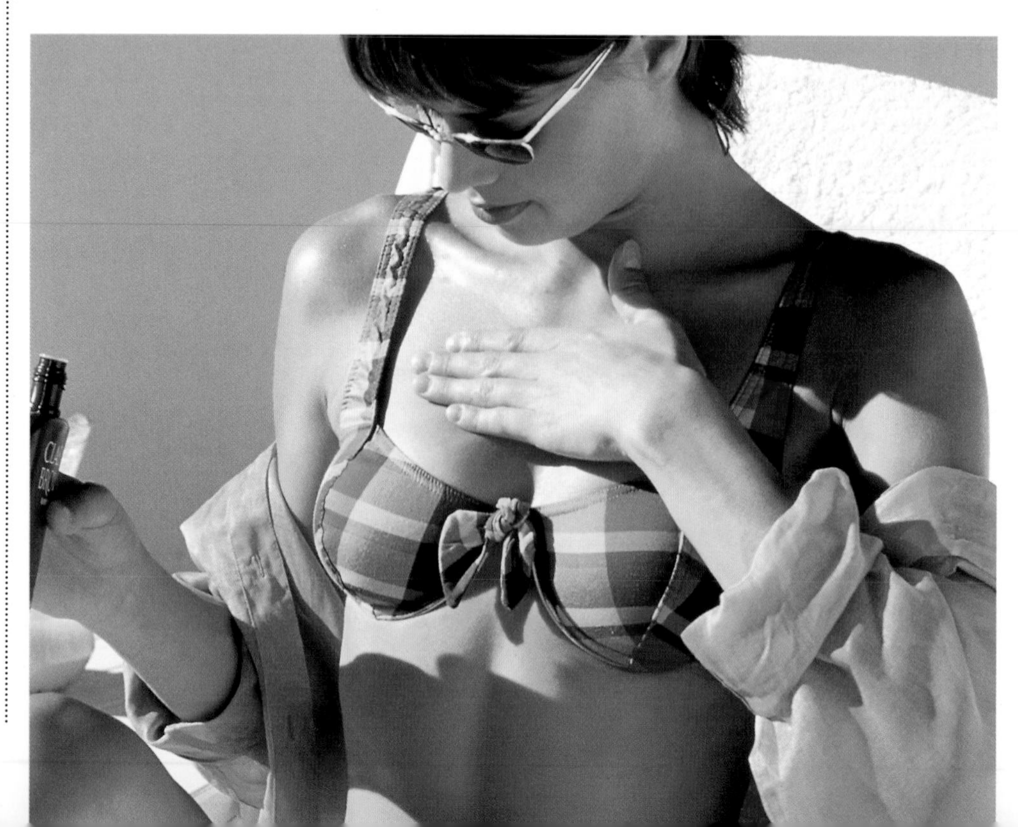

Too much sun is dangerous and the use of sun block is essential, especially in fair-skinned people.

NAUSEA AND VOMITING

For all forms of nausea and vomiting, including travel or motion sickness (car, air, and sea sickness) and morning sickness during pregnancy, take ginger. Make it into a tea (cut the root into pieces, simmer for about 15 minutes, and drink); or take it in capsules (two half an hour before traveling, or as necessary for other forms of nausea); or simply chew the raw root. Eating crystallized ginger during the journey can also be effective.

The herbs Roman chamomile and black horehound can also reduce nausea and vomiting, but do NOT take if pregnant.

Take the homeopathic remedies nux vomica together with cocculus (both 6c) for general nausea and vomiting; sepia 6c for nausea brought on by the smell of food; pulsatilla, ipecacuanha, arsenicum album (all 6c) for motion sickness; tabacum 6c if symptoms include sweating and giddiness; and borax 6c if there is anxiety.

Essential oil of peppermint can also help. Add four drops to a neutral oil, such as grapeseed, and rub onto the chest to be inhaled. Alternatively, put the drops onto a tissue or handkerchief and breathe in the vapor that way.

Elasticized bands with a sewn-in acupressure stud, which can be worn on the wrist during a journey to help keep sickness at bay, are available from many drugstores and health food stores.

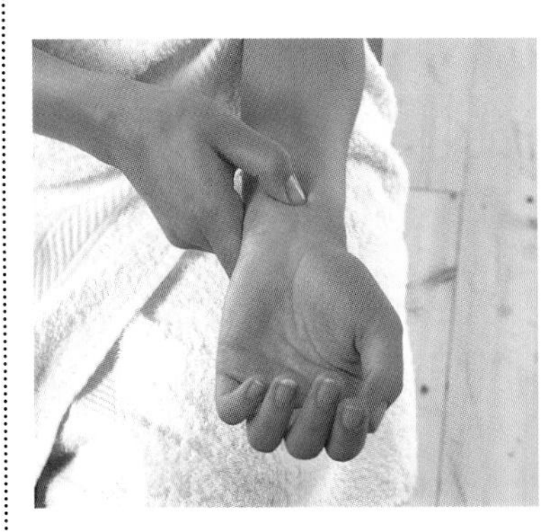

If you do not have an acupressure wristband, press a point on the wrist in line with the largest (middle) finger, three fingers' width from the wrist crease nearest the hand for several seconds.

TOOTHACHE

Apply oil of cloves to the sore area. Chewing a dried clove will achieve the same effect by releasing the anesthetic that the herb contains.

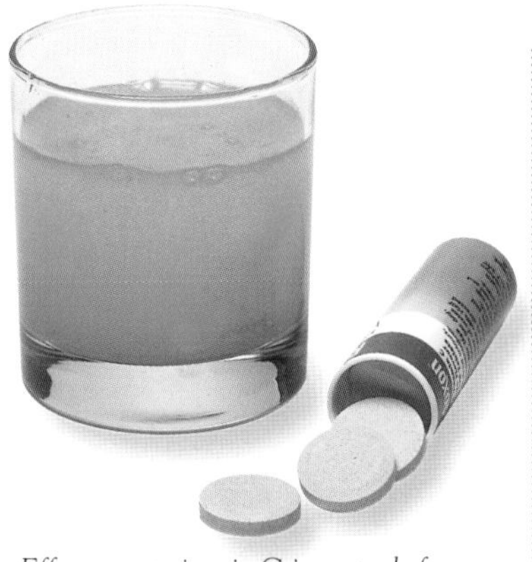

Effervescent vitamin C in water before sleep can help avoid hangover.

HANGOVER

Drink at least a pint (570 ml) of water with 1 g of vitamin C before going to sleep, and peppermint, nettle, chamomile, or yarrow tea throughout the following day. Honey (12 teaspoonfuls), alone or in warm water, may also help.

CRAMP

Press hard into the center of the painful area with the thumbs and try to stretch the muscle at the same time. While the cramp is easing, apply a hot compress—a washcloth soaked in hot water and wrung out will do. Repeat the application four or five times, then try gently working the muscle by stretching and kneading it.

Effective herbal remedies are kelp, ginko biloba, and crampbark (taken as tea), and the homeopathic cuprum 3c.

Eating plenty of dark green leafy vegetables together with shellfish, nuts, and seeds can help prevent attacks, as can daily supplementing with evening primrose or starflower (borage) oil (1 g a day), vitamin C (3 g), E (250–400 iu), calcium, and magnesium.

NOTE In hot countries, heavy sweating can cause cramp through loss of salt. Too much salt loss can lead to coma, so eat more salt with food. Magnesium supplements (500 mg a day) may be necessary too.

Homeopathic first aid

For	Remedy	Dose
Severe pain (after injury)	*Aconite*	*1 × 6c pill*
Insect bites and stings	*Apis*	*1 × 30c pill every half hour*
Accidents or injuries	*Arnica*	*1 × 6c pill every half hour*
Bruises	*Arnica*	*1–2 × 3c pills every half hour*
Burns, blisters, scalds	*Cantharis*	*1 × 6c pill*
Anxiety and general pain relief	*Chamomilla*	*1 × 3c pill as needed*
Cuts and wounds	*Hypericum*	*1 × 30c pill every hour for 3–4 hours*
Hangover, motion sickness	*Nux vomica*	*1 × 6c pill*
Nosebleed from injury	*Phosphate*	*1 × 6c pill*
Muscular pain	*Rhus tox*	*1 × 6c pill every hour*

For best effect homeopathic pills should not be swallowed but allowed to dissolve slowly under the tongue.

MENTAL AND EMOTIONAL PAIN

The subtle interrelationship between body and mind only began to be explored in any detail in the last 30 years, but studies have now demonstrated that, just as physical pain can be mentally and emotionally painful, so also can psychological pain lead to physical pain. The idea of pain being mental or emotional as well as physical is an unfamiliar one to many people, but those who suffer from it know its reality all too well.

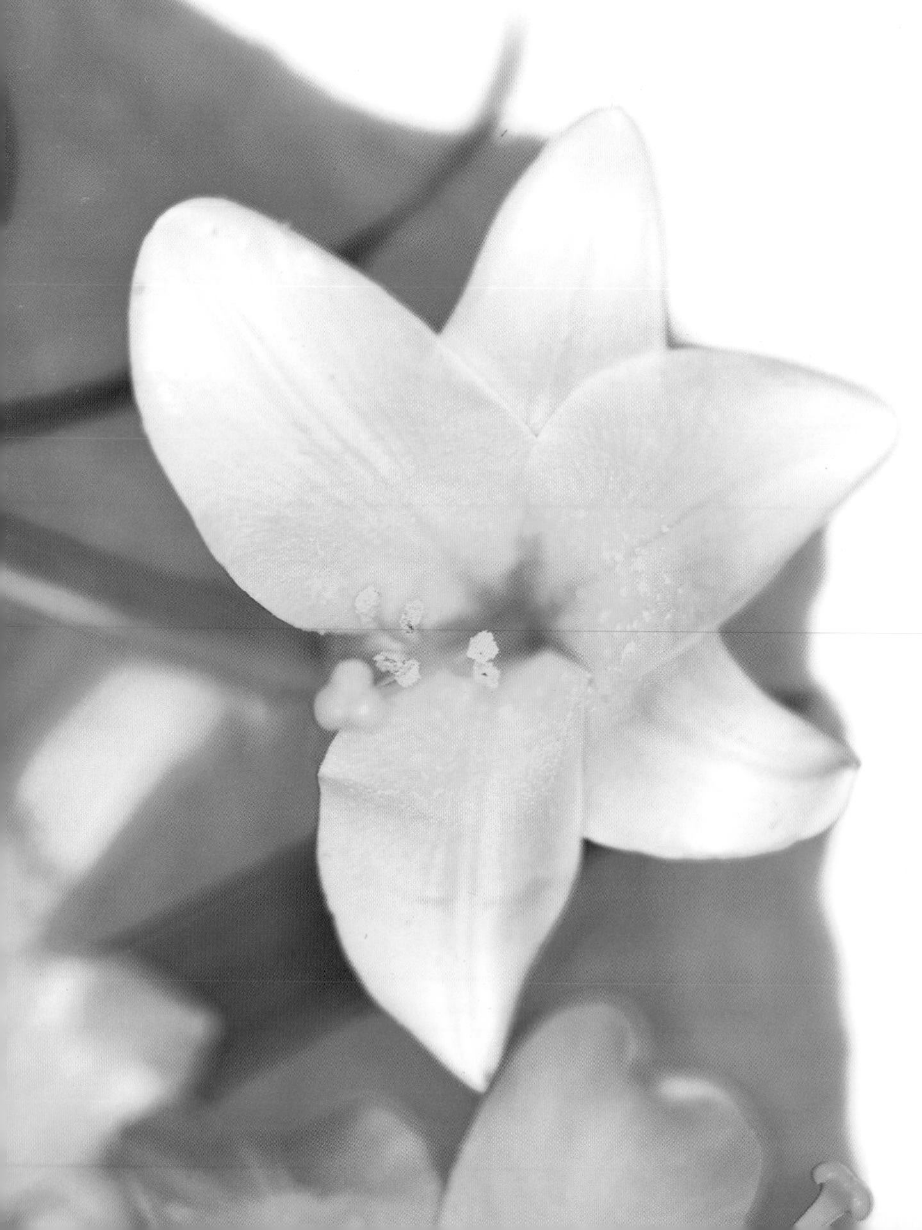

Mental and emotional pain are often depicted as originating in the head and the heart: the head as the source of mental pain, and the heart as the seat of emotional pain. But this is only partly true, because mental and emotional pain are not physical pain in the sense the word is normally used: neither is limited to just one organ, and each can affect various other organs in the body.

Mental and emotional pain (psychological pain) is what most people know as depression, an all-encompassing description that can cover anything from feeling "blue," perhaps because the weather is cold, to such extreme mental and emotional agony—from bereavement, redundancy, or a broken relationship, for example—that its victims can feel suicidal. But depression can have a physical cause as well as a psychological one —vitamin and mineral deficiency, for example, can be to blame—and the interrelationship between the physical and the psychological is both complex and crucial in understanding, and so being able to treat, the problem. Moreover, mental and emotional pain, though closely interlinked, have their own special pain "subsets"—and each of these can have a physical cause as well as a psychological one. Nightmares, fears, and phobias are examples of pain that tends to be more psychological than physical, while conditions such as manic depression and various psychoses (paranoia and schizophrenia) are more likely to have a physical cause. By comparison, dealing with a sprained ankle is a walk in the park!

Clearly, because of this, there are conditions that are not really suitable for self-help and so are not included in this book. Manic depression and psychotic illnesses, such as paranoia, autism, and schizophrenia, are excluded. Serious psychological pain (doctors tend to use the word "disturbance" or "disorder" rather than pain) is the exception rather than the rule, however, and the majority of psychological pain can be effectively treated at home, or with a little help. Even phobias, obsessions, and addictions (to food, sex, drugs, alcohol, and so on), though serious, are open to the possibility of self-help following initial treatment by specialist practitioners.

Not surprisingly, effective therapies include both physical and psychological ones. The following therapies have a good record in the treatment of most forms of mental and emotional pain, from general "blues" and anxiety to Seasonal Affective Disorder (SAD) and postnatal depression.

Psychological therapies

Self-help Meditation, visualization, self-hypnosis, biofeedback

Self-help with trained guidance Creative arts therapies (music, art, dance, drama)

From a qualified therapist only Counseling, psychotherapy, hypnotherapy

Energy therapies

Self-help Flower remedies

Self-help with trained guidance Homeopathy, healing

From a qualified therapist only Acupuncture, traditional Chinese herbal medicine

Physical therapies

Self-help Massage, aromatherapy, reflexology

Self-help with trained guidance Nutritional and dietary therapy, herbal medicine, movement therapies (yoga, tai chi, Alexander technique), light and color therapy, hydrotherapy

From a qualified therapist only Cranial osteopathy

IDENTIFYING PAIN

An important factor in successful self-help is identifying the cause of your particular type of pain. Often the cause is obvious or known to you already, but knowing exactly what is behind your problem—or even more or less knowing—is the first step toward successful treatment. Problems arise when the cause is a complete mystery, because, clearly, if the cause is unknown, effective treatment is extremely difficult, if not impossible. If you know you are in pain but do not know why or how badly, try the self-assessment questionnaire on the following page, "How depressed are you?" It will help you to get the most from this section. If you are still no wiser about your problem after completing the questionnaire, the help of a trained specialist is advisable.

Mental and emotional pain can be as painful as physical pain—and often far harder to bear, especially if on your own.

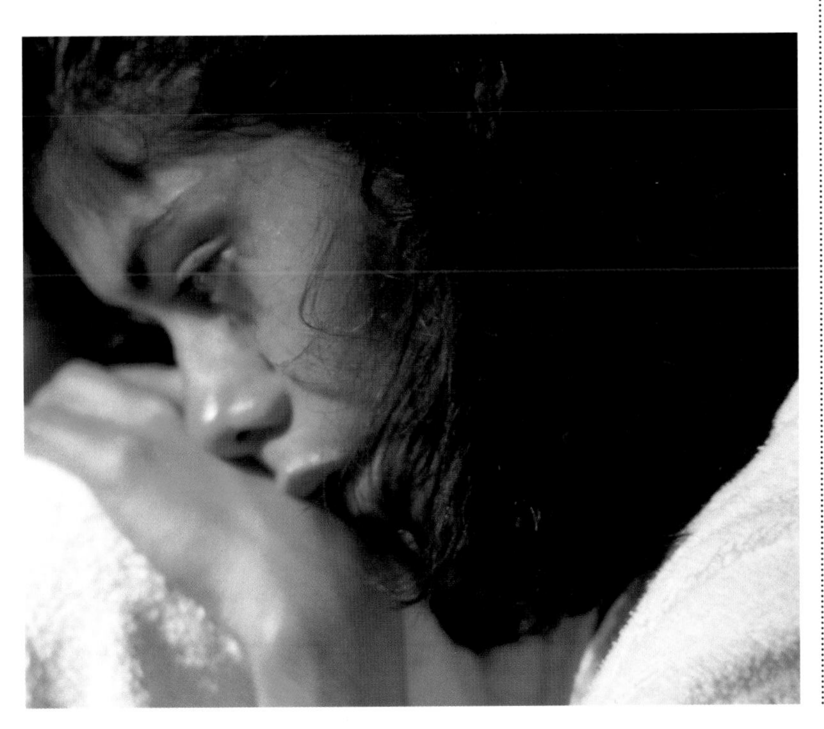

DEPRESSION

A number of approaches promote mental and emotional recovery by encouraging both relaxation and a positive image of oneself. A good way to start is with a progressive muscular relaxation exercise.

Sit in a comfortable position (it is better not to lie down or you may fall asleep!). Start with your feet by wiggling your toes. Then squeeze your feet with your hands and let them go. Now rotate your ankles. Squeeze or tense your calves, knees, and thighs in turn before relaxing. At each stage, be conscious of the difference in feeling before and after. Next clench your buttocks and relax them. Tighten the stomach muscles, and slowly breathe in before more slowly breathing out. When you reach your shoulders hunch them up and release (many people hold tension in their shoulders without realizing it). Do this a few times. Finish by screwing your face up and stretching your jaw before releasing. Relax.

At the end of this routine you should feel quite relaxed. See if you can keep this feeling of relaxation during the rest of the day. Test your body from time to time. If you think you have tensed up, run through the sequence again. It does not take long—no more than a few minutes—and is easy to fit into even the busiest routine. With practice you will find it will help you cope better and give you more stamina and clarity of mind.

Combining the relaxation exercise with any of the following therapies can produce an extremely powerful healing force.

How depressed are you?

Evidence shows that the more we know about the causes, or possible causes, of our mental and emotional pain or depression, the more likely we are to come to terms with or get over it successfully. The following self-assessment helps you to find out just how depressed you really are—so that you can begin to do something effective about it. Score the following 10 categories from 0 to 4, as shown, with your own idea of how severe each is in your case.

	None	**Mild**	**Moderate**	**Severe**	**Very severe**
Depressed mood	0	1	2	3	4
Feelings of guilt	0	1	2	3	4
Suicidal feelings	0	1	2	3	4
Problems with concentration and memory	0	1	2	3	4
Feelings of lassitude	0	1	2	3	4
Disturbed sleep	0	1	2	3	4
Loss of sexual desire	0	1	2	3	4
Loss of appetite	0	1	2	3	4
Feelings of anxiousness	0	1	2	3	4
Symptoms of anxiousness	0	1	2	3	4

After scoring each category, add the scores together to give a total (maximum 40). Any score of 10 or under classes you as "normal"—that is, you are experiencing what the great majority of people feel most of the time. To be classified as actually depressed, you must score at least 2 on the first category "Depressed mood." The higher the total score above 10, the more you should consider trying the treatments in this chapter. A score over 30 means a doctor or other specialist in treating depression should be consulted.

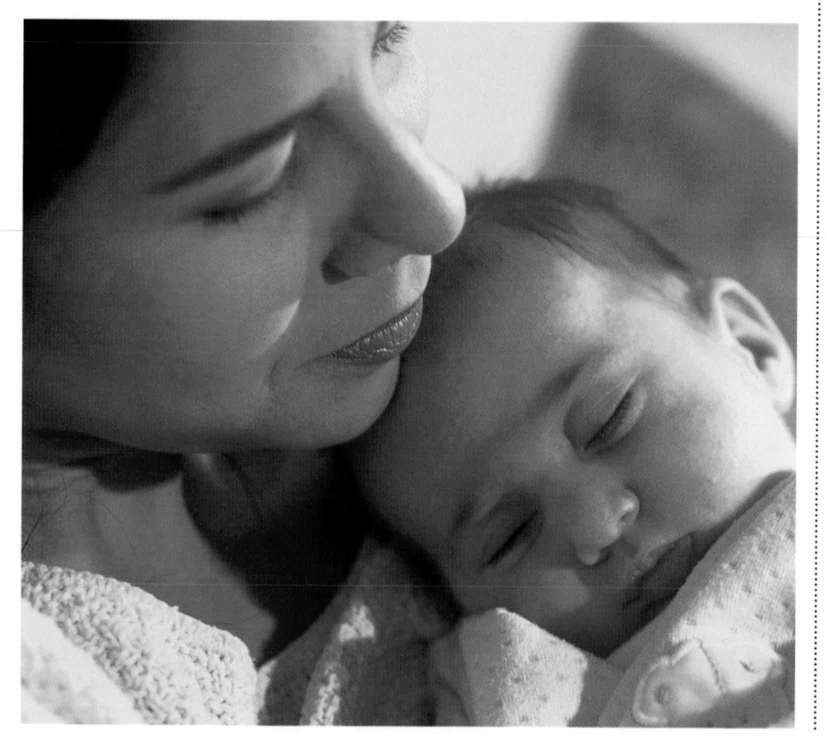

Babies know how to relax instinctively but adults are not so good at it. A wide range of techniques have been developed to help them relearn the "lost" art.

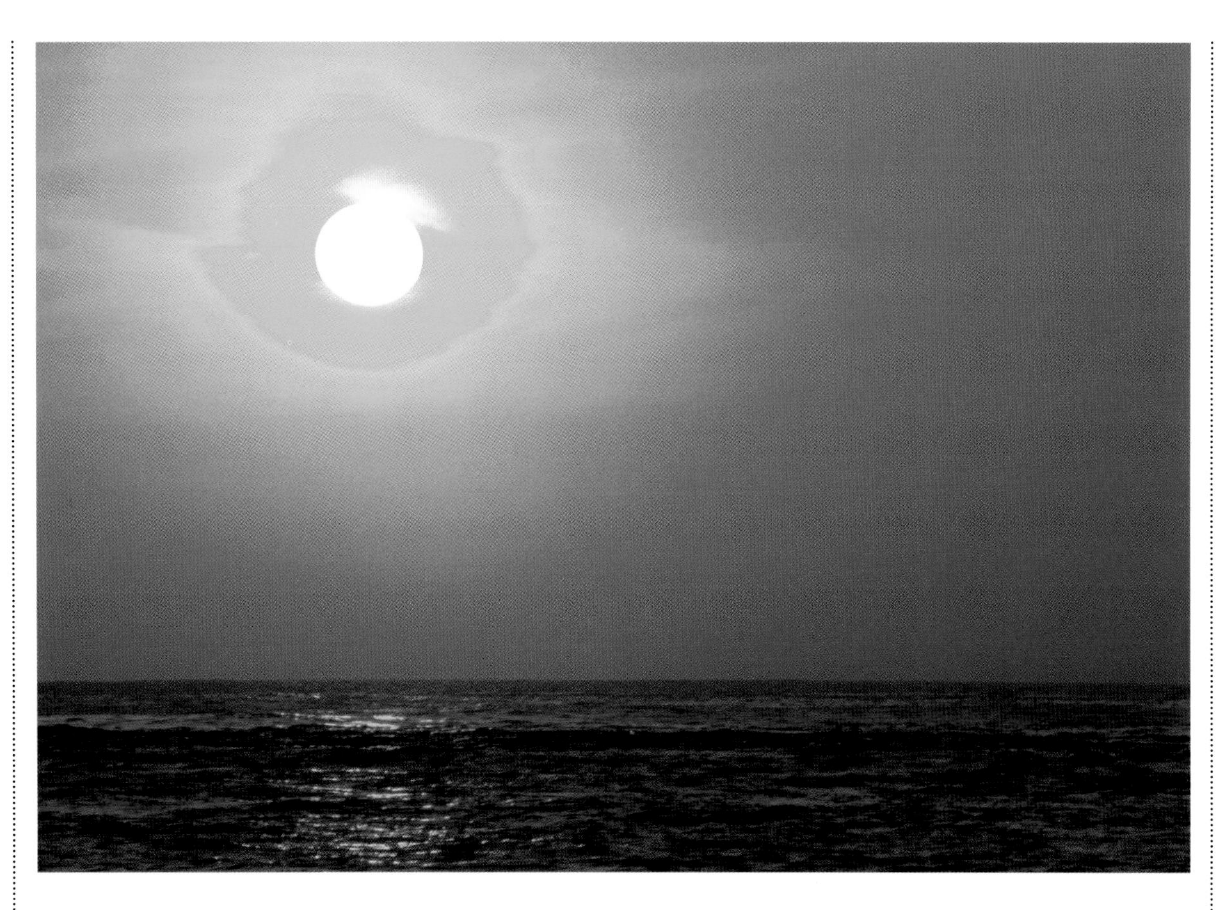

Picturing pleasant, positive images in your mind can be a powerful benefit during periods of depression.

Visualization

Focus on the pain you are feeling. Whether it is a physical or psychological pain, try and get a sense of it—a feeling for it almost. What exactly is it like (throbbing, sharp, dull)? What "shape" is it (small, wide, large)? What "weight" is it (light, heavy)? Identify it as precisely as you can. The aim is, having identified it, to decide to change it by imagining something appropriate in your mind's eye that will best deal with it. For example, a "heavy, wide, dull" pain may be seen as a large rock pressing down on that part of you; or a "sharp, thin, light" pain as a needle sticking into you. So, in the first example, you could visualize a crane or a giant gently lifting the rock off you and crushing it to powder. Or, in the second, reaching down and slowly pulling the needle out and throwing it into the sea.

Psychological pain is often harder to "picture," but not impossible. If depression is the basic problem, try to identify the cause, if it is not already obvious. Rejection, for example, may be seen as a small, lost child, crying and alone. A smiling angel may be visualized walking up to the child and taking it by the hand into a room full of warmth and light, where other people come up, also smiling, and hug and talk to the child. Equally, an aching heart may be seen as bruised, and benefit from being surrounded by purple light, or warm sea-water, or a soft hand; mental turmoil or confusion as a cage that is unlocked and lets all the chaos escape, leaving a clear, empty, silent space.

The possibilities are endless. The illogicality or unlikelihood of the image is not important. If the result makes you feel good—or at least better—then let it happen, whatever it is. Sustain the picture as long as you like, go in any direction you like, see whatever you want to see. The important thing is to think of a positive image, an image that is a solution, at least in your mind's eye.

Having found an effective image, visualize it regularly. And if it ceases to be effective, simply change it for something that is—and do that regularly. Continue until your mind is in control of the pain and not the other way around. At best, you will find that your mind can literally think the pain away. At worst, it will give other methods a better chance of helping you recover, or enable you to face life with more strength and so allow more positive experiences to come your way that will displace the old negative thoughts and feelings more completely.

Meditation

Anyone can meditate, but it takes a little practice to do it properly. That is why it is a good idea to be shown how to do it by someone experienced. The basic idea is to begin by relaxing the body and then try to do the same with the mind to reach a state of what is often termed "passive concentration." This can be a bit difficult to achieve at first, but it becomes easier with practice.

Sit upright in a comfortable and well-supported position (do not lie down, or you could fall asleep and remove the point of the exercise). Close your eyes, or if this makes you feel sleepy, try fixing your gaze on a single, simple object, such as a lighted candle or a stone. The aim is to remain mentally relaxed yet alert.

Repeat, silently or aloud, a single word or phrase over and over again. (This is known as a *mantra* in the Indian tradition, and is similar to a chant. The word often used is "Om"—a symbolic term of assent—but it does not really matter what it is as long as the sound is pleasing and your mind becomes focused on it to the exclusion of everything else.) Do not worry about stray thoughts that flit through your mind (they usually do). Do not be concerned about how well you may (or may not) be doing—it is not a test. The most important thing is to adopt a "let it all happen" approach. Experienced meditators say: "Don't push the river, let it flow by itself."

Try and retain your "passive concentration" for at least 20–30 minutes. When ready to stop, get up quietly and slowly. The effects of meditation are often hard to pinpoint at first, but regular meditators claim dramatic increases in energy, stamina, and resistance to diseases of all kinds, including the effects of pain, in the long-term. The lesson is that for meditation to be successful—and it can be extremely successful for some people—it needs to be practiced regularly.

Autogenic training

Autogenics is a form of "westernized meditation" that needs to be taught by a specialist in the first place, but once learned is ideal for self-help. The technique uses six standard exercises that involve directing your attention inward and focusing your mind on different parts of the body. You train yourself to be aware of:

- *sensations of heaviness in your body*
- *warmth in your arms and legs*
- *the calmness and regularity of your heartbeat*
- *your easy and natural breathing*
- *warmth in your abdomen*
- *coolness in your head.*

Hypnosis taped

Tapes, CDs, and videos, available from stores and mail order companies, that offer programs of self-hypnosis as well as overt hypnosis (delivered by a hypnotherapist) are claimed to overcome a variety of mental and emotional problems, from depression to addictions.

Self-hypnosis tapes are usually subliminal—that is, the message is "hidden" behind a calming background noise, such as sounds of the sea, and absorbed through the subconscious mind.

Results vary, but seem to depend as much on how the individual person responds to the particular program as on the quality of production itself. Beyond luck in choosing the tape or video that appeals, it seems to be necessary for the recipient to be willing to participate and be helped.

Tapes and CDs featuring natural sounds without subliminal hypnotic messages—falling rain, ocean waves, birdsong, wind in trees, and so on—are found by many people to be relaxing and uplifting, and can therefore be just as beneficial (audiotapes and disks much more so than videotapes).

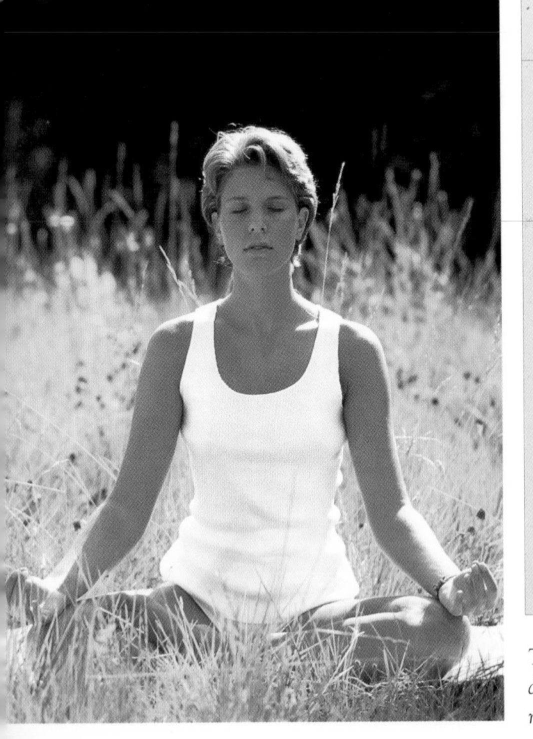

The "classic" meditation pose—but you don't have to sit like this to benefit from meditation, or "passive concentration."

Self-hypnosis

The ability of the mind to "hypnotize" or "reprogram" itself to think itself—and therefore the rest of the body—better is not only powerful but immensely effective. This has obvious implications in the natural treatment of pain, both mental and physical. The best-known recent exponent of the process of self-hypnosis is the American healer Louise Hay, who coined the term "affirmations" to describe the process.

Another, older description is "autosuggestion," credited to the Frenchman Emile Coué, who launched the technique more than a century ago with his famous phrase: "Every day, in every way, I am getting better and better." Examples of affirmations useful for mental and emotional pain are the following (they are best performed looking into a mirror):

"I am calm and confident."
"I love and approve of myself."
"I am a wonderful human being."
"I am the power and authority in my life and no one else is."
"I am strong and my mind/heart is healing itself."
"I am filled with healing power."

Affirmations can be learned easily from books, tapes, and videos, but sometimes initial guidance from a specialist teacher, or perhaps an experienced acquaintance, can put you on the right track and save time and effort.

Biofeedback

The use of a brain wave metering device to discover control of one's own mental activity, biofeedback must be learned under professional guidance. Once learned, it is an effective way of educating the mind into better habits by doing more of what is good for the body and less of what is bad.

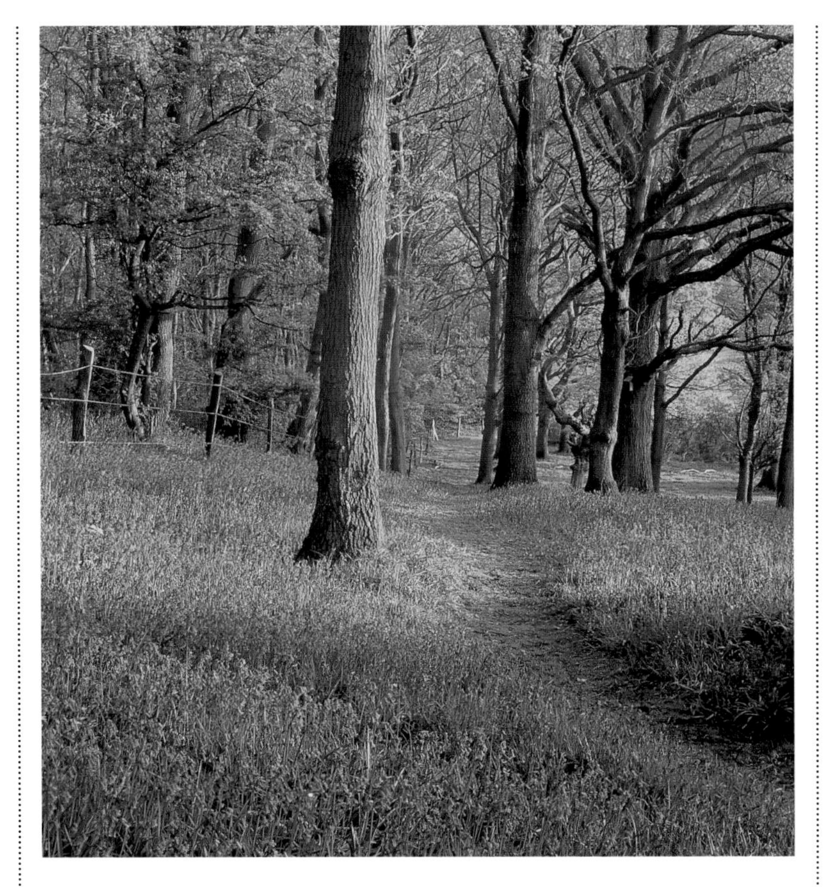

Remedies made from bluebells are just one of the many from flowers that are said to help with depression.

Flower remedies

Self-diagnosis and self-selection is very much the rule in using flower remedies for psychological pain. Bluebell, violet butterfly, and mariposa lily, for example, are recommended for depression of various kinds, but it is for the individual to decide which "feels" right. These days, with some two dozen suppliers making more than 100 remedies in over 50 countries around the world, the choice is enormous. The box below gives an idea of some of the original Bach flower remedies available for psychological pain.

Bach flower remedies for psychological problems

Cherry plum *For tension, fear, uncontrolled or irrational thought*
Crab apple *For shame at the ailment*
Gorse *For feelings of hopelessness, defeatism, and pessimism*
Mustard *For a "dark cloud" descending, feeling sad and low for no reason*
Olive *For exhaustion, feeling drained of energy*
Rock rose *For feeling suddenly alarmed or scared*
Sweet chestnut *For dejection and despair*
Willow *For resentfulness and bitterness, and always thinking "poor me"*
Rescue Remedy *A combination of five remedies (cherry plum, clematis, impatiens, rock rose, and star of Bethlehem) for shock, illness, grief, injury, or trauma*

Exercise

Any form of exercise is one of the best ways of helping with mental and emotional pain of almost any kind, especially if the exercise is energetic and distracting, so that the mind and emotions are prevented from "taking over." In addition to promoting heart and lung health, physical exercise naturally releases the so-called "pleasure hormones" (endorphins) that dampen down psychological and physical pain. Running, walking, climbing, swimming, and cycling are all excellent ways of using exercise to help with psychological pain. Exercise with someone, or alone if you prefer: the choice is yours. But exercising at the first sign of a depression can often stop it in its tracks—and you will be better physically for it too.

Any form of exercise, such as jogging, is one of the best ways to counteract the effects of mental and emotional pain.

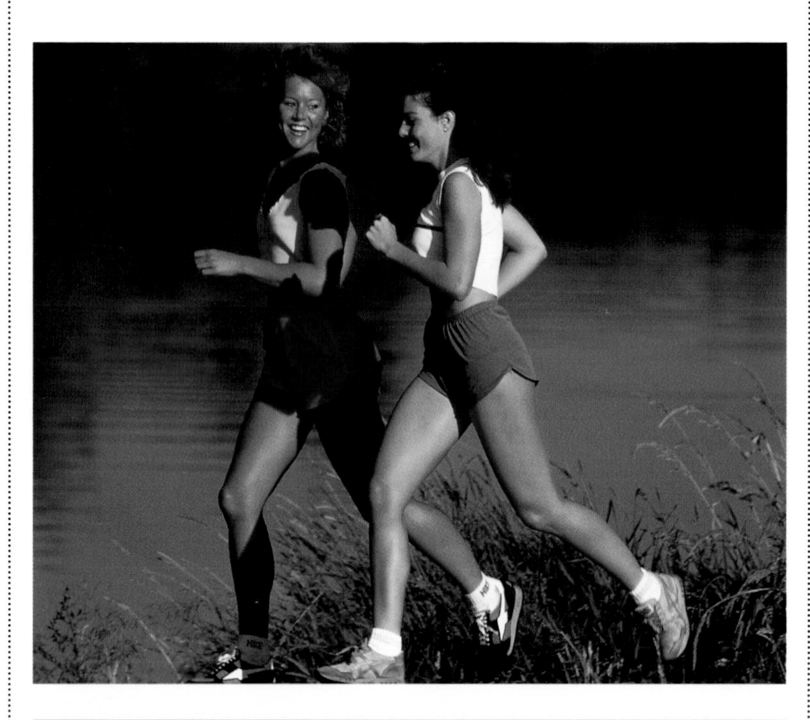

Massage

Massaging, or being massaged, is a wonderful de-stressor and psychological pain-reliever, especially if used with aromatic or essential oils. There are a number of recognized techniques taught to professional massage therapists (see pages 128–129), but using firm, flowing strokes and doing what you or your partner likes is more important than formal technique in self-help.

Aromatherapy

The range of essential oils is wide, and almost all have a useful role in treating psychological pain of all kinds, whether used in massage, inhaled, or vaporized in a burner. Oils most favored are shown below, but if you are unsure, ask at a store that supplies them (they usually also have samples for you to try), or seek the advice of a qualified clinical aromatherapist.

Essential oils for depression

Effect	Essential oils
General antidepressant	*Bergamot, frankincense*
Antidepressant and sedative	*Sandalwood, ylang ylang*
Depression with restlessness and irritability	*Chamomile, clary sage, lavender*
To lift mood without sedating	*Bergamot, geranium, melissa, rose*
Mild depression, feeling "under the weather"	*Lavender, clary sage*
Depression with lack of confidence, fear	*Jasmine, frankincense, rose*
Depression with anxiety, insomnia	*Neroli, geranium, lavender, rose, vetiver*
Emotional pain with anger	*Chamomile, ylang ylang, patchouli*
Deep emotional pain	*Neroli, rose*

For massage, mix two or three drops of the chosen oil(s) in about 1 fl oz (20 ml) of neutral carrier oil, such as grapeseed or sweet almond.

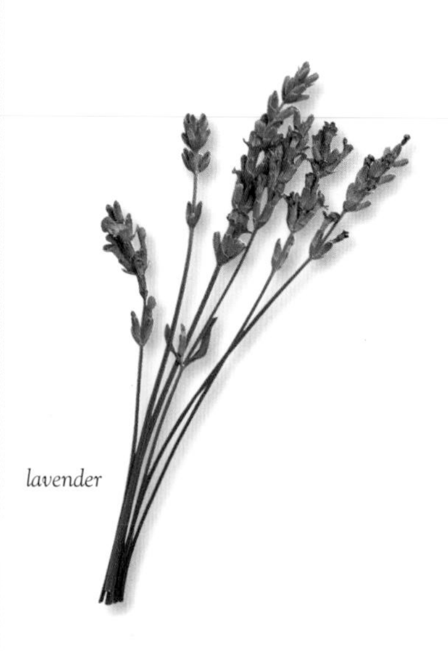

lavender

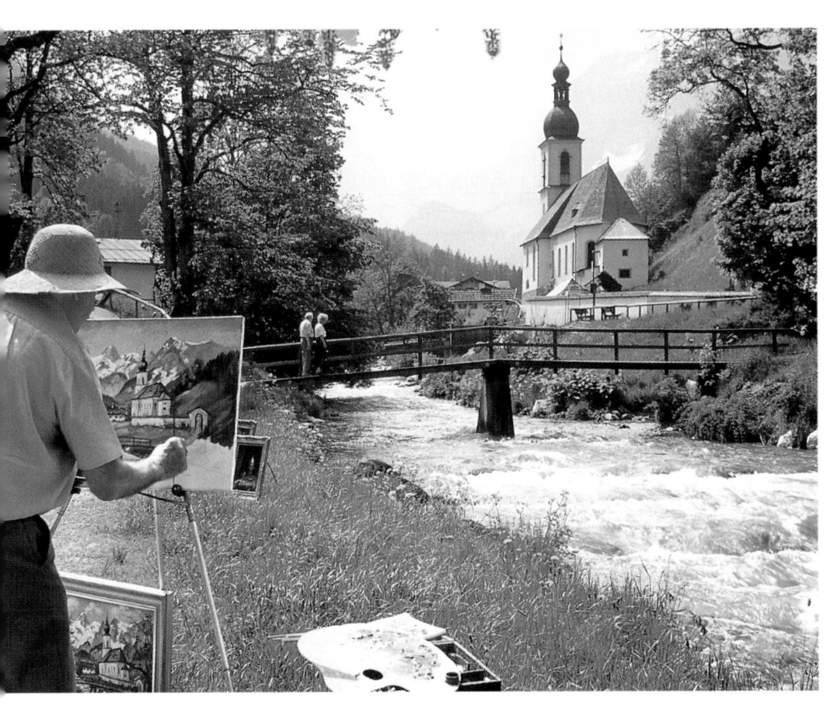

Painting—though not necessarily as well as this man—is an effective way of nonverbal expression.

Creative arts

Expressing feelings in nonverbal ways through music, painting, dance, drama, and sand play helps many people find relief from psychological pain not alleviated in any other way. Help is essential initially from a specialist in the rapidly growing field of creative arts therapy, but some of the techniques can be easily and effectively used at home once discovered. A good therapist will be available to help you further if you want it.

Reflexology

Manipulating the soles and sides of the feet is another excellent relaxer that benefits the mind and emotions as much as the body—especially, as with massage, when done with an essential oil. Because so many organs are said to correspond to so many different parts of the foot—making specific treatment complicated for a nonspecialist—a good overall massage of the entire foot, but particularly the top half including the toes, is best. For even better results, get someone else to do it to you.

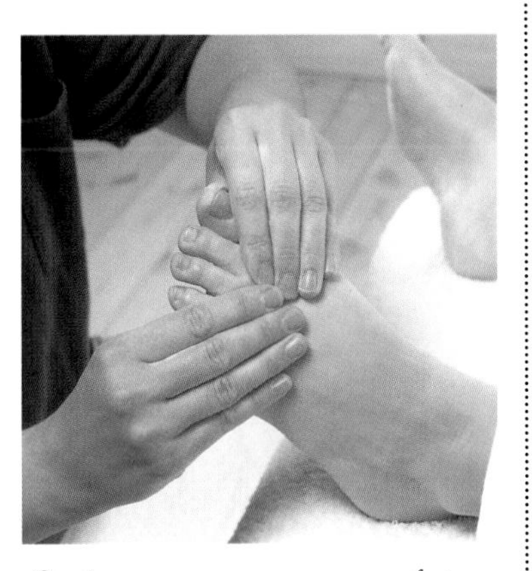

Getting someone to massage your feet can be highly soothing. Better still, visit a trained reflexologist, who will be able to pinpoint and relax areas of tension.

Sand-play is a relatively new but extremely powerful way of learning to express feelings without using words.

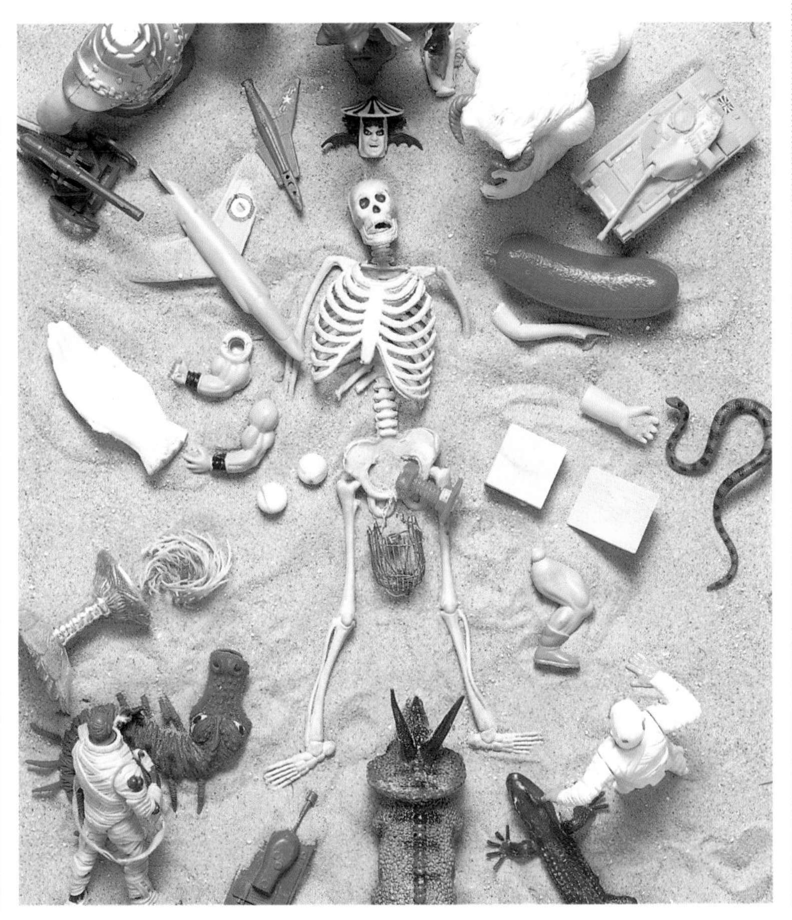

Homeopathy

There are literally hundreds of homeopathic remedies for every possible combination of psychological pain, some linked to physical pain and others not. The choice is so wide that individual assessment by a qualified practitioner is highly recommended, and this is especially so for serious or persistent situations.

It is essential to see a trained, qualified, and experienced specialist in homeopathic medicine to benefit fully from this approach. However, once the remedy pattern has been established by a professional, it is, of course, open to you to help yourself.

Healing

It is generally held that we have within us the ability to heal much of what ails us. How well we do it depends on many factors, including general health, attitudes and beliefs, and contact with deep sources of inner strength. The methods described in this book can enhance the operation of our inner healing mechanisms, but some people may wish to turn to an outside helper, or healer.

There is no inherent mystery or danger about healing, or "therapeutic touch"—it either helps or it does not. The healer's role is to help other people activate their own healing processes. Personal recommendation is the best way to find the right helper, but this is easier in some countries than others (in parts of the United States and Germany, for example, the professional practice of "psychic" healing is illegal). The important thing is to open up your own healing processes, and it is possible to obtain equally good and longer-lasting results from self-help approaches such as visualization and meditation.

Nutritional and dietary therapy

Vitamin and mineral deficiencies are commonly believed to be a cause of much depression because chemical imbalances in the body (most body chemicals come from what we eat and drink) can affect hormone levels, and hormones play a major part in mood. Finding out if this is a factor in a particular case needs the help of a specialist, who will need to carry out very careful tests over a period of time.

Though results can be extremely dramatic, interfering with the body's hormones (the endocrine system) should never be undertaken lightly. Nevertheless, eating a healthy diet and taking a good multivitamin food supplement—containing a broad spectrum of nutrients, including vitamins A, B-complex, C, E, minerals zinc, calcium, selenium, magnesium, and potassium, and a range of amino acids—is good for any psychological condition.

Daily supplements for depression

Vitamin B-complex • 50 mg
Vitamin C • up to 3 g
Zinc • 15 mg
Calcium • 500 mg
Magnesium • 200–400 mg

Herbal medicine

Hypericum, valerian, rosemary, lavender, and lemon balm are effective against depression, especially mild depression as a result of anxiety and insomnia. Hypericum, in particular, is now widely available from drugstores and health food stores following research that showed its effectiveness. It is necessary to take the recommended dose for 2–4 weeks to see any results.

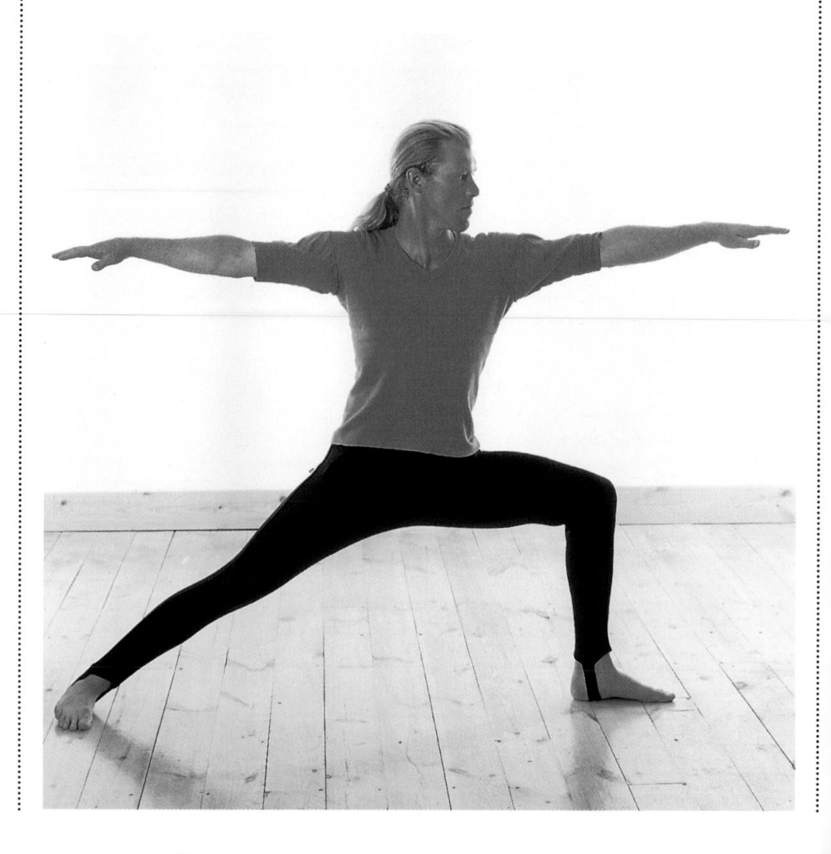

Many movement therapies can be useful in situations of mental and emotional pain. The Warrior yoga posture is said to tone the nervous system.

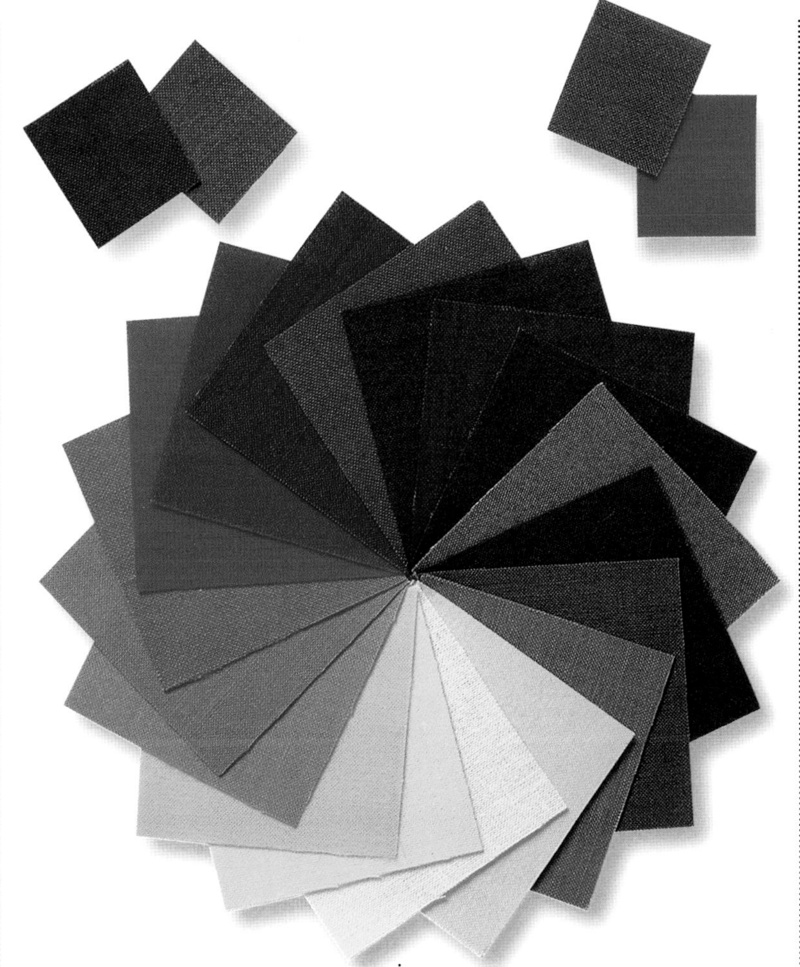

Colors are well known to affect us in a number of ways, both for good and ill. Pink, for example, is said to calm while red excites; green is said to bring harmony and tranquillity while orange can induce irritability.

Movement therapies

The eastern techniques of yoga and tai chi, and the western Alexander technique, involving physical movement with correct breathing and mental concentration, each have profound benefits for those with mental and emotional problems, because of their almost unique combination of mind and body with exercise. The range of movements is enormous, particularly in yoga and tai chi. However, it is advisable to seek guidance toward the most appropriate sequence, along with training in the techniques themselves, from an experienced practitioner initially.

Light and color therapy

Light and color are both known to have an effect on our mental, emotional, and physical state. Sunlight deprivation, for example, is the main cause of the depressive winter syndrome Seasonal Affective Disorder (SAD) by affecting the levels of the hormones melatonin and serotonin. Shades of blue are "cooling," pinks are calming, and reds "warm" or exciting. Effective treatment for SAD is a matter of either investing in lighting for home use that mimics the effect of natural daylight—known as full spectrum lighting (FSL)—or regularly visiting a center that has FSL devices. To check that you have the colors likely to be of most benefit to you, it is best to seek advice from a trained color therapist.

Hydrotherapy

Floating in a shallow bath of warm water and Epsom salts, inside an enclosed container, produces a profound sense of relaxation that many find a wonderful way to de-stress. There is the choice of lying in complete silence and darkness or with light and soft music. Flotation "tanks" are expensive to own and run, but can be found in many health and leisure centers.

Other therapies for depression

From a qualified therapist only

Counseling and psychotherapy • *page 154*

Hypnotherapy • *page 153*

Acupuncture and traditional Chinese herbal medicine • *pages 150–151*

Cranial osteopathy • *pages 153*

PHOBIAS AND ADDICTIONS

Severe psychological pain from such chronic conditions as manic depression, phobia, obsession, and addiction is not suitable for self-help, at least in the initial stages of treatment. Help is best sought from a professional. Approaches with a good record in treating all forms of severe psychological pain include:

- counseling and psychotherapy
- hypnotherapy
- acupuncture
- cranial osteopathy
- nutritional and dietary therapy
- herbal medicine
- massage
- aromatherapy
- reflexology
- yoga and tai chi.

For more information see pages 116–154.

SKIN PAIN

Skin is the largest organ of the body, weighing nearly 9 lb (4 kg) on an average adult, and covering an area of over 2 sq yd (about 2 sq m). It is also the first line of defense in any threat from outside, so it is hardly surprising that it is often the victim of aches and pains. This is especially so from accidents and injuries, but infection and illness can also cause painful inflammations from within the body that appear on or just below the skin's surface.

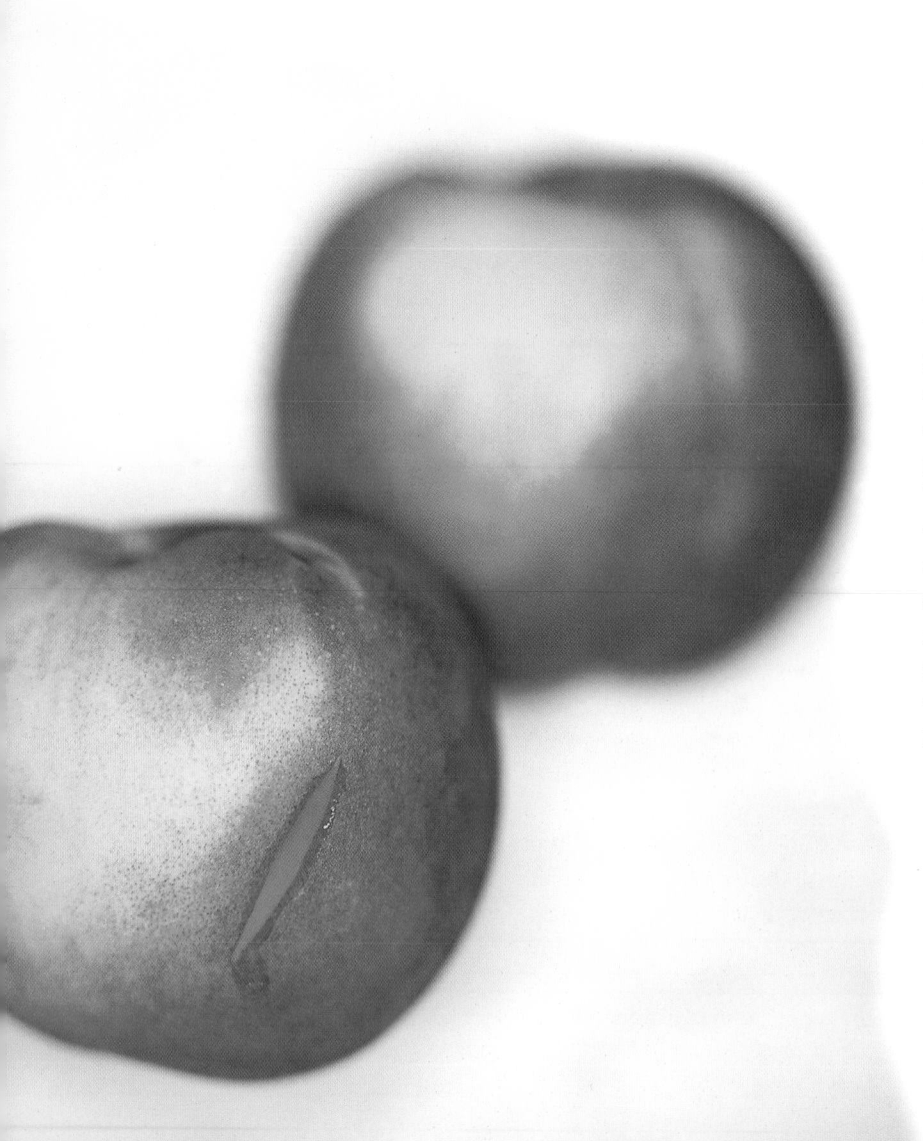

Skin consists of three layers: the outer epidermis layer, the middle dermis layer, and the innermost layer of subcutaneous fatty tissue. The innermost layer is where blood vessels run and hair roots start to grow; the middle layer is where sweat glands are found, and also the glands that produce lubrication for the outer layer of skin (sebaceous glands), as well as the web of nerve endings that send a constant stream of messages to the brain about temperature, touch, taste, and so on. The outer layer is the elastic surface that we see. Though relatively resilient, it is extremely thin and can damage easily. But it also repairs very quickly. Its entire surface is renewed every month, but this process speeds up if something happens to rub or scuff it.

HEAT RASH AND SUNBURN

Heat rash is an allergic reaction to too much heat, resulting in red and uncomfortable blotches over the surface of the skin. Children and women seem to be more susceptible than men. The symptoms, though intense, are usually short-lived and disappear when the irritant—too much heat or the sun—is avoided.

To provide relief, bathe the affected area with tincture of calendula or lavender. Chamomile lotion or sempervivum, dabbed on with absorbent cotton, can cool and soothe. Drinking tea made from lime or peppermint may also help. For sunburn, see "First Aid for Pain," page 24.

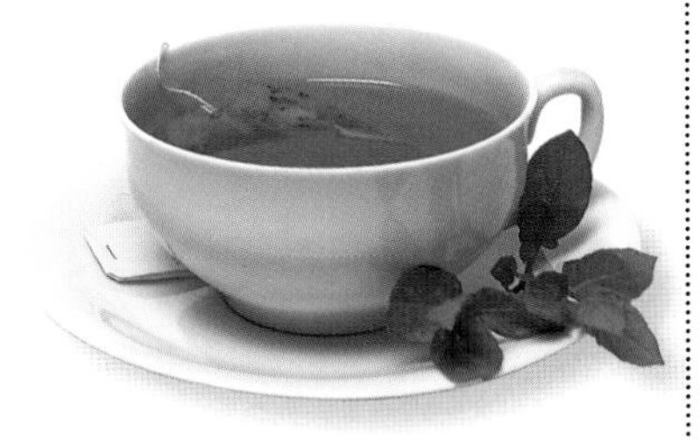

Peppermint tea may help soothe skin rash caused by excessive heat.

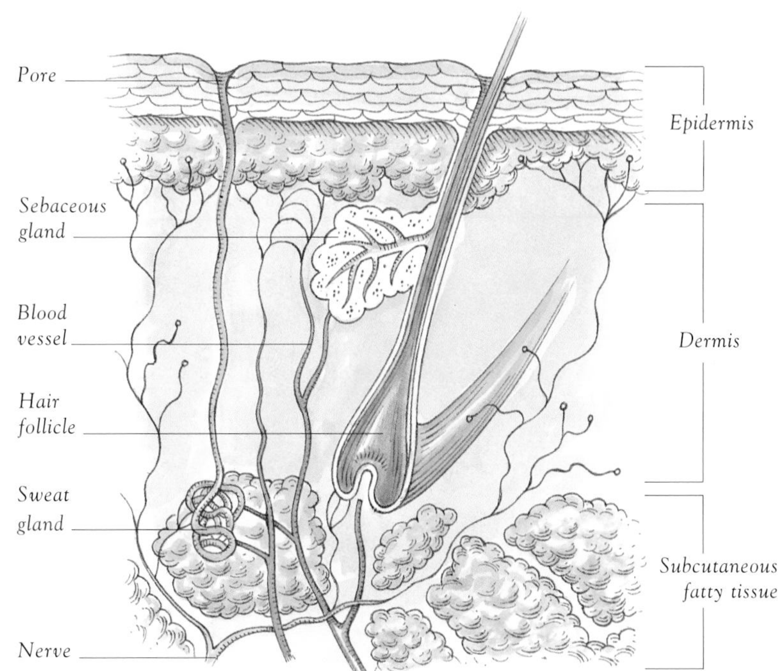

The skin performs vital protective, perceptive, and temperature and fluid control functions.

BOILS

Boils are an inflammation of the skin from a bacterial infection, producing tender, pus-filled, raised spots. They are more uncomfortable than serious, but seldom clear unless the pus is drained first.

Herbal medicine

Use a hot poultice of slippery elm paste, kaolin, or magnesium sulfate, applied over several days to bring the boil to a head, followed by tea tree antiseptic oil after the boil has burst. An alternative is a bread poultice: crumble bread into boiled milk or water, wrap the mixture in gauze, drain, and apply hot every 3–4 hours; or a hot Epsom salts pack (2 tablespoonfuls in one cup of water). While the boil lasts, take one teaspoonful of equal parts of echinacea, cleavers, and yellow dock, made into a tea and drunk three times times a day.

Homeopathy

Take hepar sulf to bring the boil to a head, and silicea after it has burst.

BLISTERS

Blisters are thin swellings of the skin, containing a watery fluid, caused by friction. Apply the natural antiseptics lavender, tea tree, or Roman chamomile oil onto the punctured blister, or dab on a mixture of hypericum and calendula. Take the homeopathic remedy rhus tox 6c every four hours for a day to prevent any worsening and rub on aloe vera gel. The tissue salt kali mur, taken as a supplement, and garlic may also help.

CHAPPING

Usually the result of prolonged exposure to cold and wet, chapping mainly affects hands, which become red and tender. Glycerin mixed with rose water and rubbed well into the hands is the favorite remedy, but mudpacks made from clay-rich earth may also help.

CHILBLAINS

Reddish-blue swellings that itch and burn, usually on the hands and feet, are the result of extreme cold and poor circulation. Mix the white of an egg and a tablespoon of flour with glycerin and honey, work it into a paste, and spread it over the affected part (do not rub). Leave it in place, covered by a cloth or bandage, for 24 hours, and keep it warm. Vitamin E-rich foods, such as seeds, nuts, wholegrains, green leafy vegetables, and wheatgerm, and the herb echinacea can also aid recovery.

For burning and itching skin, try the homeopathic treatment rhus tox cream twice daily, agaricus every three hours, or carbo veg if chilblains feel worse in a warm bed (6c three times daily for two weeks). For cracked skin: tamus ointment and petroleum 6c three times daily for two weeks.

WHITLOW (FELON)

A whitlow, or felon, is an inflamed growth, exuding pus, usually appearing on the fingers, around the nails, but also on the toes. The standard treatment is Morrison's paste (magnesium sulfate).

TINEA (RINGWORM/ ATHLETE'S FOOT)

Tinea is a fungal infection of the skin, misleadingly known as ringworm. It is most commonly experienced as "athlete's foot," but can also affect any other part of the body where warm, damp conditions can encourage fungus growth. The most common symptom is intense itching, but local pain can be felt if the condition is severe.

Keeping the affected area clean and dry is the most effective treatment, so a high standard of personal hygiene is important. In cases of athlete's foot, let plenty of fresh air get to the feet and wear cotton (never nylon) socks.

Aromatherapy

Essential tea tree oil, applied undiluted, can help. For athlete's foot, add 2 drops each of oils of lavender, tea tree, and tagetes to a bowl of warm water and soak the feet for 10 minutes each night. An alternative is a compress of the same oils on the affected area, kept in place with a bandage or sock overnight. In the morning, wash and dry the feet, repeat the compress, but add a tablespoonful of calendula oil, and leave in place during the day.

Hydrotherapy and herbal medicine

Among a number of treatments that can be effective when used on the affected area are propolis or calendula cream, vitamin C powder, or roll cotton (cotton wool) soaked in honey and cider vinegar and left on overnight. For athlete's foot, use a daily footbath of golden seal root or a mixture of 10 oz (30 g) each of red clover, sage, calendula, and agrimony with two teaspoonfuls of cider vinegar. Bathe the feet for half an hour, dry well, and powder with arrowroot or powdered golden seal root. For severe cases, begin with regular cleaning with roll cotton (cotton wool) soaked in hydrogen peroxide, followed by the treatments above.

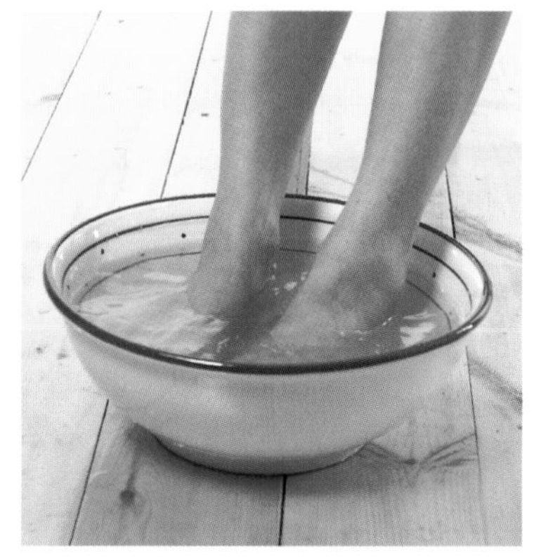

Soaking feet daily in an infusion of golden seal root can help athlete's foot.

HIVES (NETTLE RASH/URTICARIA)

Intensely itchy raised red patches on the skin, sometimes with pale centers, characterize hives—also known as nettle rash or, medically, as urticaria. It is caused by an allergic reaction to a number of foods (including eggs, milk, citrus fruit, strawberries, and shellfish); drugs, such as antibiotics; insect bites and stings; and emotional stress. The rash, which usually affects the face, neck, and trunk, may last for a few hours or some days.

An infusion of chamomile or chickweed relieves the itching, vitamin E cream helps skin recovery, and vitamin C bolsters against further attacks. The homeopathy treatments rhus tox, apis, or urtica urens (all 3c) can also help. In each case, dissolve one tablet under the tongue every hour until the symptoms subside.

CAUTION In rare cases the swelling can affect the throat and restrict breathing. In this situation urgent medical help is essential.

ECZEMA/DERMATITIS

Eczema is a widespread and sometimes severe skin condition from touching or eating/drinking a substance the body reacts against. This is usually described as an "allergic reaction." "Contact" eczema is also known as dermatitis. Symptoms in both cases, though, are the same: intensely itchy, red skin that can become cracked, raw, and painful. Of more than a dozen different types of eczema, the most common is atopic or infantile eczema, seen mainly in children (atopic means having an inherited tendency). Examples of substances that can "trigger" eczema are detergents, dyes, plants, some foods and drinks, animal hair and feathers, and house dust. Emotional stress is a known psychological trigger. A tendency to eczema is lifelong and there is as yet no cure, but a wide range of natural approaches can help.

Long-term relief can be achieved with careful diet and nutrition, but a variety of other natural remedies can help bring immediate relief. Consult a professional therapist for all types of

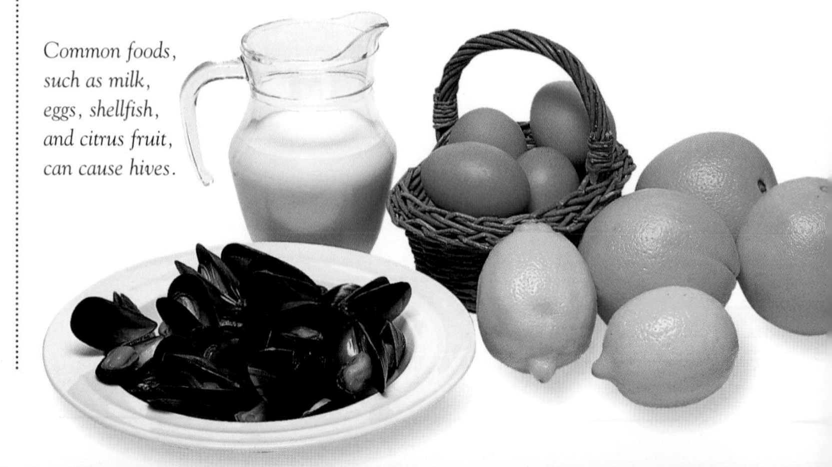

Common foods, such as milk, eggs, shellfish, and citrus fruit, can cause hives.

eczema. Results will depend on the type of eczema and individual response. Never use skin creams containing lanolin to treat eczema.

Nutritional and dietary therapy

Identifying and eliminating allergens (substances that cause an allergic reaction) is the first and most important step in the treatment of eczema. Sometimes allergens are easy to identify: for example, a reaction caused by animal fur. But if not, identification is normally done either by having an allergy test (see page 62), or by following an "exclusion diet" (see page 62). The following "good eating" tips may help:

Eat LESS

- *Dairy products, the most common food allergens*
- *Animal fats, sugars, and salts*
- *Processed food, and foods with additives and preservatives*

Eat MORE

- *Vegetables, vegetable oils, and oily fish such as tuna and mackerel*

Regular supplementation with gammalinolenic acid (GLA) can be beneficial for eczema. The best-known form is evening primrose oil (EPO), but starflower (borage) and blackcurrant seed oils both contain high levels of GLA. The doses may need to be as high as six capsules a day, and benefits may not be apparent for three months or so, but good results have been reported. Other supplements with a good record in helping eczema over the long term (three months or more) are beta carotene (the natural precursor of vitamin A), vitamins B, C, and E, and the micro-minerals zinc, selenium, and magnesium.

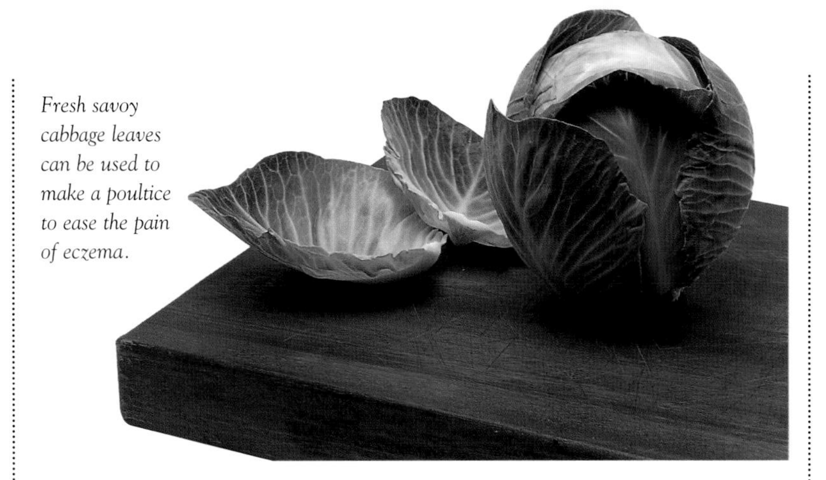

Fresh savoy cabbage leaves can be used to make a poultice to ease the pain of eczema.

Herbal medicine

A poultice of savoy cabbage leaves can be very effective. Clean, warm, and crush the leaves, then layer them on the area and bind in place with a bandage. Repeat morning and night. Herbal teas said to relieve eczema symptoms include calendula, chickweed, walnut leaf, nettle, chamomile, blackberry, raspberry, and loganberry. The dried herbs parsley, dandelion root, red clover, and golden seal may also help. Mix a teaspoonful of each with honey and use on bread as a spread. A teaspoonful of golden seal, mixed with hot water to form a tincture and painted on the skin, can also offer relief.

Hydrotherapy and aromatherapy

Dissolve two tablespoonfuls of sodium bicarbonate in warm water and bathe the affected area. Apply calamine lotion, preferably containing arachis oil. Rub on essential oils of fennel, chamomile, geranium, hyssop, juniper, or lavender (12 drops to 1½ fl oz/ 50 ml carrier oil). If the affected area is dry, use calendula as a carrier oil; if moist, use a neutral carrier, such as grapeseed oil. Apply morning and night.

Homeopathy

Graphites, petroleum, rhus tox and sulfur may help eczema, but always seek professional advice first.

Chinese "miracle cure"

A combination containing 10 different Chinese herbs in a "tea," used by a Chinese herbalist in London, England, made the headlines in 1993 as a "miracle cure" for atopic eczema. It was subsequently researched by a British company, and following successful trials, patented under the name Zemaphyte. Many Chinese medical herbalists claim a similarly high success rate with others of the more than 4000 herbs used in traditional Chinese medicine, so this could be an avenue worth exploring.

CAUTION *The range of Chinese herbs contains many that are extremely potent and not yet properly researched. Great care must be taken in choosing a practitioner.*

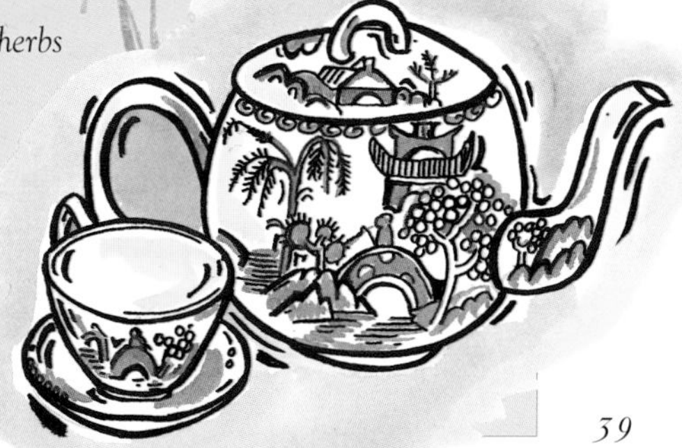

PSORIASIS

Psoriasis is a skin disease characterized by dry, reddish patches covered with silvery scales that can develop on any part of the body (usually the head, lower back, elbows, and knees) as the result of an abnormally high rate of skin cell reproduction. It is not contagious, and pain is usually psychological, though severe forms can involve cracks in the skin and, in rare cases, a painful type of arthritis, affecting legs, hands, and spine. The cause is unknown, but it appears to be an inherited tendency that stays once it starts, coming and going at intervals. Attacks are classically triggered by stress and illness.

Naturopathy

Natural sunlight, containing ultraviolet A and B rays, is the best of all treatments for psoriasis, but except in unusual places, such as the Dead Sea, exposure must not be long (10–30 minutes, depending on skin type). To improve skin health, some naturopaths recommend fasting for 48 hours, drinking water or freshly pressed fruit and vegetable juices—a combination of carrot, celery, beet, cucumber, and/or grape is best, taken as often as you want. If drinking only water, do not exercise, and take plenty of rest. If doing a juice fast, exercise moderately. To encourage cleansing, take Epsom salts or castor oil in orange juice, two days before starting the fast, and the morning of the first day of the fast.

Nutritional and dietary therapy

Eat a healthy diet with plenty of fresh fruit, vegetables, and salads, and reduce intake of animal fats as much as possible. Oily fish, such as mackerel, salmon, sardines, and herring, is recommended. Bitter melon is an old remedy for psoriasis that might be of help, and so are avocado and sauerkraut.

Supplementing with a daily tablespoonful of cold-pressed extra virgin olive oil, flaxseed (linseed) oil, or canola oil may help—or, better, take capsules of essential fatty acids (EFAs) containing gammalinolenic acid (GLA) and eicosapentenoic acid (EPA), such as starflower (borage) oil, evening primrose oil, and fish oils. Other supplements that might help during an attack are vitamin A (10,000 iu three times daily for six days), vitamin B complex (100 mg twice a day with meals), vitamin D (400 iu a day), spirulina (an algae rich in micro-minerals), zinc (15–20 mg a day), and the tissue salts silicea, nat sulf, kali phos, ferr phos, and calc sulf.

Herbal medicine

A type of berberis (*Mahonia aquifolium*) has recently shown success in treating psoriasis, but a more traditional treatment is dandelion root and burdock with red clover flower as blood cleansers. Nettle is also said to help psoriasis by "purifying" the blood. Other useful herbs are echinacea (for the immune system), yellow dock (boil 2–3 leaves per quart/liter of water, and drink), garlic, and sarsparilla.

Homeopathy

The remedies sulfur 6c (for dry, red, itchy patches), petroleum 6c (dry, rough, and cracked skin), and graphites 6c (oozing plaques) can help alleviate acute attacks. Take 3–4 tablets daily for 14 days.

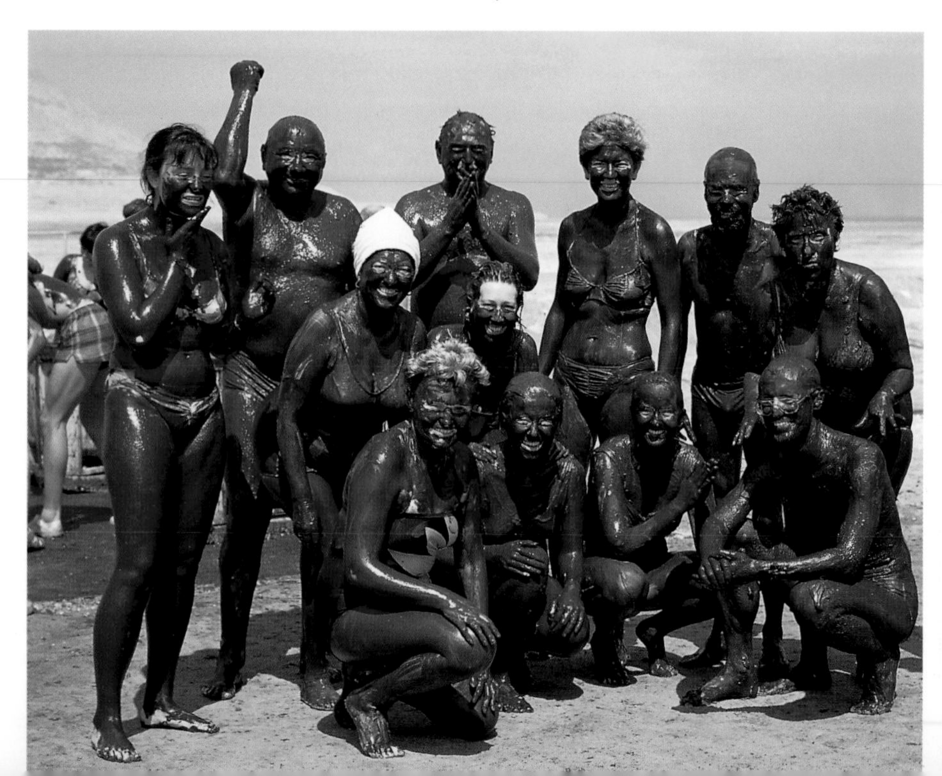

The Dead Sea resorts between Israel and Jordan have an unequaled reputation for treating psoriasis. At 1300 ft (400 m) below sea level, the atmosphere naturally filters out the harmful rays and leaves only the beneficial UVA and UVB rays. This, coupled with bathing in the Dead Sea itself and the mud around it—both high in minerals good for skin nourishment—provides the almost perfect psoriasis treatment.

Castor oil treatments for psoriasis

Pack

Soak a cloth in castor oil, so that it is wet but not dripping. Apply to the affected area, and cover with plastic. Place a heating pad on top, starting at medium heat and increasing to high. Leave on for an hour. Remove, and clean the skin with two teaspoonfuls of sodium bicarbonate in a quart (1 liter) of warm water. Repeat four times a day.

Bath

Fill the bathtub with warm water. Add half a cup of castor oil and mix thoroughly. Soak in the mixture for 30 minutes, rubbing your body all over, then wash off with shampoo. The tub will be very slippery, so be careful when getting in and out.

Aromatherapy

The essential oils bergamot and lavender, added to a bath or rubbed on in a neutral oil or lotion, may help. Sandalwood vaporized in a burner can also be beneficial.

Reflexology

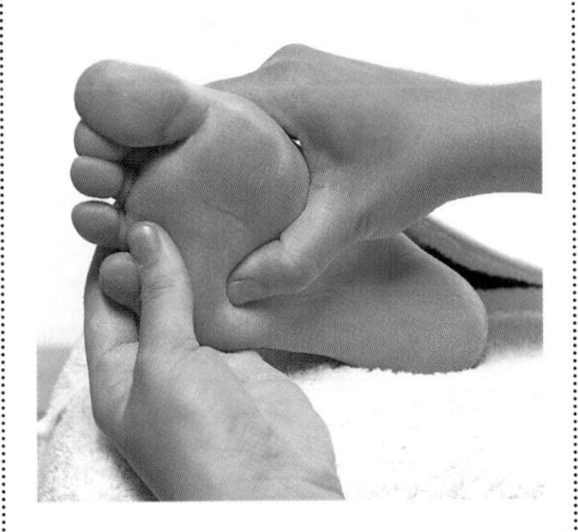

Massaging the reflex points linked to the liver, kidneys, and lungs are said to help psoriasis, along with those of the solar plexus and diaphragm (shown above).

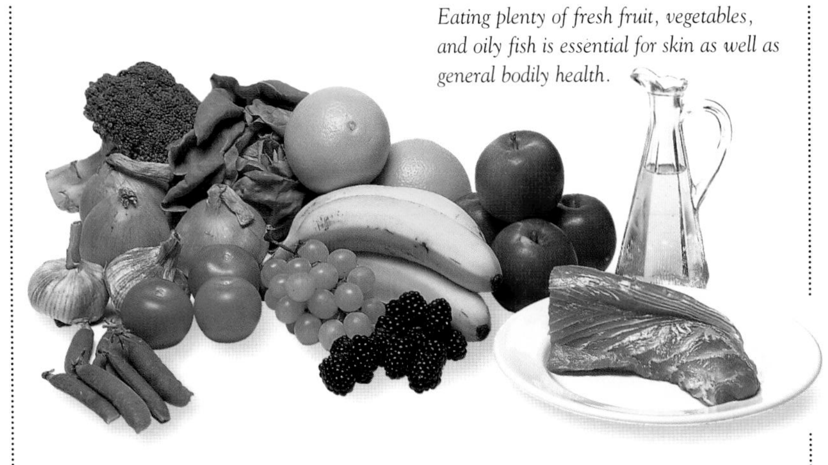

Eating plenty of fresh fruit, vegetables, and oily fish is essential for skin as well as general bodily health.

Relaxation

Reducing stress levels and learning to relax is important in preventing psoriasis, which is why approaches such as meditation, visualization, and biofeedback can help. Bathing and listening to relaxing tapes and CDs can also help.

SHINGLES

This is an extremely painful, blistering rash that normally occurs around one half of the midriff (although the neck, face, and sometimes the eyes can be affected) as a result of inflammation of nerve roots. Shingles is caused by the same herpes zoster virus that provokes chickenpox, and is often the result of a weakened immune system coinciding with a period of emotional stress. It is most common in older people.

Hydrotherapy

Bathing in a warm to hot bath of sodium bicarbonate (one to two cupfuls to a bath) eases irritation. An alternative is an oatmeal bath: hang a 1 lb (450 g) bag of unground oatmeal under the running water and when the bath is half full, mix in a few tablespoons of raw, finely ground oatmeal. Again, the water should be warm to hot. Use the wet oatmeal bag as a sponge to dab the affected areas. Spend 30 minutes in the bath every day.

Nutritional therapy

A multivitamin, containing vitamins A (as beta carotene), B-complex, C, E, the mineral zinc, and the amino acid lysine can help.

Aromatherapy and herbal medicine

The essential oils geranium, sage, and thyme, mixed together, and rubbed, or dabbed, gently onto the affected area can help, if used at the first signs of a rash. Mix three drops of each oil into 1 fl oz (30 ml) of neutral carrier oil, such as grapeseed. Apply aloe vera to alleviate the rash, either as a gel or a liquid (straight or diluted, as required).

Homeopathy

Used early on, the remedies rhus tox 6c (for red, itching, and blistered skin), apis (burning), and mezereum (pain and itching) are most effective—the last two as a cold liquid or lotion.

Other therapies

From a qualified therapist only

Acupuncture, for eczema, psoriasis, and shingles—especially for the alleviation of pain following rash (post-herpetic neuralgia) • *pages 150–151*

CANCER PAIN

Cancer—a disease in which the cells of the body "rebel" and multiply out of control—is feared as much for the belief that it is always painful as for its erratic, unpredictable, and hard-to-treat nature. But the truth is that most cancers do not cause pain—at least initially—which is why it is difficult to detect some forms in the early stages.

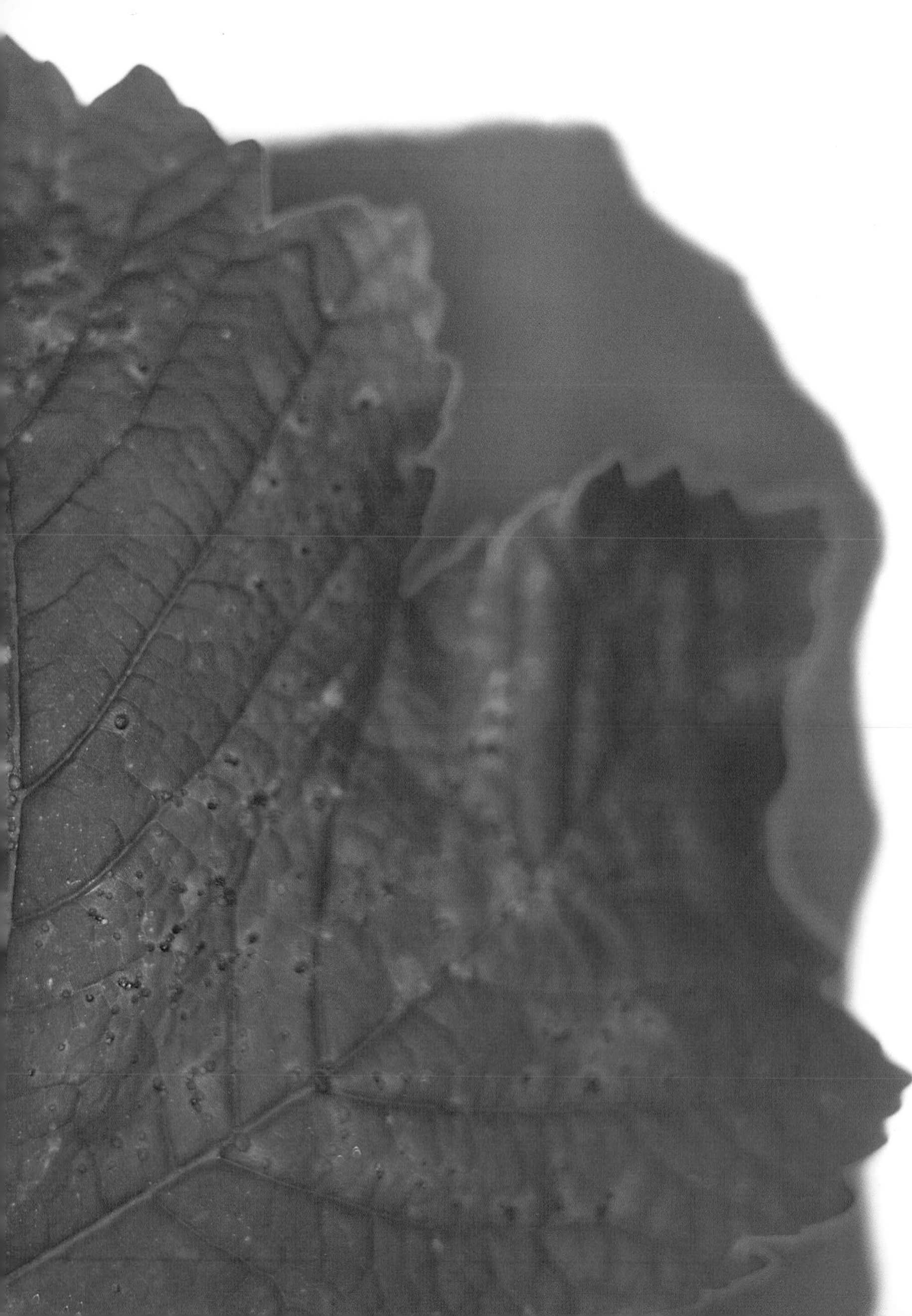

There are no precise statistics, but various estimates have suggested that as few as half of all those with cancer feel pain. Some cancers—liver cancer is the best example—cause minimal pain even in the advanced stages. Cancer can, and does, give rise to pain, but the significant fact is that when the pain eventually makes itself felt, it is more usually the result of the cancerous growth pressing on a nerve or interfering with some other bodily function than the cancer itself giving pain.

Mind and emotions have been shown to be as important in the effective treatment of cancer as treating just the body—and may even be more so. The alleviation of cancer pain is a matter of combining various psychological and physical approaches to marshal and make best use of the natural mind-over-matter powers that we all have. Helping yourself is possible to a very large extent in cancer, but the following suggestions are meant as a complement to any conventional medical treatment rather than as an alternative to it.

CAUTION It is illegal in many countries for anyone who is not a medical doctor to treat cancer or to claim to treat cancer.

Nutritional therapy

Vitamins and minerals do not have the painkilling properties of some herbs, but a complex supplement of 17 micro-minerals developed by the Hungarian doctor Jøszef Béres in the early 1970s is claimed to have dramatic pain-relieving effects. Called "Béres Drops Plus," the combination is said to work by restoring the body's natural mineral balance, but it is not yet widely available in the West.

Aromatherapy

Massaging with essential oils is one of the best ways to counter cancer pain, especially if you can find someone to do it to you. Use geranium, jasmine, juniper, or Roman chamomile. Vaporizing essential oils of lemon, lemon grass, and/or lavender may also help.

CAUTION It is not recommended to massage over the site of the tumor, or where treatment has made the body tender or sore.

Reflexology

The same principle applies to reflexology as to massage, except that reflexology offers the advantage of massaging areas of the body affected by tumors indirectly via the feet. You can identify the part of the foot to be manipulated by referring to the "foot map" on page 145. The same oils useful in massage can be applied to the feet, and again it is better if someone does the manipulating for you, making sure they use firm but not sharp pressure (thumbs are best for this) for 5–10 seconds at a time.

Acupressure

The principles and techniques of acupressure, including its Japanese equivalent shiatsu, follow on from the above two therapies in cancer pain relief. Applying finger, thumb, knuckle, or even whole hand pressure to points that relate to the affected part or parts of the body can be very effective (refer to the "body maps" on page 143). Pressure should be steady and deep (though not hurtful), and last for about 20 seconds at a time.

Herbal medicine

A wide range of herbs can help in cancer pain, depending entirely on the symptoms and the individual. The most important are Jamaican dogwood, lady's slipper, passionflower, skullcap, and valerian. But the advice of a qualified medical herbalist should be followed. If not consulting a trained therapist, always take medicinal herbs as tablets or capsules in the controlled doses supplied by druggists and health food stores.

Homeopathy

Nux vomica (3c or 6c, taken three times daily for a month) is said to relieve discomfort, particularly nausea, caused by conventional cancer treatments.

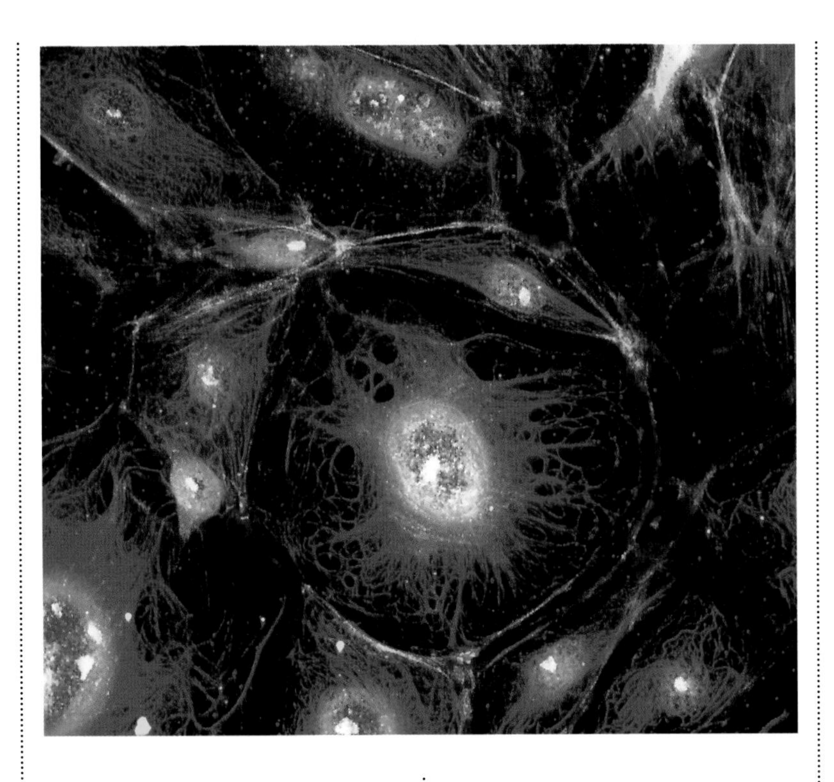

Cancer cells magnified 400 times.

Mind-body therapies

Psychological techniques combine de-stressing and relaxation with positive thinking. The self-help techniques most successful in overcoming pain in cancer are:

- meditation, including autogenic training (see pages 138–139)
- visualization (see page 137)
- creative arts therapies, especially music and painting (see pages 140–141)
- counseling and psychotherapy (see page 154)
- hypnotherapy (see page 153).

Other therapies

From a qualified therapist only

Acupuncture, for relieving some of the painful after-effects of conventional cancer treatment, such as surgery and chemotherapy • pages 150–151

TENS, and more particularly GigaTENS • pages 123

HEADACHES AND MIGRAINES

Headaches (and to a lesser extent, migraines) are a widely experienced form of pain—and the most common type of "referred pain." This means that although a pain in the head can obviously result from a bang on the skull, the more usual cause of a headache is a problem elsewhere in the body. Muscle tension in the neck and shoulders, for example, or in the case of migraine, an allergic response to food are frequently to blame.

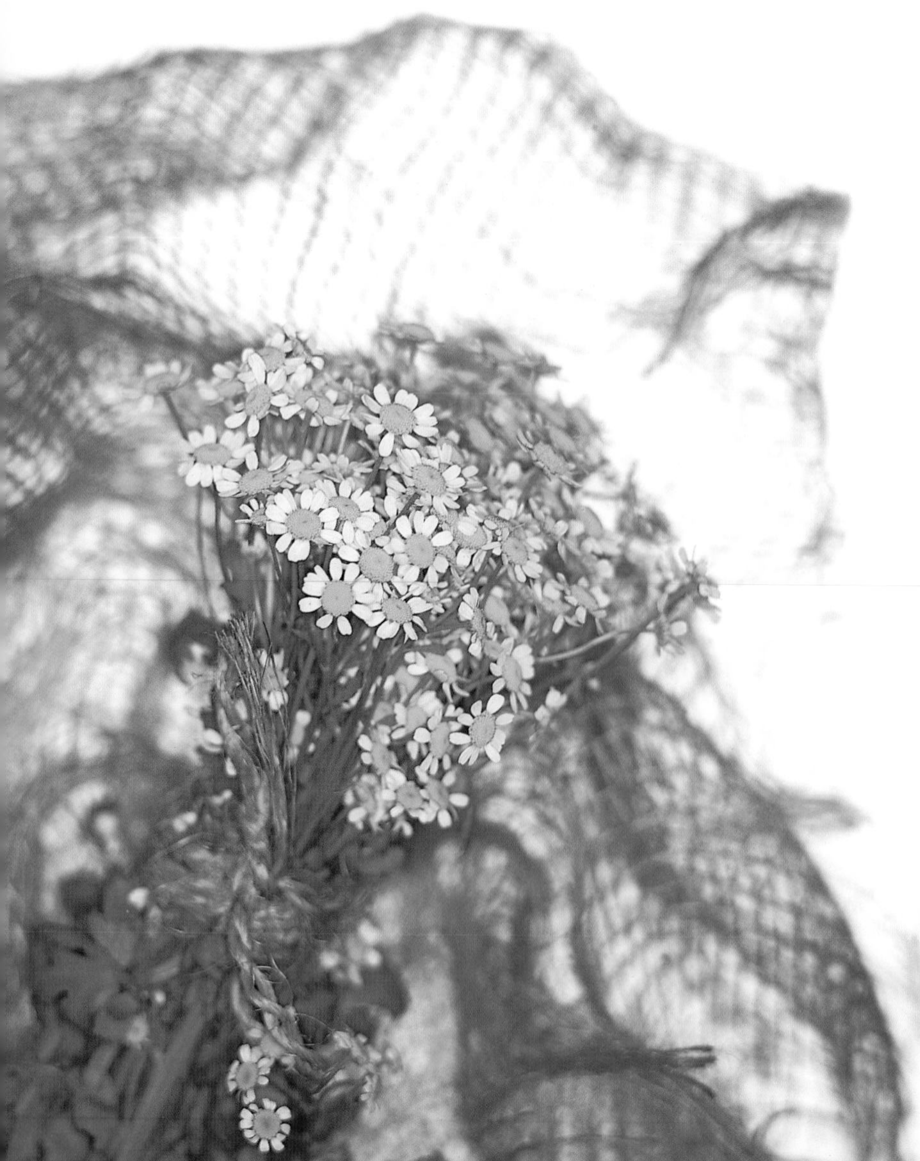

The good news is that headaches and migraines both respond extremely well to a wide range of natural methods of treatment—in fact, many doctors today would recommend them before standard drug treatments.

Common causes

- *Stress*
- *Food and drink (especially alcohol, coffee, oranges, cheese, and chocolate)*
- *Eyestrain*
- *Overwork (particularly work requiring mental effort)*
- *Muscular stress and strain*
- *Illness and infection*
- *Depression*
- *Drugs*
- *Injury*

CAUTION

Prolonged or frequent headaches should be reported to a qualified medical practitioner.

HEADACHES

Most headaches are of the type often referred to as "tension" headache, because they are caused by tension in the muscles and tissues of the head, neck, and shoulders—usually as a direct result of the stresses and strains of everyday living. Overeating and drinking are also common causes of tension headache. These common headaches, whether stress- or food-related, are the easiest to treat naturally. Headaches as a result of more serious conditions, such as infection, are harder to assist, but help is still possible with care.

Warning

Seek immediate medial attention if head pain is caused by:

- *concussion*
- *stroke*
- *cerebral hemorrhage*
- *cancer*
- *meningitis*
- *poliomyelitis.*

Acupressure

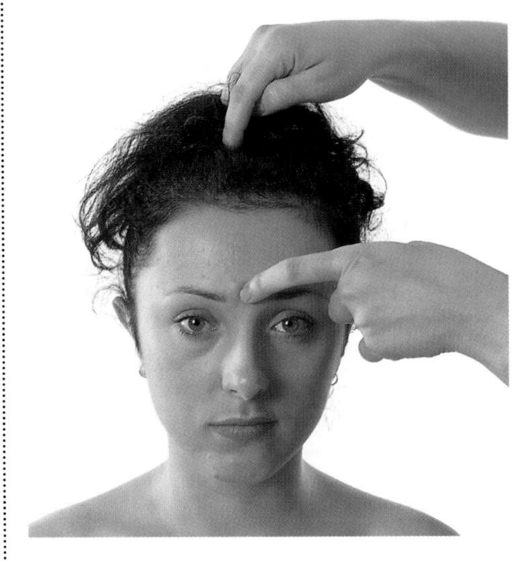

one

Using both hands, apply gentle fingertip pressure to a point midway between the eyebrows and another immediately above, on the top of the head. Hold the pressure for about five seconds and then relax.

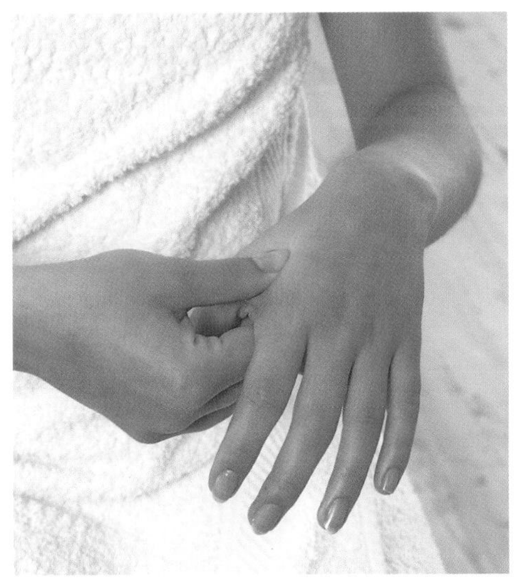

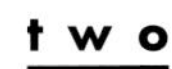

two

Another point worth trying is the soft pad between thumb and first finger, either hand. Use the thumb of your other hand to apply the pressure. Again, a few seconds of gentle pressure is all that is needed.

CAUTION This method is not recommended during pregnancy.

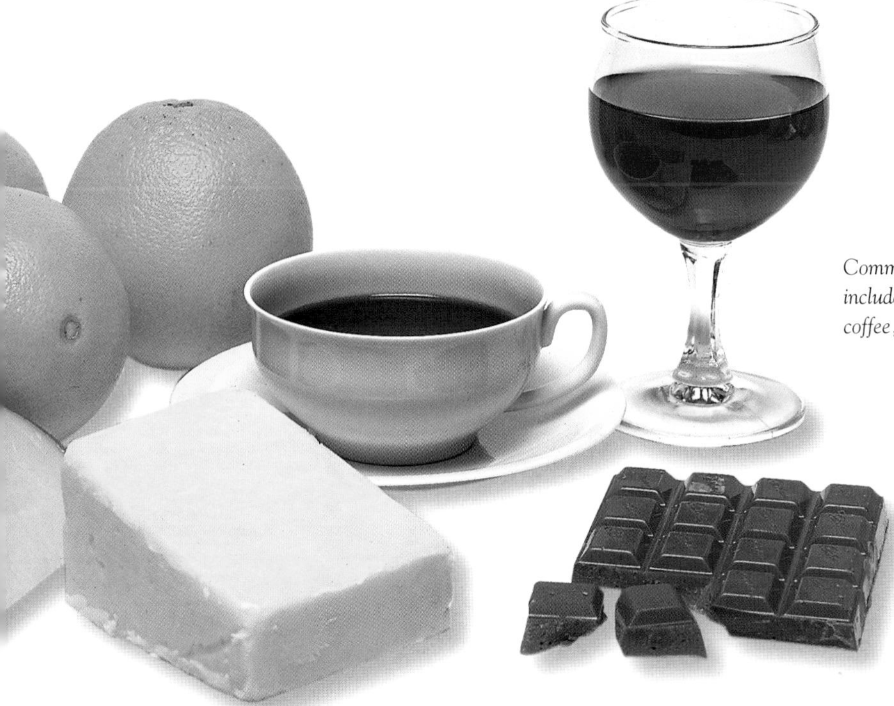

Common food causes of migraines include chocolate, cheese, oranges, coffee, and alcohol.

Aromatherapy

For headaches caused by colds, flu, or breathing problems, such as sinusitis and bronchitis, inhale steam from hot water infused with Olbas oil, or a mixture of essential oils such as eucalyptus, juniper berry, peppermint, wintergreen, and cajuput. A pleasant and relaxing alternative is to add a few drops of the oils of melissa, rosemary, or marjoram to a hot bath, and soak.

Hydrotherapy

Sitting or lying in a quiet and restful position with eyes closed is an effective first step to relieving headache. Keeping warm is also important. Water therapy acts to treat the symptoms of tension headache, and relaxing techniques to remove the underlying causes. For immediate relief, soak a washcloth in cold water, wring it out, and lie down with it over the forehead and eyes. Rest with eyes closed for as long as possible. Resoak the cloth as often as needed to keep the head cool.

Relaxation

Consciously getting your body to relax and noting the change is a very effective way of relaxing that is not only useful for preventing and removing headaches but for pain caused by tension in any part of the body.

Herbal medicine

The bark of the willow tree and the plant meadowsweet contain natural painkillers effective against headache (aspirin was developed from them). Other useful herbs are valerian (a sedative), chamomile, passiflora, ginger, lavender, and rosemary. Pour hot water onto a teaspoonful or two of the dried herb in a cup, and drink as a tea.

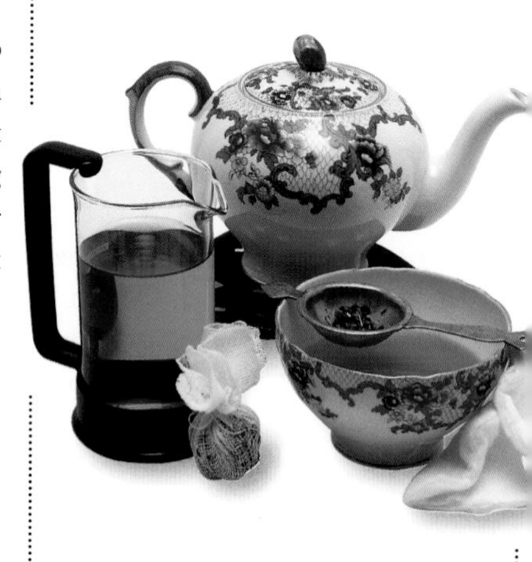

Herbs known to help remove headaches are best drunk as infusions (teas).

CAUTION Self-medication with wild plants is not recommended without guidance from a qualified herbalist, because many herbs are strong and can be dangerous if taken in excess. One of the best ways to treat yourself with herbs is to take ready-made tablets or capsules, which are widely available from reputable health food suppliers and drugstores.

Massage

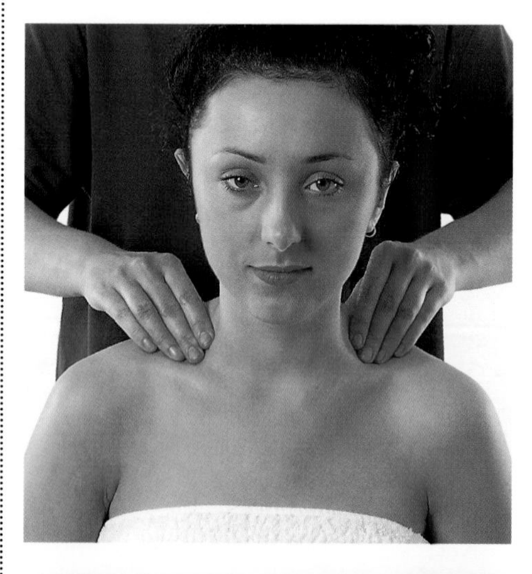

one

Make sure you are in a comfortable position—sitting in a hot bath is ideal—and massage the back of the neck, shoulders, and temples. Better still, get a friend to do it for you.

two

Use relaxed but positive strokes on the shoulders and fingertip pressure on the back of the neck and temples. For a better effect, lubricate your hands with a neutral oil (such as grapeseed), infused with three or four drops of an essential oil, such as lavender, chamomile, basil, or peppermint.

Alexander technique

The technique—which teaches correct posture by "re-educating" the head to sit correctly on the shoulders—must first be learned from a trained teacher but it is then easy to use yourself at home. Practiced on a regular basis, the Alexander technique is effective for the prevention of headache as well as their treatment.

Therapeutic touch

Get a friend to stand behind you and "stroke" either side of your head with their hands held about an inch (2–3 cm) away from your hair. Ask them to wish or will your headache away as they stroke. Close your eyes and visualize the headache going away as they do it. Continue for as long as you think it worthwhile, but 10–15 minutes will normally yield results.

Reflexology

Apply determined fingertip or thumb pressure to the bottom, sides, and top of the toes of both feet (the toe is said to link to the head in reflexology). Concentrate on areas where the toes are tender, pressing until the tenderness wears off. Do the same to the area where the toes join the foot (said to correspond to the neck). Treating yourself is not ideal, or easy, but it can be done—though the help of a friend is better. For best results, consult a trained therapist.

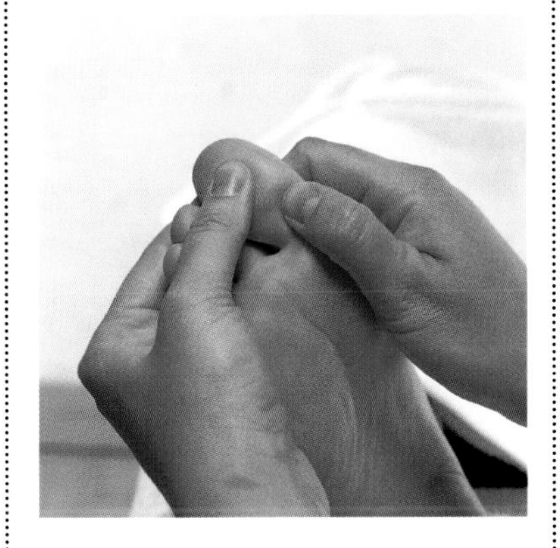

Massaging the big toe is the reflexology equivalent of massaging the back of the neck and shoulders, and is particularly useful if you can't find anyone to massage your back for you.

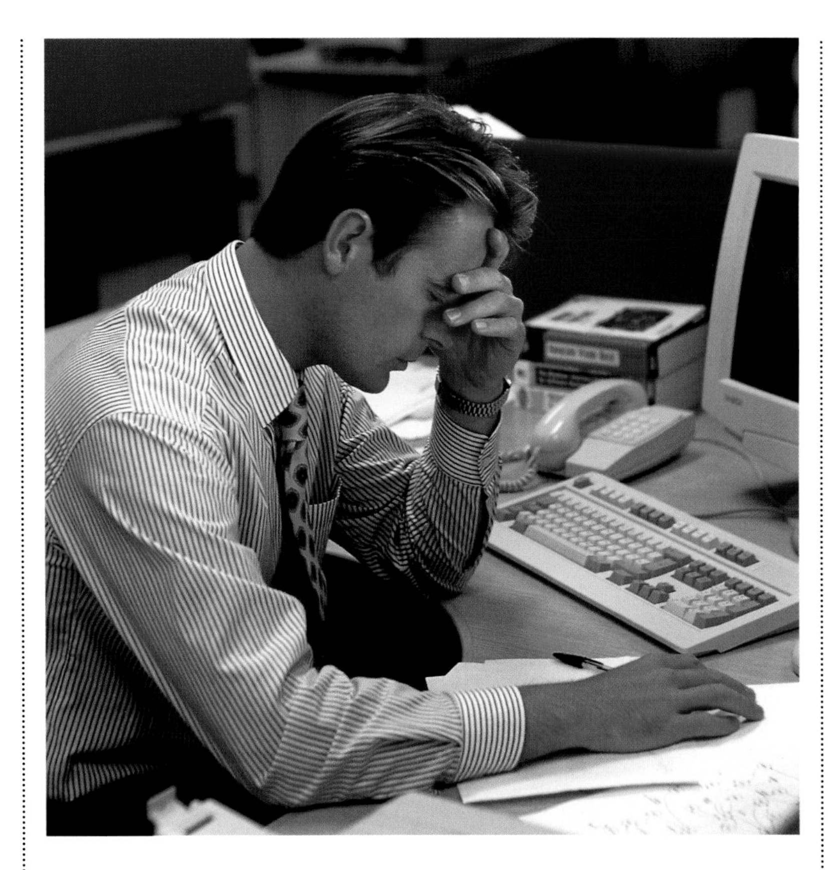

Working too long in front of a computer monitor can cause eyestrain and trigger both headaches and migraines. Using a filter over the screen and taking regular breaks can help prevent attacks.

Homeopathy

Homeopathic treatment for headaches depends on the cause or causes (or an assessment of the likely cause or causes if not known). For example, pulsatilla can help a headache from overeating and drinking, but gelsemium or ignatia are best if the pain arises more from emotional fear or excitement (see table below).

Treating headaches using homeopathy

Cause of headache	Remedy	Dose
Overeating, feeling bloated	*Pulsatilla*	*6c, one every hour until better*
Indigestion, constipation	*Nux vomica*	*6c, one every night and morning*
Fear, emotional excitement	*Gelsemium, Ignatia*	*6c, one every hour until recovered*
Heat exposure, sunstroke	*Belladonna*	*6c, one every hour until better*
Injury or fall	*Arnica*	*6c, one every hour until better*

CAUTION *Homeopathic remedies can be a useful first aid treatment in emergencies, but a consultation with a qualified homeopath is advisable, particularly for recurring or chronic headache.*

MIGRAINES

Classic migraine is much more than just a bad headache. It is a severe and often disabling pain in the head—usually on one side only—accompanied by sometimes alarming symptoms such as altered perception, a feeling that the skull is in the grip of a tightening vise, pins and needles or numbness, nausea and vomiting, and an inability to do anything. Symptoms can come and go and last for hours—sometimes even days. No two people usually experience the same symptoms, and one person can experience different symptoms on different occasions.

Migraines—which have been compared to an electrical storm going on inside the head—arise from the dilation or constriction of small arteries in the head region. Many different factors seem to cause them, but those most often reported are extreme stress, disco lights and noise, menstruation (women suffer from migraine much more than men do), and eating or drinking "trigger" foods, such as chocolate, cheese, oranges, coffee, and red wine.

Self-hypnosis

The technique of warming the fingers by using the power of your mind has been shown to produce lasting benefits for many sufferers of chronic migraine. The technique, which is a form of self-hypnosis, involves willing your fingers to a temperature 96°F (35.6°C) by concentrating. It is not easy but can be done—and is said to work for 85 percent of people.

Reflexology

The same reflex points used to ease headaches can work for migraine sufferers also.

Relaxation

Therapies such as meditation, tai chi, and yoga are effective for prevention in the long term by teaching the body how to relax and "harmonize" within itself. All three are best learned from a qualified teacher first.

Nutritional, dietary and herbal therapies

The herb feverfew is well known to be effective in preventing attacks. One fresh leaf a day (eaten either in a salad or sandwich) is the recommended amount if you are prone to regular bouts of migraine. But it is not nearly so effective if an attack has already started. An alternative to eating the raw leaf is to take 125 mg capsules or tablets (available from most good health food or drugstores).

Vitamin C (ascorbic acid), the B vitamins (especially vitamin B3, niacin), and the mineral magnesium are also said to help not only prevent attacks but alleviate the symptoms. If you do not want to go to the expense of consulting a qualified nutritionist for individual advice on optimum dose levels, take a good-quality multivitamin containing these ingredients. Another supplement said to help is royal jelly. Beneficial foods include carrots, celery, beet, cucumber, spinach, and parsley. For best effect they should be juiced and drunk.

Acupressure

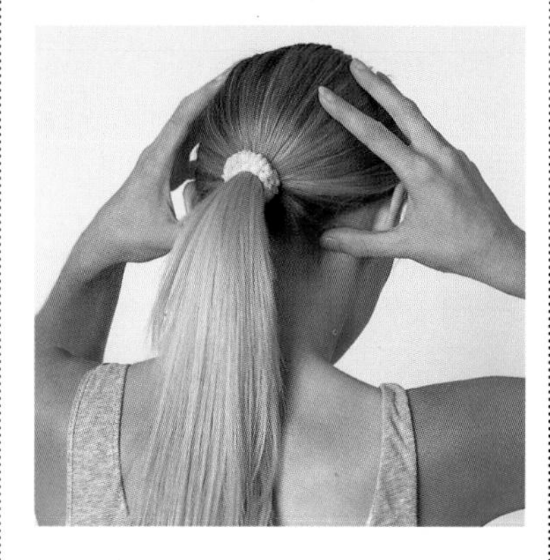

A number of pressure points are effective, the majority of which are on the upper back, shoulders, and the back of the neck. Try pressing the back of the head, under the base of the skull, halfway between the ear and the midline, in a hollow in the neck muscles. Press slightly upward and toward the opposite eye.

Homeopathy

For acute attacks, tablets of natrum mur, lycopodium, nux vomica, silicea, or spigelia (6c dose, taken hourly) can be beneficial, but self-help is not normally recommended for migraine, because the treatment depends on your particular circumstances and symptoms. Homeopathy is most effective if individually tailored to your needs by a qualified practitioner.

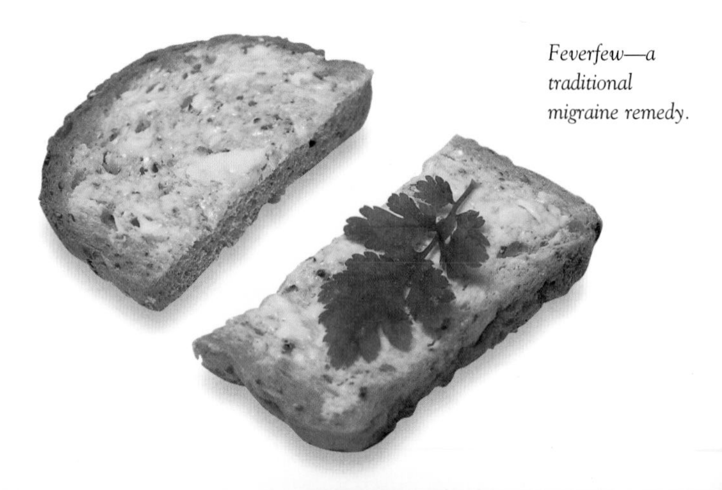

Feverfew—a traditional migraine remedy.

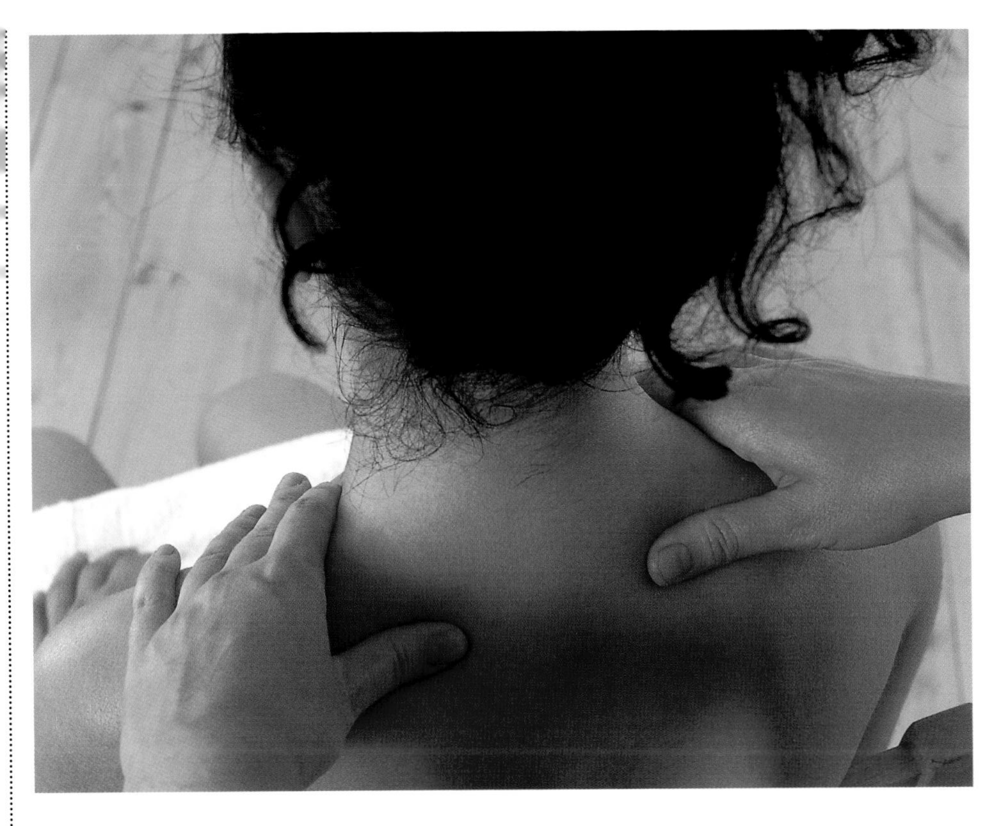

Stress can trigger both headaches and migraines by causing tension in the neck and shoulders. Firm massage, using the thumbs for extra pressure, can quickly disperse tension and bring rapid relief.

Massage and aromatherapy

Massage of the head, neck, shoulders, back, feet, and hands can sometimes bring relief, but you will need the help of a friend. The massage should be soothing rather than vigorous—use long, smooth strokes—and be continued as long as you find it comfortable or it brings relief. If trying aromatherapy use the same oils as for headaches (see page 46).

Hydrotherapy

As immediate first aid for migraine pain, apply a warm washcloth or compress to the back of the neck and the side of the head affected (both sides if necessary). Lie or sit somewhere comfortable, and if light is a problem close your eyes (or darken the room with the drapes. Keep the washcloth in place—warming it by running hot water over it and then wringing it out—for as long as it brings relief.

Making waves

A device developed in Britain during the 1980s that makes use of low-level electromagnetic waves claims to have a success rate of around 80 percent in reducing the incidence of migraine. The device, invented by UK electronics engineer and migraine-sufferer Steven Walpole, gives out minute electromagnetic impulses every few seconds to "correct" the deficiency in the sufferer's brain waves that is said to cause the migraine. So, for example, correcting a deficiency in theta brain waves, which are involved in pain control, reduces pain.

The device is small enough to be worn like a large watch or pendant, but has to be specially programmed by a trained practitioner, using a computerized brain frequency analyzer, before it is effective. Available in Europe, North America, South Africa, and Australia under the brand names Trimed and Empulse, the device is claimed to work for other kinds of pain relief also, including arthritis, back pain, and sciatica, as well as a variety of allergic reactions.

Other therapies

From a qualified therapist only

Acupuncture • pages 150–151
Osteopathy and chiropractic • pages 152–153
Hypnotherapy • page 153
Counseling and psychotherapy • page 154

EYES, EARS, MOUTH, NOSE, AND THROAT PAIN

The head not only houses the brain, the body's "central computer," but also most of its sensory organs: that is, the organs that register sight, sound, taste, and smell. The only sense not confined to the head is the fifth sense—touch, which occurs through nerve endings in the skin all over the body. Unlike headaches and migraines, which are felt in the head but whose root causes are often elsewhere in the body, the source of aches and pains in the sensory organs is mostly specific to each organ.

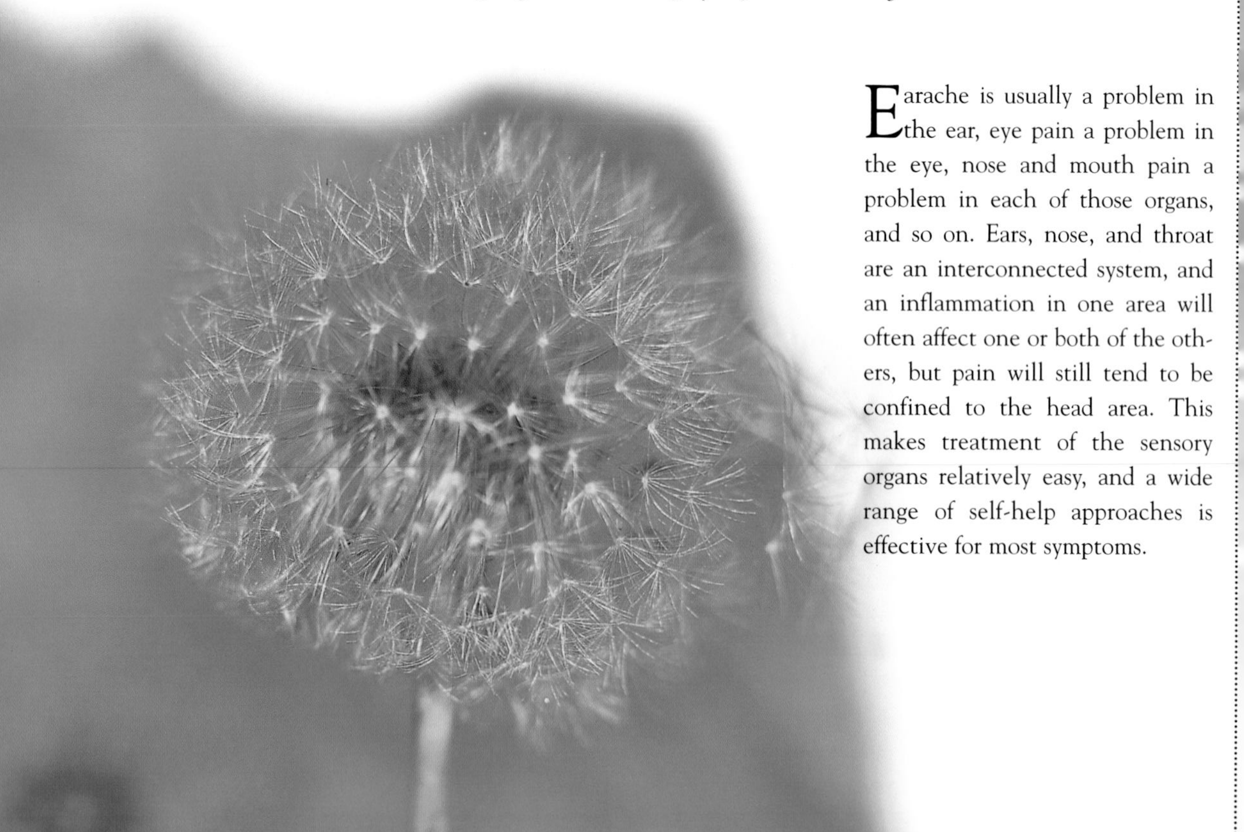

Earache is usually a problem in the ear, eye pain a problem in the eye, nose and mouth pain a problem in each of those organs, and so on. Ears, nose, and throat are an interconnected system, and an inflammation in one area will often affect one or both of the others, but pain will still tend to be confined to the head area. This makes treatment of the sensory organs relatively easy, and a wide range of self-help approaches is effective for most symptoms.

A network of cavities links organs at the front of the head, especially the nose, mouth, and throat, and all can be affected if one becomes infected or inflamed.

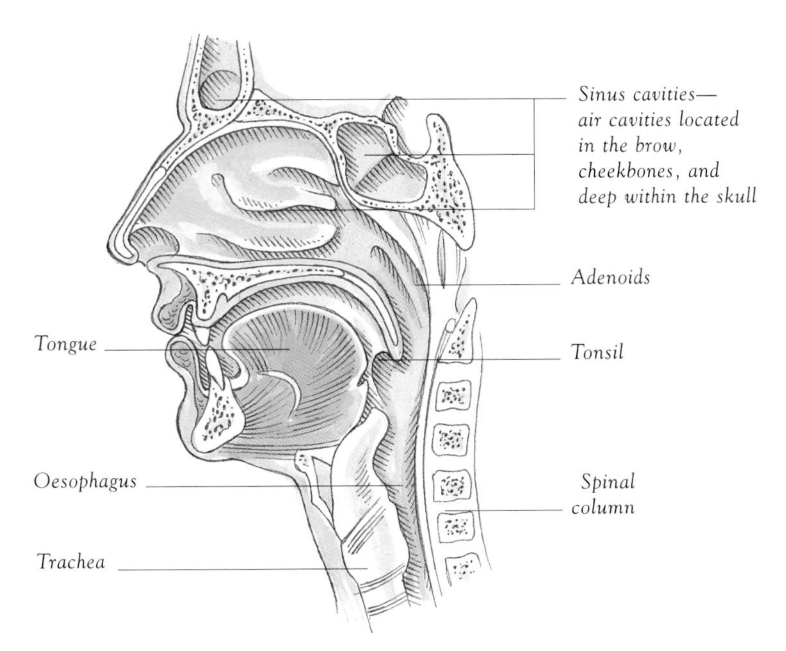

COLDS AND FLU

Colds and flu are the most common and still one of the most elusive viral illnesses of the human race, producing a variety of uncomfortable and often "achy" symptoms. In colds, symptoms are mainly in the head, especially in the ears, nose, and throat, while flu can be felt throughout the body, particularly in the joints, chest, and lungs.

Most colds are not serious enough to be a real bother, and go away of their own accord after about a week. Flu is more serious, and requires bed rest in its early stages. Natural therapists insist that the symptoms of neither should be suppressed, however, particularly if a raised temperature is involved; the fever should be encouraged to come out through sweating. The following approaches can help accelerate recovery.

Herbal medicine

Echinacea, garlic, ginger, and lemon are all effective at combating infection (echinacea is best taken as either a tincture or capsule). A hot tea of equal parts of elderflower, peppermint, and yarrow is also beneficial drunk at least three times a day. Add boneset if there is a fever.

Naturopathy

Rest, keep warm, and drink plenty of fluids (6–8 glasses a day), especially if there is a fever and sweating. Mix honey and lemon (or cider vinegar) in hot water and drink regularly. Regular inhaling with mixtures such as Olbas oil (containing eucalyptus, juniper berry, menthol, clove, wintergreen, cajuput, and mint oils), either sprinkled on a handkerchief or tissue, or added to steam and breathed in, helps clear nasal passages and ease breathing.

Nutritional and dietary therapy

Take vitamin C with bioflavonoids (6–10 g a day), zinc (15–20 mg a day), vitamin B-complex (best as a multivitamin, with iron), and cod liver oil (EPA). If hungry (loss of appetite is normal and aids recovery), concentrate on fresh fruit, nuts, seeds, grains, and vegetables.

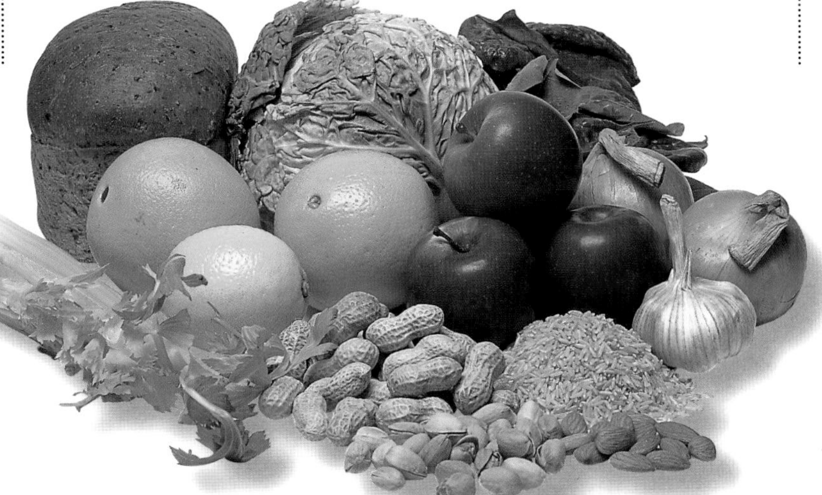

A healthy diet of fresh fruit, vegetables, and nuts always helps in the fight against illness, but especially those of the ears, nose, and throat.

EYES

The first resort whenever eye symptoms arise should be to consult an eye doctor. However, there are suitable home remedies for less serious eye problems such as eyestrain.

EYESTRAIN

A few simple exercises can help relieve eyestrain. First, blink rapidly, then follow by "palming" the eyes. To "palm," sit comfortably, rub your hands together vigorously to generate heat, and place them over the eyes. Hold them there for several minutes.

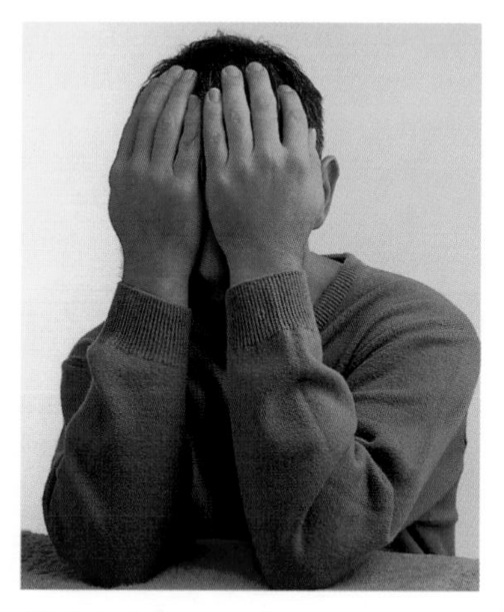

"Palming" the eyes relieves eyestrain.

Herbal medicine

Grate a raw potato and place enough on the closed eyelid to cover the entire eye. Cover with gauze and leave in position for 1–2 hours. Alternatively, bathe the eye with euphrasia, either using an eyecup (eye-bath) or soaking some roll cotton (cotton wool) in the liquid and applying it to your eye for around 20 minutes every hour while the pain lasts.

Homeopathy

For tired muscles, take arnica 6c; for aching eyes, natrum mur 6c; for burning or strain after reading, ruta 6c may help.

CONJUNCTIVITIS

Conjunctivitis, or "pink eye," is inflammation of the membrane inside the eye tissue (conjunctiva), causing redness, pain, and, often, a sticky discharge. Infection is usually the reason, but an allergic reaction, smoke, and chemical sprays can also be to blame.

Herbal medicine

Wash the eye several times a day with a mixture of one tablespoon of golden seal root powder, one teaspoon of salt, and 250 mg vitamin C, added to 2 pints (1 liter) of clean water. Let the mixture settle before using.

Homeopathy

Bathe the eye three times daily in 1 part euphrasia tincture to 10 parts boiled water, and take five tablets of ferrum phos 6c dissolved in hot water four times a day. Other helpful remedies (all at 6c) are belladonna; for the early stages of inflammation: aconite; for severe pain with itching and blistering: apis; for burning, sensitive eyes: euphrasia; for sticky lids: mercurius corrosivus; for discharging, itchy eyes: pulsatilla; and for hot, watery eyes: arsenicum album.

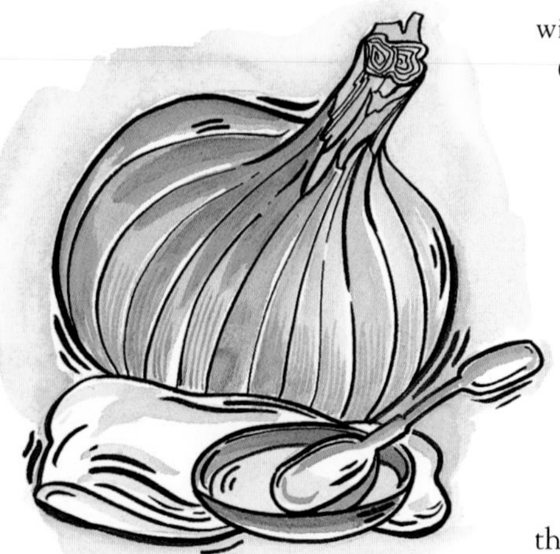

An onion or mustard poultice behind the ear can help earache.

EARS

Problems such as earache are particularly common in children, and they may be linked to infections in other areas, for example tonsillitis.

EARACHE (OTITIS)

Pain in the ears can be caused simply by loud noise and exposure to cold, windy conditions, or, more seriously, by infection. A heating pad or wrapped hot-water bottle held over the ear will ease the pain.

CAUTION Infection of the inner ear (otitis media) is a serious condition and medical help should be sought if it is suspected. Antibiotics may be advisable, particularly in children with a high fever. Untreated, it can lead to meningitis.

Nutritional and dietary therapy

If pain is recurrent, reduce intake of dairy products, drink 6–8 glasses of water every day, and cover ears in windy conditions. Regular supplementation with vitamin C, zinc, and garlic can also help.

Herbal medicine

Put 2–3 drops of warmed almond or castor oil into the ears and seal with a small swab of cotton. Other effective drops are oils of garlic, hypericum, or mullein. A couple of drops of tinctures of pennywort, chamomile, yarrow, hyssop, or lobelia can also help. An alternative is a hot onion or mustard poultice placed behind the ear and left until the ache eases. If infection is the cause of the ache, take echinacea tincture every two hours: 30 drops (half a teaspoon) for an adult; half that dose for a child.

Homeopathy

For restlessness and irritability: chamomila 3c. Following measles or whooping cough: pulsatilla 3c. In early stages or recurrent earache: ferrum phos 3c/6c, or aconite 3c. With flushed face: belladonna 3c. For discharging ears: hepar sulf 3c. Following infection: silicea 12c.

TINNITUS

A constant background noise in the ear, usually described as "ringing in the ears," that you can hear but nobody else can. There is no single known cause, but some likely sources are depression, stress, anxiety, infection, high blood pressure, drugs, and congestion (with wax).

Herbal medicine

"Ear candles" are said to be particularly beneficial, though you will need someone to help. The "candles" are thin, hollow tubes, containing traces of herbs, that are placed in each ear in turn and burned slowly down to the ear. It takes about 10 minutes to do one ear. Wax and other impurities are drawn into the tube, and the smoke from the herbs is said to have a healing effect on the ear cavities. The technique is simple to perform and painless. The herb ginko biloba can also help, taken either as a capsule or as a tincture of equal parts with black cohosh.

Acupressure

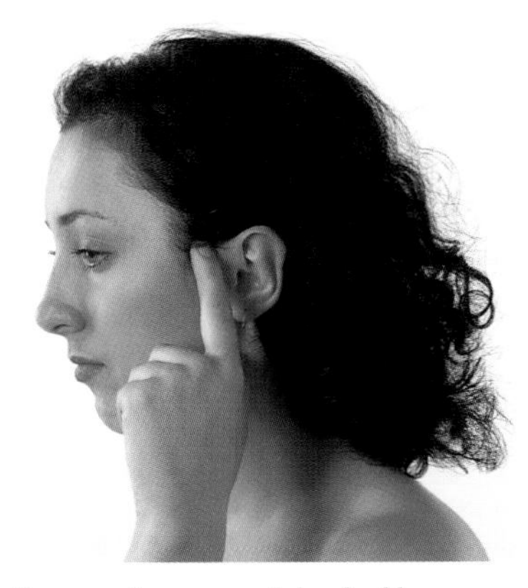

Press a point on top of the cheekbone about a finger's width from the ear to relieve ringing in the ears. Hold your finger in this position for a few seconds and release. Do as often as comfortable.

Hydrotherapy

Inhaling steam containing the same herbs that help clear noses and sinuses can help ringing in the ears (see "Sinusitis," pages 53–54).

Homeopathy

For pain with giddiness and a "roaring" noise: salicylic acid 6c. For ringing, tinkling, or hissing noises: cinchona off 6c.

Yoga and meditation

Head and neck exercises, such as slowly rotating the head and trying to touch your shoulders with your ears, can benefit by improving circulation. Meditation may also help.

NOSE AND SINUSES

Natural remedies are ideal for a sore nose, which can be treated by gently rubbing aloe vera gel or vitamin E cream on the sore area.

SINUSITIS

Sinusitis is inflammation of the sinuses, often as a result of catarrh coupled with an infection. It can go from being a short-term problem to a long-term one, and so needs careful treatment. Chronic sinusitis can not only be excruciatingly painful but make thinking straight every bit as difficult as in migraines.

Hydrotherapy, and nutritional and dietary therapy

Aim to prevent attacks by reducing or avoiding foods such as dairy products, bananas, peanuts, coffee, alcohol, and hot, spicy foods, and seeing if there is an allergic cause of any underlying catarrh (see "Allergy Tests," page 52). Steam inhalation with eucalyptus and/or pine oil (or, for a stronger effect, menthol) will help alleviate the immediate symptoms. Gargling and washing the nasal passages with a teaspoonful of salt in warm water can clear catarrh. Supplement with vitamin C, B-complex, and zinc.

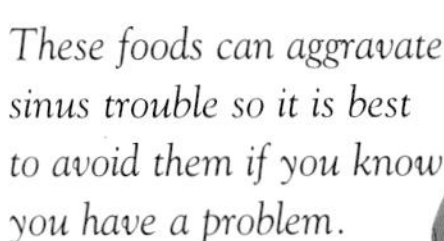

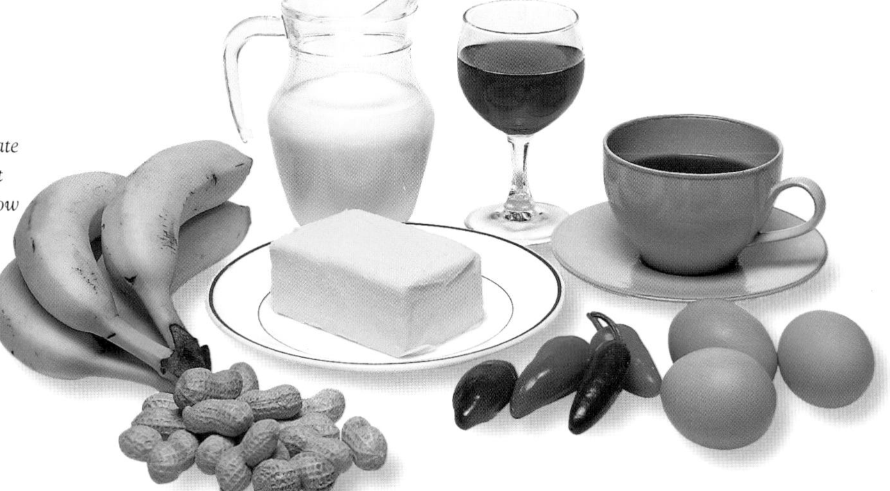

These foods can aggravate sinus trouble so it is best to avoid them if you know you have a problem.

Aromatherapy and herbal medicine
Massage the whole area of the nose, eyes, cheekbones, and temples with a mixture of essential oils of peppermint (9 drops), eucalyptus (6 drops), and lavender (10 drops). Drink a tea of equal parts of echinacea, golden rod, golden seal, and marshmallow leaf every two hours. Garlic and horseradish also help.

HAYFEVER

Hayfever (allergic rhinitis) is an allergic reaction to a number of environmental factors but particularly pollen, grass seeds, and dusts. It results in inflammation of the linings of the nasal passages, causing sneezing, a running nose, itchy eyes, and a sore throat.

Hydrotherapy and nutritional therapy
Wash the nasal passages with salt in warm water and supplement with 1–2 g daily of vitamin C with bioflavonoids (an antihistamine) and vitamin B-complex.

Herbal medicine and homeopathy
Drink a cup of tea made from two parts elderflower to one part each of ephedra, eyebright, and golden seal, twice daily. Tincture of licorice (½–1 teaspoonful in warm water, twice daily) is said to help if started a month before "hayfever season." The homeopathic treatments arsenicum album 6c, sabadilla 6c, and allium cepa 6c relieve itching eyes and sneezing.

Acupressure

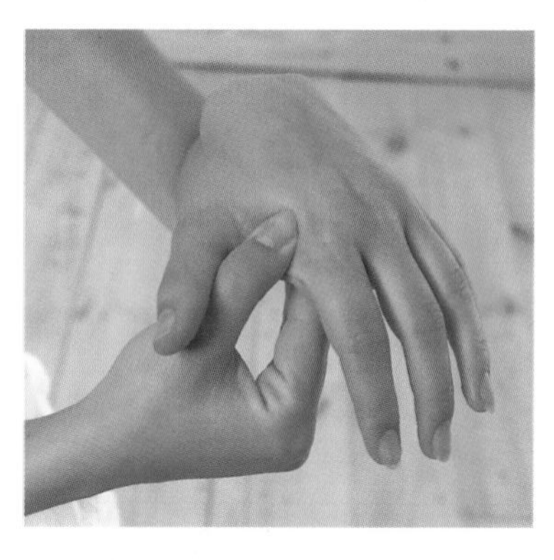

Press the point in the webbing between thumb and first finger for hayfever. Do NOT use this method during pregnancy.

MOUTH, TEETH, AND TONGUE

The most important step to keeping a healthy mouth is to maintain a regular hygiene program, including regular visits to the dentist.

TOOTHACHE

Toothache is usually a sign of the need for dental work to repair or fill a hole made by decay, so a visit to the dentist is advisable if the ache lasts more than a day or so.

Herbal medicine
Soak a swab of cotton in oil of cloves—a natural nerve anesthetic—and place it on the hole, or dab it around the sore tooth. Alternatively, chew a raw clove on the sore spot. Cinnamon oil, peppermint extract, or brandy, on cotton, are substitutes. The herbs white willow bark and meadowsweet are natural painkillers, but are best taken as tablets available through health food or drugstores.

Hydrotherapy and homeopathy
An ice-pack held to the face over the sore area (a bag of frozen peas is ideal) can bring relief. The following homeopathic remedies can also help. For throbbing and/or burning pain: aconite 3c. For nerve pain, especially in children: chamomila 3c or 6c. For pain with tearfulness: pulsatilla 6c or calcarea phos 6c.

Electronic devices
TENS, intasound, and massage devices are all effective against toothache. Treatment needs to be for three-quarters to one hour.

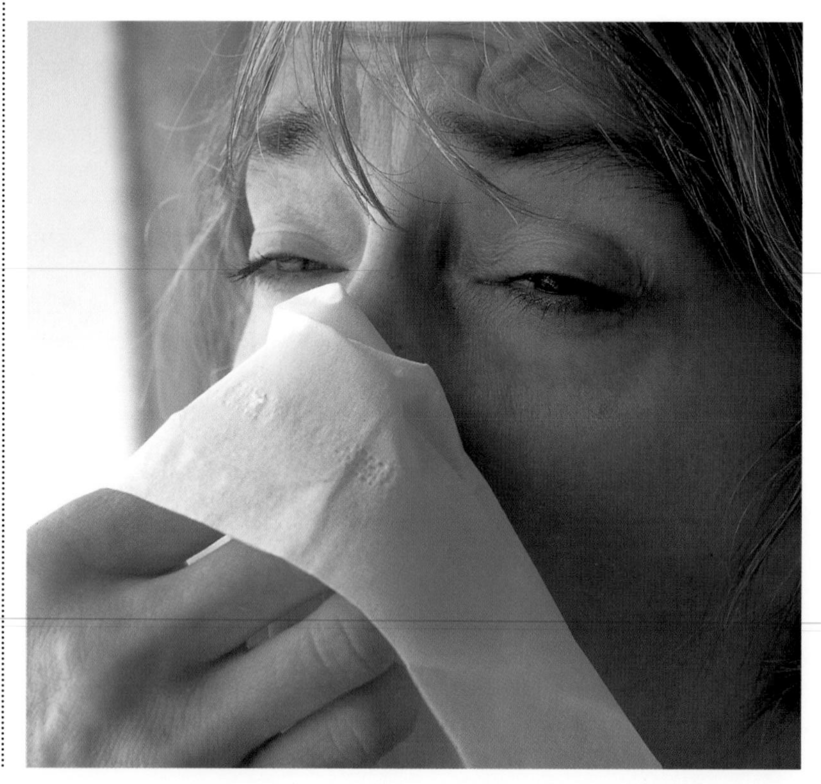

Streaming eyes and running nose are classic symptoms of hayfever. Late spring and early summer are times for sufferers to be particularly on their guard.

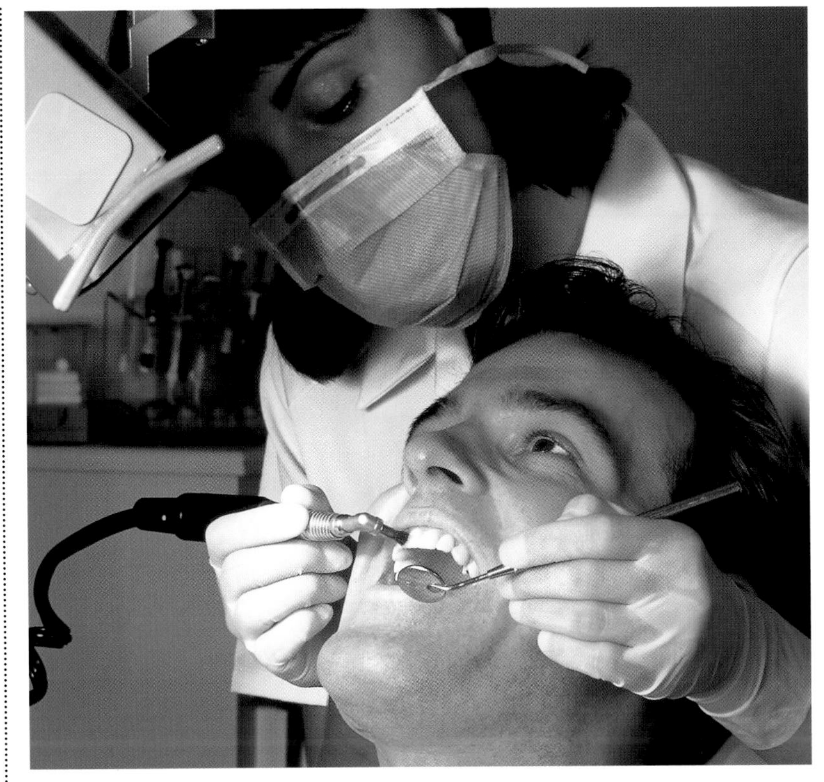

Having a regular dental check is the best way to prevent painful tooth decay. This applies to children as well as adults.

GINGIVITIS

Gingivitis is inflammation of the gums, usually from poor tooth and gum care, causing sore and bleeding gums and, in extreme cases, loose teeth. Regularly rub the gums with lemon juice, salt, or sodium bicarbonate, then rinse out thoroughly. Follow with a mouthwash of the tinctures of calendula, myrrh, and wild indigo, or hypericum in warm water. If bleeding from the teeth is heavy, take the homeopathic treatment phosphorus 30c (1 tablet every 10 minutes, and then hourly as necessary).

TOOTH ABCESS

An abcess is a small, pus-filled boil in the root of the tooth, also known as a gumboil. Treatment is normally from a dentist, who will usually perform surgery to drain the pus or remove the tooth, and prescribe antibiotics for the infection. The hydrotherapy measures that are recommended for toothache may also help to alleviate the pain of tooth abcess.

Homeopathy

Start with belladonna 200 every hour, followed with silicea when the abcess has been drained. Hepar sulf 30 or 200 is recommended for a less serious abcess (again followed with silicea). Hypericum 30c and hypericum as mouthwash (see "Gingivitis," left) can help after a tooth has been taken out.

Herbal medicine

After dental work, rinse the mouth with hot water mixed half-and-half with calendula tincture.

Oils of juniper, peppermint, or cloves applied to the gums will give relief from toothache.

FACE AND JAW PAIN

Face pain may be caused by toothache or by inflammation of the nasal and sinus cavities. Jaw pain may in fact be a psychological problem—teeth-grinding is a frequent cause—but it can also be due to the head sitting awkwardly on the shoulders, which can produce increased strain on the joint between the jaw and the skull.

Hydrotherapy

For face pain from inflammation, a covered hot-water bottle can help; a cold compress, using a pack of frozen peas, can ease pain from toothache. For jaw pain, alternating hot and cold compresses can provide some relief, but the problem is long-term and needs treatment by a specialist in musculo-skeletal correction.

Alexander technique

This technique specializes in correcting the head–body alignment, often a source of jaw pain. It must be learned from a teacher, but can be done on your own after that.

Relaxation

Since tension is often a major factor in face and jaw pain, therapies that help relax the face muscles and joints can be highly effective. Examples are meditation (especially autogenics), biofeedback, and massage with essential oils.

COLD SORES

The virus herpes simplex is behind cold sores: highly contagious blisters brought on by a number of factors but especially stress, too much sun, cold, lowered immunity, and fever. The virus is usually picked up in childhood and lies dormant in the body for years before being triggered. Cold sores are common on the lips but can easily be spread elsewhere by touch. The same virus also causes genital herpes.

CAUTION Avoid contact with the skin while the sore is still moist. Even using the same towels or pillowcases can spread the infection. Wash immediately if you touch an affected area or are touched by one—and consult a doctor at once if sores emerge near the eyes: they can be extremely painful unless treated early.

Naturopathy

In the early, more painful stage, an ice-cube applied intermittently to the sore can reduce the discomfort. Lemon juice diluted in cold water and dabbed on can also help. Alternatively, try vitamin E cream or vitamin E oil on a cotton swab, held in place for 15 minutes. In the longer-term, switching to a healthy diet (as much fresh fruit, vegetables, live yogurt, and fiber as possible, and no sugar, refined foods, and alcohol) will benefit. So will supplements that boost the immune system, particularly vitamins A, C with bioflavonoids, E, B-complex, the minerals zinc, selenium, magnesium, and calcium, the amino acid lysine, and acidophilus.

Herbal medicine

Licorice root has antiviral qualities that are said to be effective against the herpes virus. The essential oils of tea tree, lavender, geranium, or thyme can also be dabbed on.

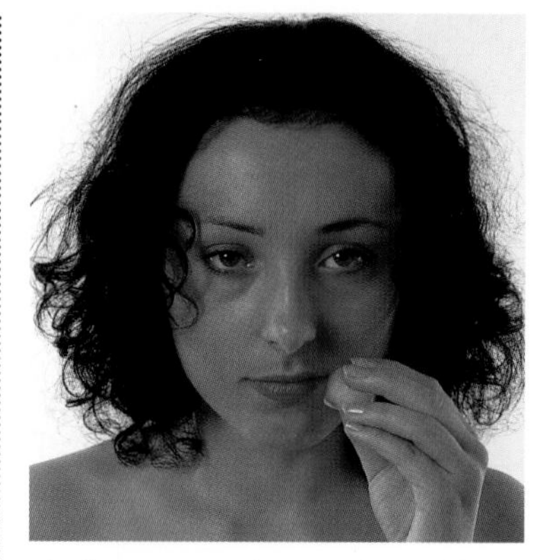

Applying an ice-cube can relieve cold sore pain in the early stages.

Homeopathy

Rhus tox, hepar sulf, or natrum mur may help. Start with a dose (30c or 6c) every four hours for two days, then once in the morning and again in the evening for three days.

MOUTH ULCERS

The cause of mouth ulcers is uncertain, but is most likely a combination of factors, particularly stress, diet, and nutritional deficiency. The virus that causes cold sores (herpes simplex) is to blame in some cases, but accidentally biting yourself and badly-fitting dentures can also lead to ulcers. First-choice treatment is to rub aloe vera gel onto the ulcer, but a mouthwash of calendula, myrrh, and thyme will also help. Alternatively, mix clove and tea tree oil with glycerin, and dab on. Take a good multivitamin with vitamin B-complex, vitamin C, and zinc.

CAUTION See your dentist or doctor if mouth ulcers do not clear up within two weeks.

THROAT

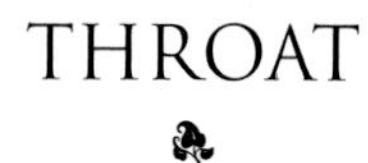

Throat problems are often an indication of infection, so prompt action early on can help prevent it developing more seriously.

SORE THROAT

A sore throat (pharyngitis) is inflammation of the pharynx, the area at the back of the mouth. The term is also used to cover inflammation of the adenoids, tonsils (tonsillitis), and the voice box or larynx (laryngitis). Laryngitis is characterized by hoarseness and loss of voice. If the soreness is not obviously caused by shouting too loudly, it may be a sign of infection.

Homeopathy

For inflammation and pain: belladonna 30c, hepar sulf 6c, arsenicum album 6c, or apis 6c. For tightness: lachesis 6c, lycopodium 6c, or phytolacca 6c.

Nutritional and herbal therapies

Gargling provides immediate relief. Choose from sea salt in warm water; cider vinegar, honey, and lemon; red sage; thyme; propolis; echinacea; or spilanthas. Or chew licorice root or suck tablets of slippery elm. Garlic and echinacea extract boost immunity. Teas of marshmallow, elderflower, and catmint alleviate symptoms and promote recovery. Vitamins A, E, and C with bioflavonoids and zinc, and fish oil (EPA) boost immunity.

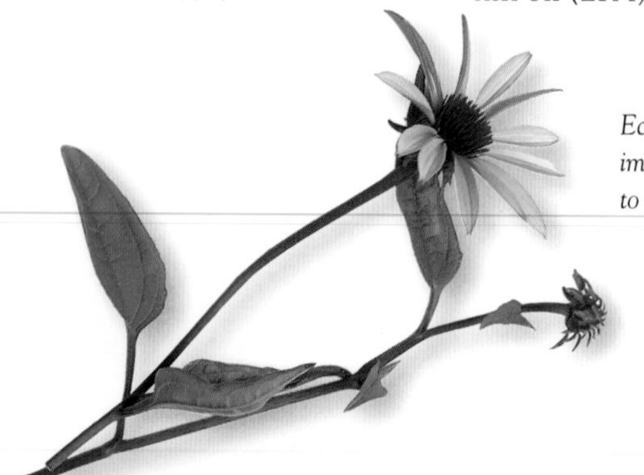

Echinacea boosts immunity and can help to ease a sore throat.

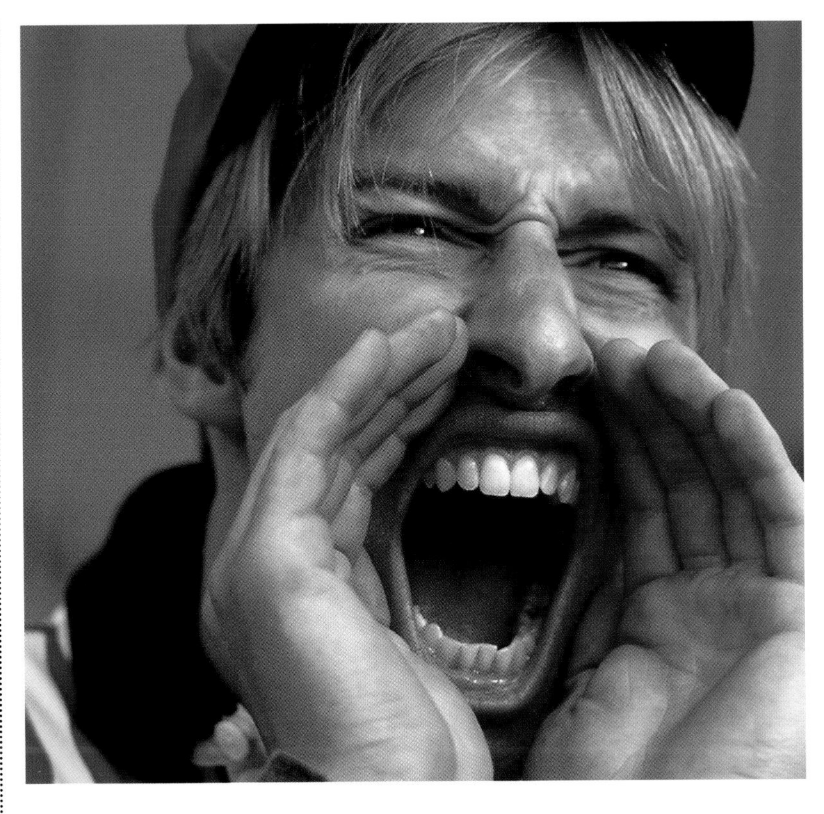

Shouting can cause a sore throat by inflaming the larynx, but the more usual cause is inflammation from an infection.

CAUTION Recurrent infection damages the tonsils by building up scar tissue and can lead to a dangerous condition, particularly in young children, known as quinsy, in which the throat threatens to close completely and prevent breathing. In this situation immediate medical help is essential.

Antibiotics are advisable in cases of severe bacterial—but not viral—infection. A course of antibiotics should always be followed by a course of probiotics (acidophilus or bifidophilus with plain, live yogurt) to replace the healthy bacteria destroyed.

TONSILLITIS

Tonsillitis is almost always caused by an infection, but also by viruses. Symptoms are a sore, red, swollen throat, fever, headache, swollen neck glands, and a dry cough.

Homeopathy

For infected tonsils, difficulty in swallowing, and discharge: mercurius solubilis 30c. For fever with bad breath: mercurius solubilis 30c. For sudden attack with fever, swelling, and stiff neck: belladonna 30c. One tablet every hour for 12 hours, followed by one three times daily for two days, is recommended. Individual prescription is advised in cases of recurrent tonsillitis.

Herbal and dietary therapies

Bed rest and taking plenty of fluids is recommended, especially diluted fruit juices, warm broths, and light soups. To ease the pain, gargle with tea made from a teaspoonful of powdered ginger (it will also promote sweating). Neat tincture of golden seal, sprayed onto the tonsils with a small hand-spray, will promote rapid healing, and powdered root of licorice dissolved in warm water and drunk will help relieve coughing. An alternative is gargling with and then drinking a tea of 1 oz (30 g) of fresh red sage (ordinary sage will also do), or a cup of hot water mixed with a few drops of grapefruit seed extract.

Other therapies
From a qualified therapist only

Eye, ear, mouth, nose, and throat pain may also be relieved with the following:

Cranial osteopathy • *pages 153*
Acupuncture • *pages 150–151*

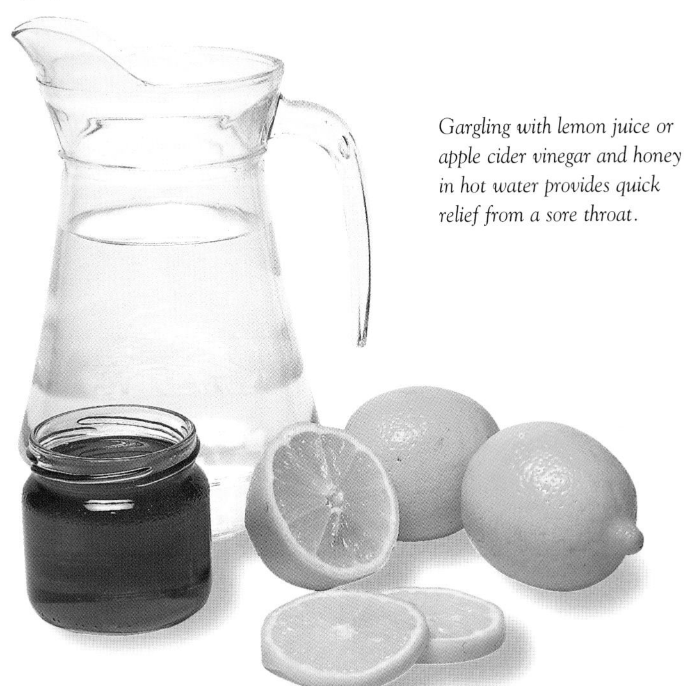

Gargling with lemon juice or apple cider vinegar and honey in hot water provides quick relief from a sore throat.

CHEST AND LUNG PAIN

The chest houses not only the lungs but also the heart, and together they form one of the most important parts of the body: the circulatory and respiratory systems. The two systems link up to circulate vital oxygen throughout the body via the bloodstream. But though they work complementarily, each has its own particular problems.

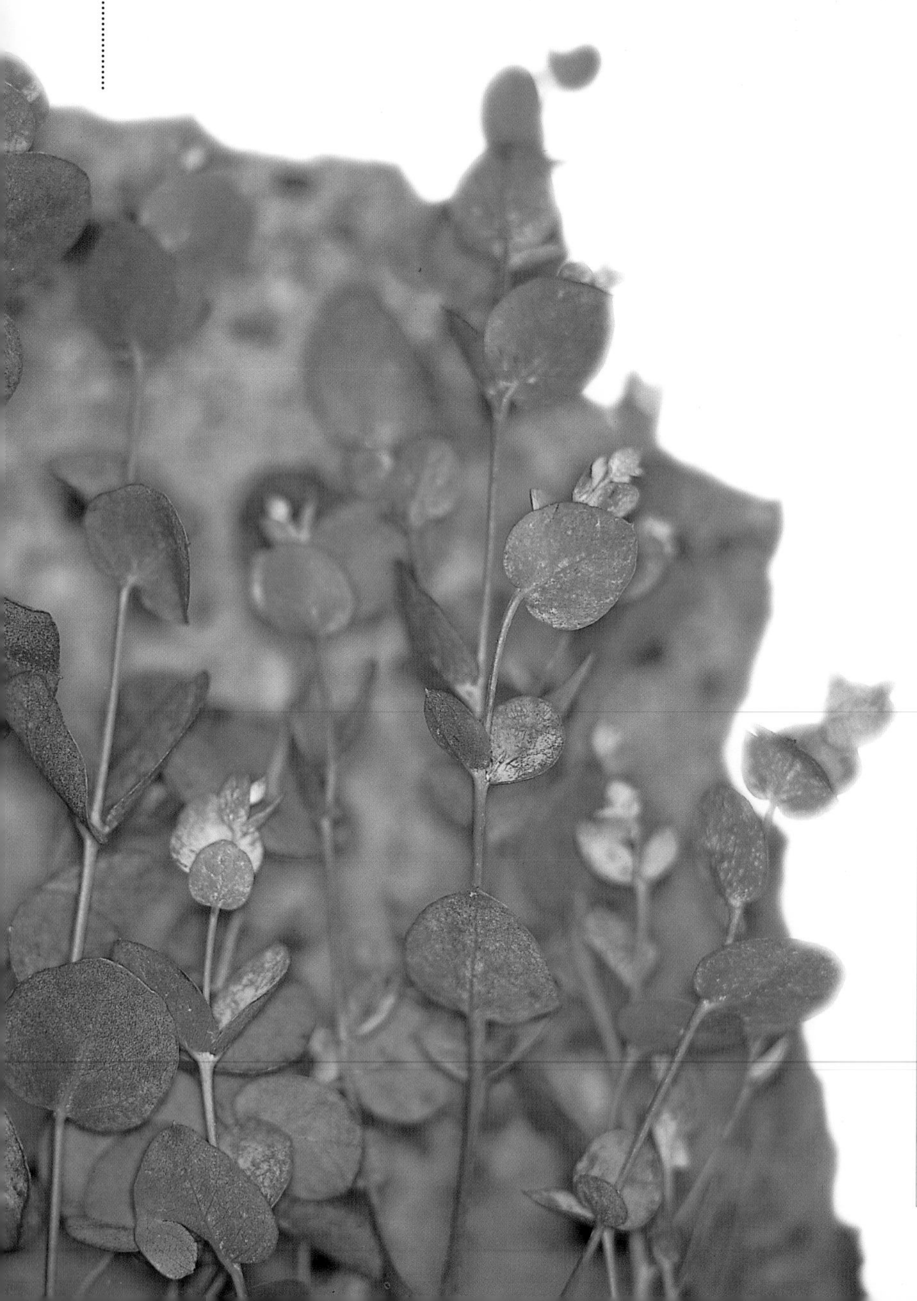

This section deals with treatments for the respiratory (breathing) system, then describes treatments for the circulatory system (the heart and blood supply).

COUGHS

Coughing is a natural way of getting rid of anything that interferes with breathing—dust, smoke, etc. Unless caused by an infection (flu, for example) or inflammation in the respiratory tract (such as bronchitis), it is usually uncomfortable more than painful. It will normally clear itself when the problem is resolved, but see a doctor if it lasts more than two weeks, or is accompanied by pains in the chest, fever, or blood in the mouth.

Warning

Seek immediate medical help if pain in the chest/lung area is:

- *severe*
- *prolonged*
- *accompanied with any breathing difficulty*
- *involves coughing up blood.*

The chest contains the heart and lungs, and together they bring vital oxygen to every part of the body.

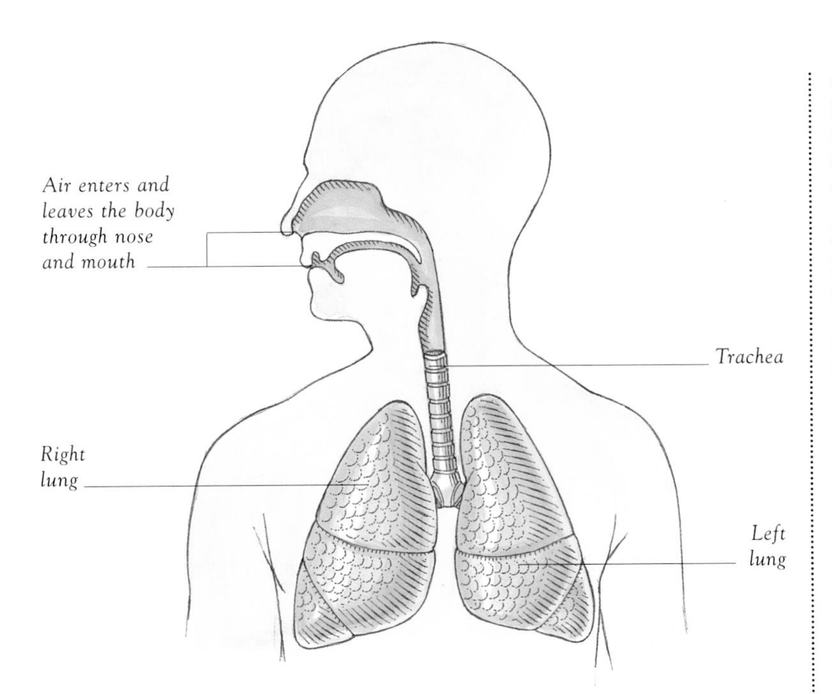

Herbal medicine

A hot drink of lemon juice, honey, and glycerin is a good throat soother, and a hot apple cider vinegar compress on the throat and upper chest can help loosen phlegm. White horehound is the best of a wide range of herbs that help alleviate coughs. Others are mullein, wild lettuce, yarrow, angelica, elecampane, licorice, and elderflower. For children, wild cherry bark is good. Make a tea and drink a spoonful three times a day. There are also a number of herbal cough mixtures available, mainly through health food stores.

Nutritional and dietary therapy

Garlic capsules (two, three times a day) and a good multivitamin complex with beta carotene (vitamin A), B-complex, C, and zinc are recommended for the relief and prevention of coughs.

Aromatherapy

Steam inhaling with various essential oils (choose from eucalyptus, cypress, hyssop, bergamot, and chamomile) is beneficial, especially in the early stages. Inhale for about 10 minutes using three or four drops of the chosen oil in boiling water. Massaging chest and back with the diluted oils of eucalyptus, thyme, sandalwood, frankincense, or myrrh can also help.

Homeopathy and biochemic tissue salts

A number of cough remedies are available from drugstores, health food stores, and specialist suppliers. They include the homeopathic treatments bryonia, aconite, pulsatilla, rumex, and arsenicum album, and the biochemic tissue salts ferr phos and kali mur. Follow the doses on the labels.

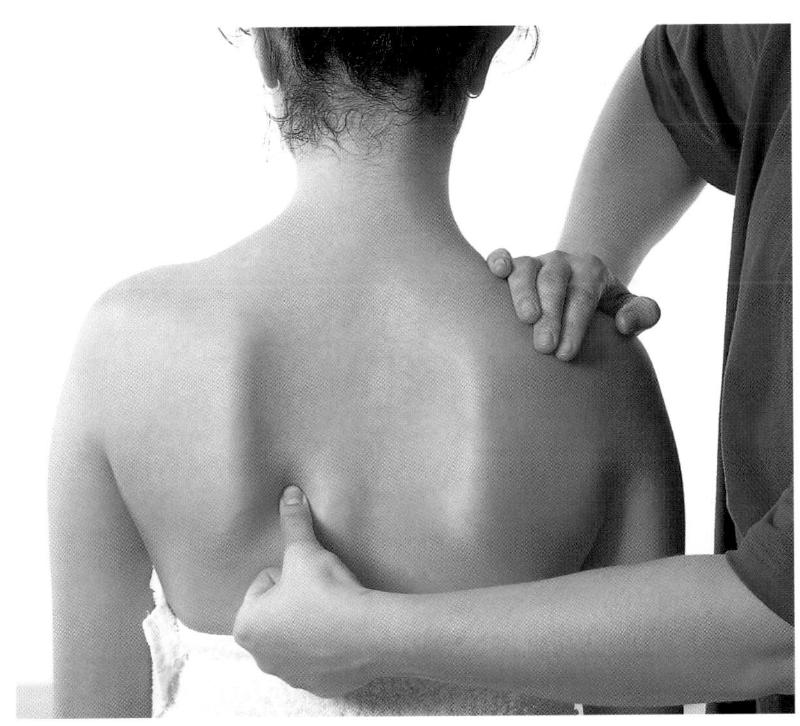

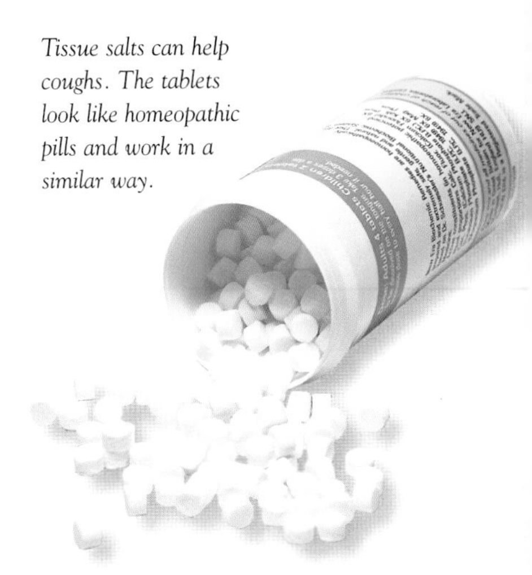

Tissue salts can help coughs. The tablets look like homeopathic pills and work in a similar way.

Pressing the acupressure point on the back by the heart, between the spine and shoulder blade, can relieve muscle spasms caused by coughing. Hold the pressure for about five seconds and repeat as needed.

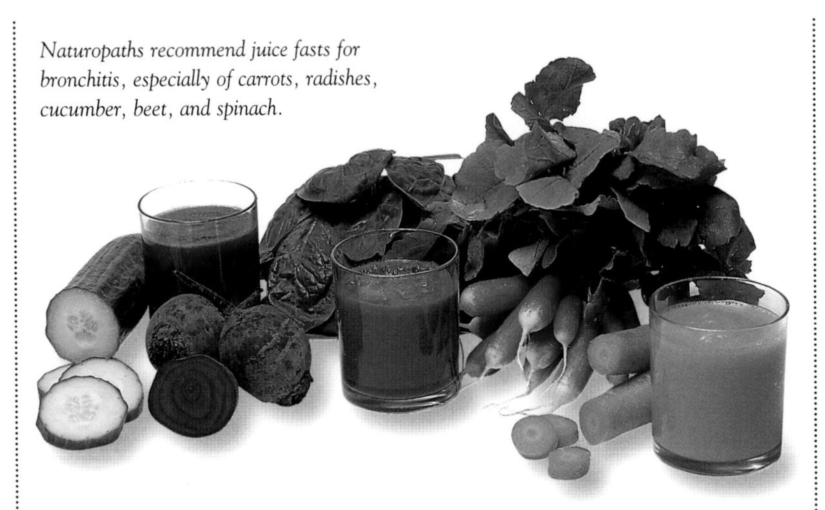
Naturopaths recommend juice fasts for bronchitis, especially of carrots, radishes, cucumber, beet, and spinach.

BRONCHITIS

Bronchitis is inflammation of the bronchii, the tubes that connect the windpipe to the lungs, and is caused by either viral or bacterial infection. It is more serious than infection of the throat (trachea), known as tracheitis. Symptoms include coughing, wheezing, shortness of breath, phlegm, tightness in the chest, headache, and fever. The condition will normally clear, with treatment, in about 10 days, but chronic bronchitis is harder to clear and extremely serious, needing special medical attention. Antibiotics may be advisable in severe cases of bacterial (but not viral) infection.

Hydrotherapy and aromatherapy

Bed rest in a warm room is advisable in the early stages. Avoid irritants, such as smoke and dust. Steam inhalations provide the best immediate relief, especially using the essential oils of eucalyptus, hyssop, cedarwood, and sandalwood. Five or six drops of one of these in a bowl of hot water will do. Around a dozen essential oils can help various symptoms of bronchitis, and individual advice from a qualified clinical aromatherapist is recommended for maximum benefit. A Swiss preparation known as Olbas oil, available from health food stores and some drugstores, is an easy alternative (it contains oils of eucalpyptus, mint, cajuput, menthol, wintergreen, juniper berry, and cloves). A warming compress (known, confusingly, as a "cold compress" in parts of Europe) can also be effective at removing tightness and soreness in the chest.

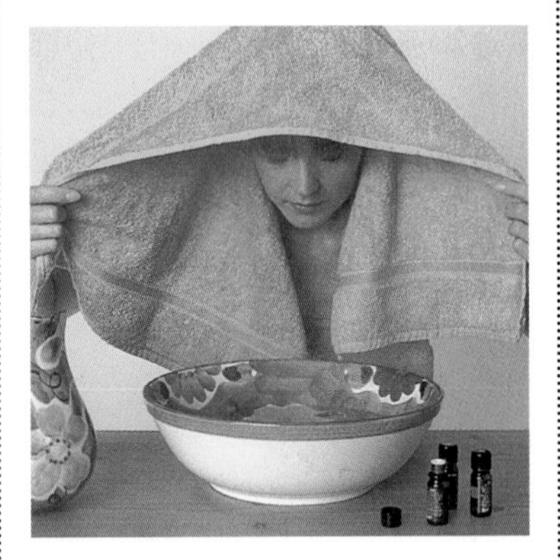
Coughing can be eased by inhaling steam from water mixed with oils of eucalyptus, hyssop, cedarwood, and sandalwood.

Nutritional and dietary therapy

An all-juice diet for the first two to three days is recommended. Taking plenty of liquids is more important than eating in the first 48 hours. Good juice diets are carrot and radish; carrot, beet, and cucumber; or carrot and spinach. Avoid dairy products, sugar, and eggs, which are believed to promote mucus, and eat hot, spicy foods that free up mucus. Examples are garlic, onions, horseradish, mustard, and chilis. Supplement with vitamins A, B-complex, C with bioflavonoids, E, zinc, and selenium.

Self-help for the lymph system

These measures can help the immune system fight infection or inflammation by boosting the efficiency of the lymph system that lies behind it.

Eating/drinking fennel or fenugreek *Swollen nodes (or glands) are an indication that the lymphatic system is not clearing toxins as efficiently as it should. Increase fluids, especially by drinking fennel or fenugreek tea, eating fennel (raw or lightly steamed), or adding sprouting fenugreek seeds to a bowl of raw vegetables.*

Mini-trampolining or rebounding *Exercise works as a pump to the lymph system, stimulating the fluids to circulate and to be excreted through the bloodstream. Rebounding, or bouncing, affects every organ and cell in the body for the better. For a fraction of a second at the top of the bounce on a trampoline, the body is weightless, improving lymph drainage, and the elimination of toxins and wastes, via the jugular vein at the side of the neck.*

Dry skin-brushing *Using a long-handled brush, preferably one with firm natural hair bristles, make long strokes over all skin surfaces toward the center of the body.*

Congestion-clearing cocktail for adults

- *4 black peppercorns*
- *4 cardamom pods*
- *4 cloves*
- *1 cinnamon stick*
- *a few slices of fresh ginger root*
- *a good squeeze of lemon juice and/or whisky*
- *honey*

Simmer (do not boil) the herbs in a pint (570 ml) of water for 15–20 minutes. Strain, add the lemon juice (and/or whisky), and sweeten with honey.

Herbal medicine

Garlic (fresh or capsules) and echinacea (tablets or tincture) can both prevent and fight infection. Teas of elecampane, licorice root, and ginger can help clear mucus and are warming. Take three times daily, hot or cold, as preferred. There are more than a dozen herbs effective for bronchial infection, and advice is best sought from a qualified medical herbalist for a prescription based on individual symptoms.

Homeopathy

Bryonia, aconite, sulfur, phosphorus, arsenicum album, and pulsatilla are recommended, but an individual prescription from a qualified homeopath is necessary, especially for chronic cases.

ASTHMA

Asthma is a chronic breathing problem from severe inflammation of the bronchioles—tubes in the lungs that deliver oxygen to the bloodstream and return carbon dioxide from it—as a result of allergic reaction. The allergic causes of asthma are similar to those for eczema and hayfever. Asthma that starts in childhood often clears spontaneously during adolescence but adult asthma is usually long-lasting. There is no known cure while the allergy lasts, but a number of natural therapies have a good record of alleviating symptoms and helping promote recovery.

CAUTION Severe asthmatic attacks are potentially life-threatening, and immediate medical help must be sought, especially if the person affected starts to develop blue lips and a cold and clammy skin.

Yoga

Improving posture can help asthma by helping the chest expand fully. Helpful postures include the Fish, the Shoulder Stand (see page 95 for both), the pelvic tilt (see page 72), and the Cobra (see page 103).

Herbal medicine

Ephedra, ginseng, euphorbia, chamomile, elecampane, and thyme are said to ease breathing. Mullein, marshmallow, butterbur, slippery elm, and passionflower can soothe and help clear the mucus membranes. Take any of these herbs as either tinctures or teas 3–4 times a day, as needed. For teas, always use the dried herb (leaf, flower, or root), not the fresh plant.

Reflexology

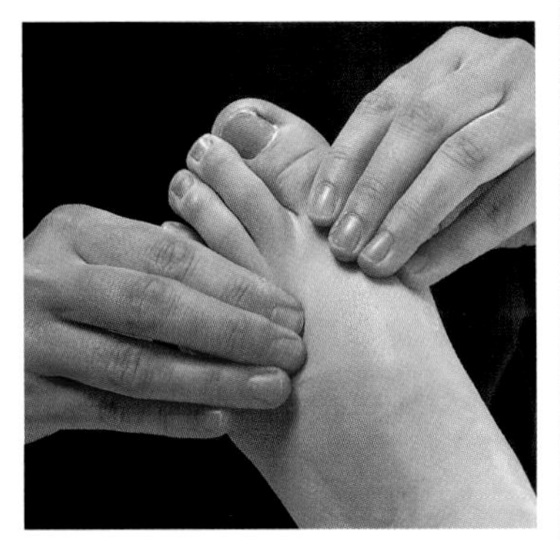

The front part of both feet, from the arch to the toes, contains the reflex points for the respiratory system. Manipulating these areas is said to help the disease-fighting function of the lymphatic system, and is therefore beneficial for bronchitis, asthma, pleurisy, and tuberculosis. Concentrate on the areas that feel tender, working them until the tenderness goes.

Warning

Asthma, pleurisy, pneumonia, emphysema, and tuberculosis are potentially life-threatening conditions, and medical help should be sought immediately.

The approaches described here are effective at alleviating symptoms, but are not a cure and not a substitute for treatment by a doctor.

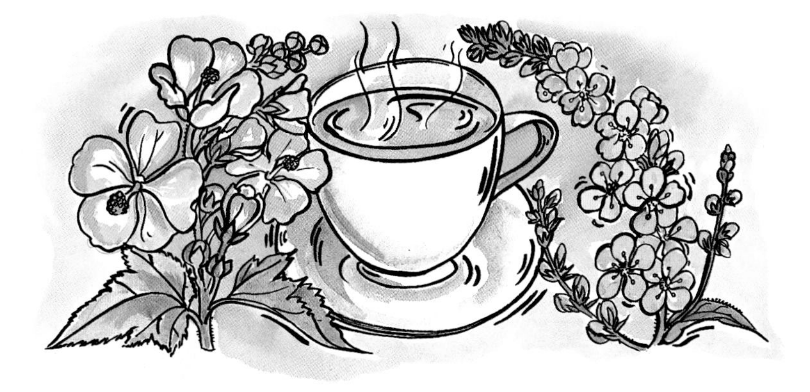

Marshmallow and mullein are two of the herbs recommended to relieve asthma.

Nutritional and dietary therapy

For prevention, identify food allergens by keeping a daily diary of exactly what you eat, and when, and follow your findings with an exclusion diet (see right). Eating a healthy diet and avoiding known allergens, such as dairy products, food additives, and colorings is a priority. For treatment during an attack, try raw juice diets, such as carrot, celery, spinach, and grapefruit, or radish, lemon, garlic, comfrey, horseradish, carrot, and beet. Cider vinegar with honey in a glass of warm water, three times a day, can also help. Supplementing with propolis (bee pollen), omega-3 and omega-6 essential fatty acids (EFA), cold-pressed olive oil, vitamins A (or beta carotene), C, E, and B-complex, and minerals magnesium, calcium, selenium, and manganese is also recommended.

Naturopathy

The main aim of the naturopathic approach is to identify the cause(s) of the allergic reaction, support the immune system in dealing with them, and remove them from the sufferer. The dust of the house mite is suspected of being the most common allergen, but identifying other allergens is difficult. Possible food allergens can be identified by an exclusion diet (see above) but environmental allergens are harder to isolate. There are several forms of allergy test available but none, as yet, is considered reliable.

Regular use of ionizers and humidifiers can help with breathing affected by air conditions. Alternating hot and cold foot baths, dry skin-brushing (see page 60), and mustard compresses and hot mud packs on the chest are also said to be beneficial.

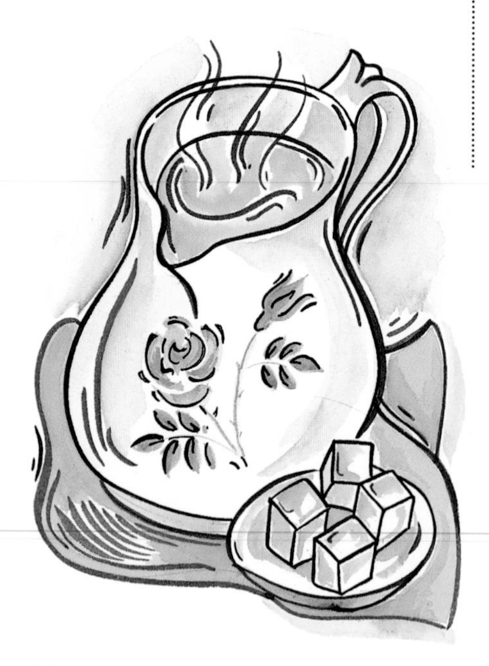

A series of hot and cold foot baths, used alternately, will bring relief from the symptoms of asthma.

How to carry out an exclusion diet

The aim of an exclusion diet is to see what foods or drinks, if any, you are allergic to by cutting them out of your diet completely for a given time and observing the results. You should cut out only one food at a time, and wait for at least five days for results. Begin with any food you suspect of causing a problem. If you have no suspicions, start with dairy products (the most common food allergens), followed by eggs, wheat, citrus fruits, and the nightshade (Solanaceae) family of foods (for example, tomatoes, peppers, and potatoes). Reintroduce the suspect food after a week and carefully note any reaction over the next 24 hours. If none, try again with another food.

CAUTION *Never cut out an entire group of foods—proteins, starches, carbohydrates, or grains, for example—for any period without consulting a qualified dietician or nutritionist, and never carry out an exclusion diet on very young children without expert advice.*

Acupressure

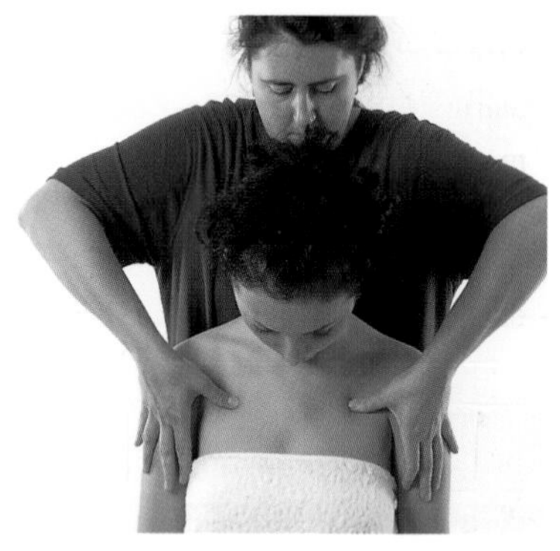

Relax the neck, letting the head drop onto the chest, and with the thumbs press the point on the front of the shoulder where it joins the chest for two minutes.

Aromatherapy

The essential oils of bergamot, camphor, eucalyptus, lavender, hyssop, and marjoram are recommended for an asthmatic attack. Mix two drops of each oil into a

Allergy tests

A variety of allergy tests is on offer—including blood testing, electrical testing (Vega and MORA), muscle testing (applied kinesiology), and pulse testing—but none is regarded as reliable by experts, because the tests are either not based on recognized scientific principles, have not been fully researched, or rely too much on the subjective judgment of the tester.

carrier oil and massage gently over the back and chest. To help mucus drain, lie with the head slightly lower than the lungs. An alternative combination is eucalyptus, juniper, wintergreen, peppermint, and rosemary. For asthma brought on by stress, lavender or frankincense are said to be calming.

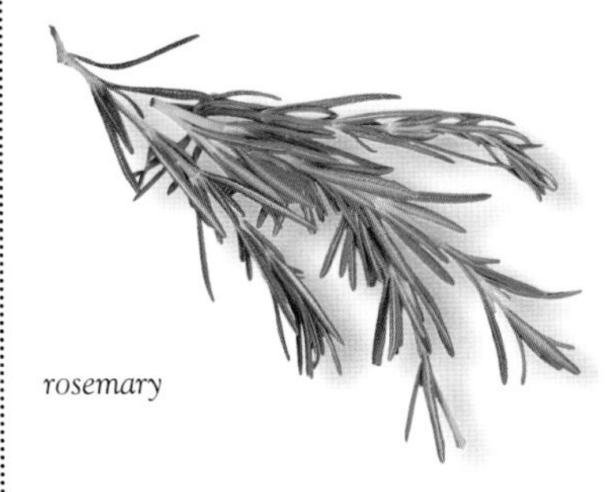

rosemary

Relaxation and flower remedies

Stress and anxiety are important features in asthma. Visualization, meditation, and biofeedback can be effective in preventing and managing attacks. Bach Rescue Remedy can help at the start of an attack.

PLEURISY

Pleurisy is inflammation of the pleura, the delicate membrane between the lungs and the walls of the chest. The most usual cause is viral infection, but it can also result from pneumonia and injury of adjoining organs. Breathing produces sharp, stabbing pains in the chest and shoulders from the fluid buildup in the membranes, and there is usually also a high fever.

Hydrotherapy

Bed rest and taking plenty of fluids is recommended. Hot compresses applied to the back and chest will bring relief and promote recovery.

Nutritional and dietary therapy

Hot soups and broths, especially containing the spice turmeric, garlic, and cloves, and chewing the rind on the inside of citrus fruits are all beneficial, and so are drinks of juiced carrot, celery, and parsley (or carrot and pineapple, or carrot, beet, and cucumber). "Toast water," a traditional remedy of powdered wholewheat toast boiled in water with butter and salt, and drunk while warm, is said to relieve pleurisy pain. The supplements vitamin C (2–3 g), A (50,000 iu), EFAs (fish oils, evening primrose and starflower/borage oils), and bromelain (pineapple enzyme) also help to promote recovery.

Herbal medicine

Mix equal parts of the tinctures of pleurisy root, echinacea, and elecampane, and take a spoonful a day. Drinking a tea of half-and-half dried mullein and pleurisy root as often as needed can also help.

Massage and aromatherapy

Massaging the back and chest with the oils of black pepper, pine, myrrh, rosemary, angelica, sage, or tea tree can bring effective relief.

"Drumming" on the back with cupped palms helps loosen mucus that collects in the lungs in pneumonia.

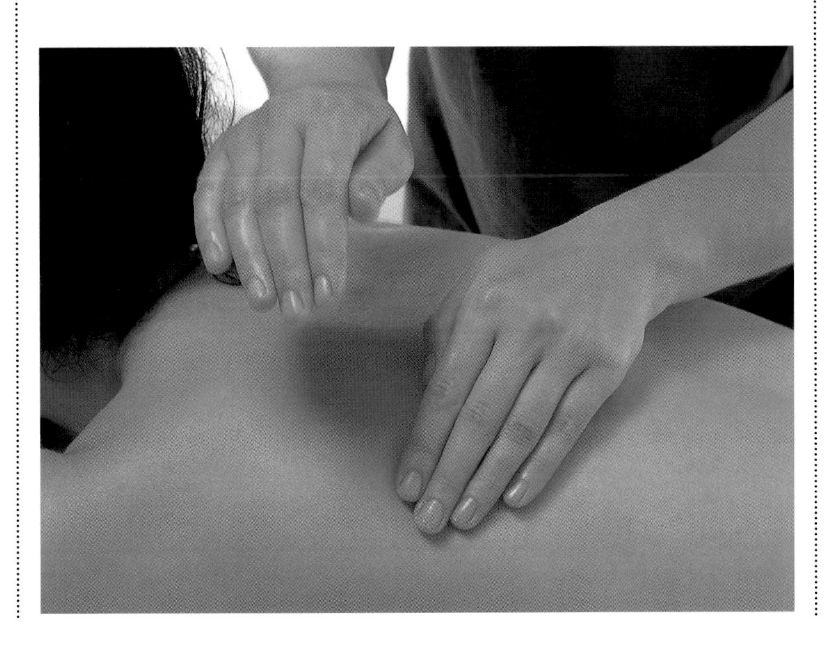

PNEUMONIA

Pneumonia is an infection of one or both of the lungs, caused by a virus or bacterium. Symptoms are chest pains, breathlessness, a cough with colored phlegm, fever, and chills. Bacterial pneumonia is more serious than viral, and can be life-threatening for the very young and the very old. Bronchopneumonia is often the final stage in people dying of old age and cancer, and is sometimes a feature of AIDS.

CAUTION Immediate antibiotics are advisable in severe cases of bacterial pneumonia.

Hydrotherapy and massage

Rest and various hydrotherapeutic methods are recommended in cases of pneumonia, including a warming compress, covering both the back and chest (also known as a "pneumonia jacket"). This should be combined with a cold compress on the forehead, and the feet in a bowl or basin of hot water. The treatment should be followed by having someone "drum" on the back with cupped hands to loosen mucus in the lungs, and (in normally strong people only) a cold friction rub.

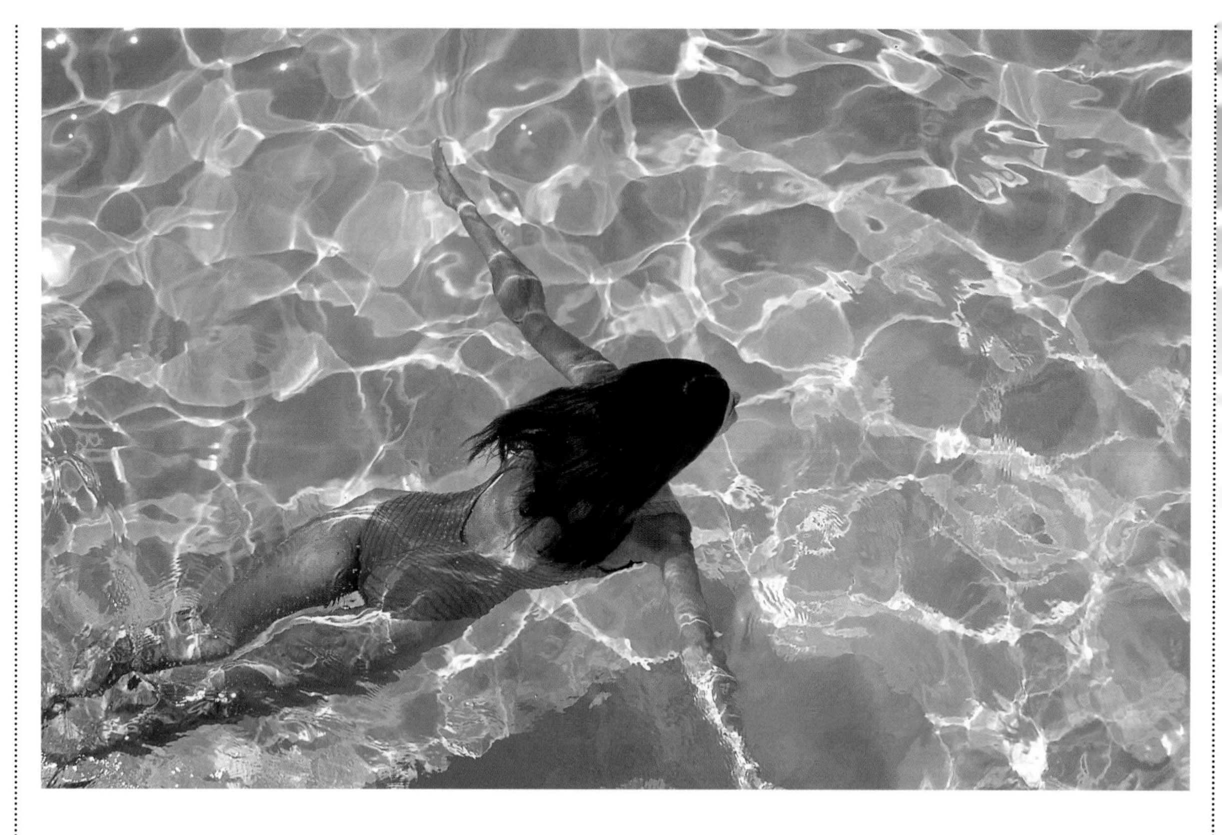

Swimming in warm water is one of the best forms of gentle exercise for those with breathing problems.

Nutritional and dietary therapy

Eat plenty of fresh fruit and vegetables (including raw garlic, chili, and cayenne peppers), and avoid dairy produce and sweet foods. Fresh diluted pear juice is claimed to have decongestant qualities, and regular drinks of fresh juiced carrot, spinach, parsley, garlic, and cumin are said to help. Supplement with large daily doses of vitamins A (preferably as beta carotene), C with bioflavonoids (6–10 g), and zinc. Other useful supplements are propolis (bee pollen) and acidophilus/bifidophilus (probiotics).

Herbal medicine

Lobelia and thyme loosen phlegm, echinacea and garlic fight infection, and elderflower and yarrow reduce fever. They should be taken as teas made from the dried herb, or tinctures. Other useful herbs are ipecacuanha, hypericum, and juniper. It is best to get a prescription from a qualified herbalist for something as serious as pneumonia.

Massage and aromatherapy

Massage the back and chest with equal drops of essential oils of camphor, eucalyptus, pine, lavender, lemon, and tea tree, diluted in a neutral carrier oil.

EMPHYSEMA

Emphysema is a progressive, and presently incurable, disease of the lungs in which the tiny air sacs (alveoli) that transfer oxygen breathed in to the bloodstream become damaged and so fail. Damage is most often because of heavy smoking or prolonged exposure to polluted air (coal miners are frequent sufferers, for example), but people who suffer from chronic bronchitis and asthma can also be casualties of emphysema. Men are far more prone to it than women. The progress of the disease is gradual, usually over a period of many years, and symptoms include breathlessness, which becomes increasingly severe over time. Death is often from heart failure.

Movement and hydrotherapy

Stopping smoking and performing gentle exercise are the most vital aspects of natural therapy to keep the lungs working and flexible. Good exercise options are swimming, tai chi, and yoga. Using ionizers and humidifiers can also help. "Pneumonia jackets" and drumming the back with cupped hands (in the same way as for pneumonia) can bring relief from excess mucus.

Massage and aromatherapy

Massage the chest with cedarwood, pine, peppermint, and eucalyptus. Steam inhaling with basil, cajuput, eucalyptus, hyssop, or thyme (or evaporating them in a burner) can also help. Experiment to get the right combination. Six drops of each oil is enough.

Herbal infusion for emphysema

An infusion of licorice root and comfrey is good for emphysema.

Mix ½ oz (15 g) of each dried herb in about 1 pint (570 ml) of water, and simmer for about 15 minutes. Drink four tablespoonfuls of the warm liquid four times a day.

Nutritional and dietary therapy

Drinking regular mixtures of juiced vegetables, such as garlic, carrot, spinach, celery, wheatgrass, watercress, potato, and barley, or fruits, such as grapes, oranges, lemons, and blackcurrants, is effective. Avoiding mucus-forming foods, such as dairy products, and eating spicy foods, such as garlic, horseradish, mustard, onions, and chili peppers, can also be beneficial. Supplementing with vitamins A, B-complex, C, E, zinc, co-enzyme Q10, and lecithin helps: a good wide-spectrum multivitamin will have most of these ingredients.

Relaxation

Relaxation techniques, such as meditation, visualization, and biofeedback, can help ease the tension that often makes emphysema worse than it need be.

TUBERCULOSIS

Tuberculosis (TB) is a severe and potentially fatal bacterial infection caused by the organism mycobacterium tuberculosis. Though it is a systemic disease (it can affect any part of the body), it most often affects the lungs, causing pain, breathlessness, fatigue, loss of appetite and weight loss, fever, night sweats, and coughing blood. Despite a worldwide vaccination campaign that saw TB fall to an all-time low between 1944 and 1985, cases have risen dramatically since and are now at record levels—due, it is believed, to increased movement of people from infected areas, the rise of HIV, and declining levels of immune system functioning in the industrial world generally.

NOTE Immunization with the BCG vaccine is the preventive treatment of choice among doctors, but it is only partly effective in some people. Moreover, it limits diagnosis because, once vaccinated, a person will normally register permanently positive in tests.

Naturopathy

Specialist care is essential in TB, and the traditional mountainside clinics common before 1940 remain the "natural" treatment of choice. This means being able to breathe clean, dry air, with plenty of rest, preferably in sunshine. Various compresses (applied by a trained hydrotherapist) can bring relief, as can hot packs of eucalyptus oil, alcohol, and grapes. Supervised fasting may also be recommended in certain cases.

Nutritional and dietary therapy

A diet with fresh fruit (especially pears and bitter melon) and raw vegetables is recommended, coupled with plenty of protein foods and garlic. Supplement with EFAs, vitamins A, B-complex, C, E, magnesium, calcium, and zinc. Avoid added salt in food. The juice of the common stinging nettle is also said to be effective. Equal parts of juiced carrot and raw potato (with the settled starch removed), mixed with a teaspoonful of olive or almond oil and honey, and beaten to a froth are also said to be beneficial; drink a glassful of this remedy, three times daily.

Herbal medicine

The herb echinacea is an effective immune system booster, especially taken as a tincture with elecampane and mullein (a teaspoonful three times daily). Licorice and citrus seed extract can also help.

Massage and aromatherapy

Gently massaging the whole body can be both palliative and curative. Use diluted essential oils of eucalyptus, tea tree, cypress, juniper, peppermint, ginger, rosemary, marjoram, and neroli.

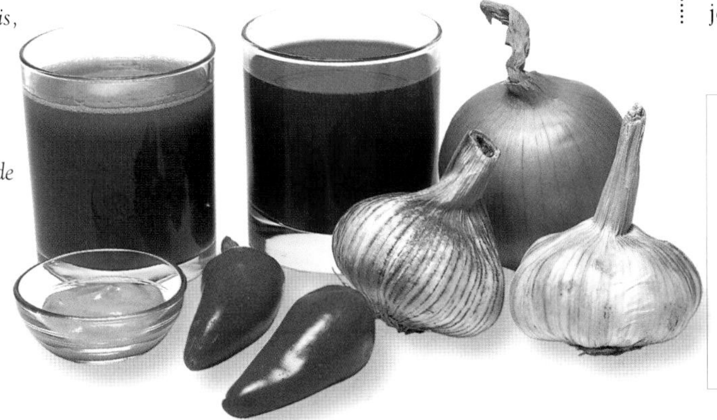

Raw garlic, chilis, and onions can help breathing problems. An alternative is to drink juices made from them.

Other therapies
From a qualified therapist only

Osteopathy • pages 152–153
Acupuncture • pages 150–151
Psychotherapy • page 154
Hypnotherapy • page 153

NECK AND BACK PAIN

The neck and back—meaning the spine and spinal cord, together with the large muscles, tissues, and the organs attached to them—is one of the most important and sensitive parts of the body. The neck not only supports the head but surrounds some of the most critical nerves and blood vessels, while the back not only holds us upright but controls posture—the way we stand and walk.

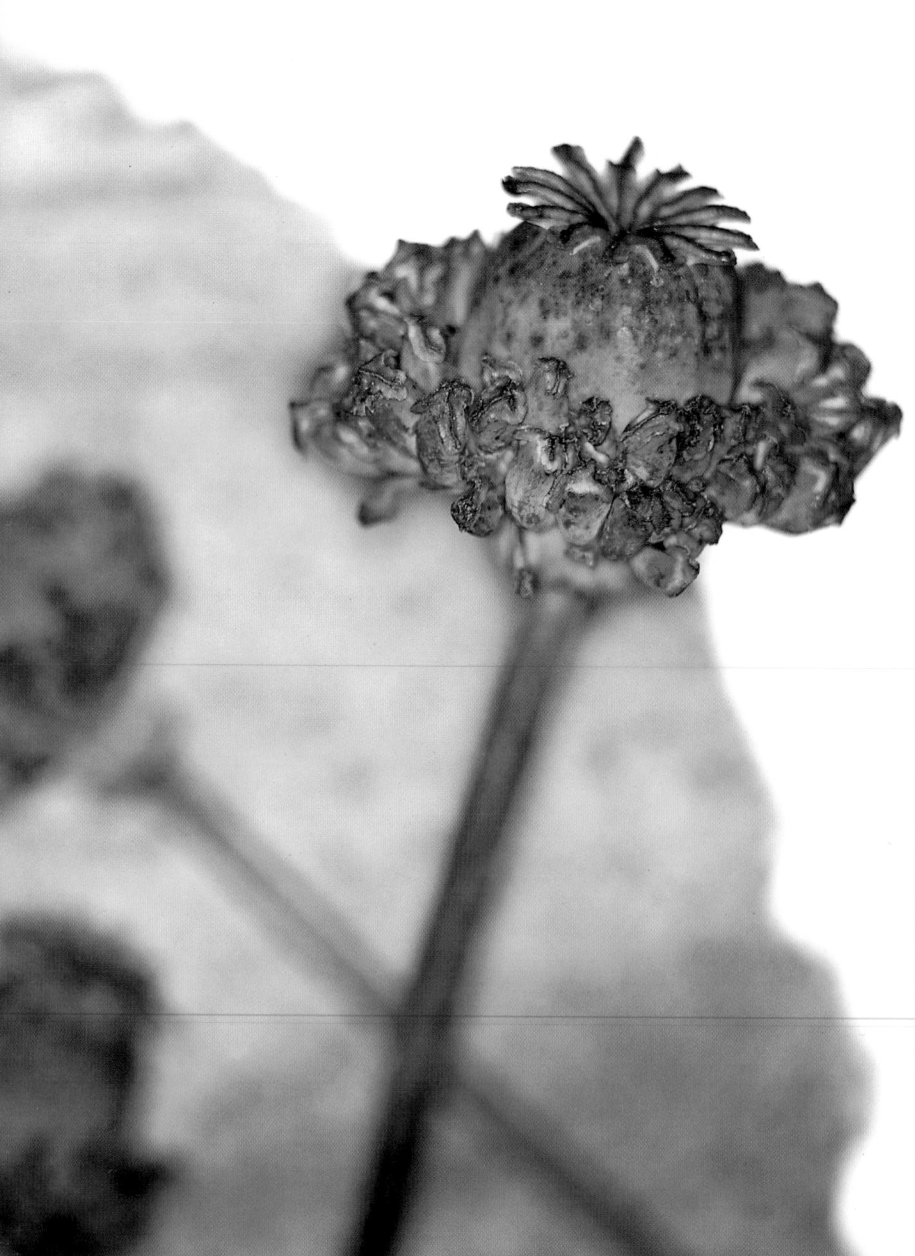

Our posture affects our health in many ways. Poor posture can cause problems not only with our backs, hands, arms, and legs but less obvious parts of our body too, such as ears, eyes, brain, throat, mouth, blood, bladder, and bowels. It can also be responsible for many so-called psychosomatic complaints, from tiredness, depression, and headaches to poor breathing, constipation, and incontinence.

Warning

Seek immediate medical help for neck/back pain as a result of:

- *accident or injury*
- *no obvious reason, especially if accompanied by:*
- *feverishness or very high temperature*
- *severe headache with vomiting and nausea*
- *sudden loss of appetite and weight loss*
- *extreme tiredness*
- *loss of bladder or bowel control*
- *pins and needles in the loins*
- *weakness in the legs and/or foot-dragging.*

A physical problem with the back can affect the mind and emotions as well as the body. On the other hand, good posture means that muscles work more efficiently, breathing is deeper and less strained, blood is stronger and richer in oxygen, the immune system is more effective and, generally, we will feel more balanced, energetic, and healthier.

The problem of poor posture is not confined to any one group of people. Most people spend a lifetime with a body that is unbalanced—the result of poor eating and living habits, lack of exercise, wearing the wrong shoes, sitting around too much, and not sitting properly. All these things lead to muscle tightness and imbalances that in turn create abnormal weight distribution and stresses and strain on other, hidden, parts of the body—often far from the root of the problem.

The work we do, our temperament, the genes we were born with, and the diseases we experience can all affect our posture. But posture is something we can do a very great deal to correct, regardless of its origins (though some problems, such as inner ear infection that can cause a loss of balance, may need drug treatment as well).

Standard conventional therapy for back pain involves the taking of drugs, such as muscle relaxants, anti-inflammatories, antidepressants, corticosteroids, and tranquilizers—none of which should be a first-resort treatment, and all of which have side-effects (some of them serious). Natural therapy, by contrast, concentrates on alleviating immediate symptoms with such approaches as hydrotherapy, massage, TENS devices, and acupuncture, and long-term removal of causes by correcting poor posture and maintaining good posture.

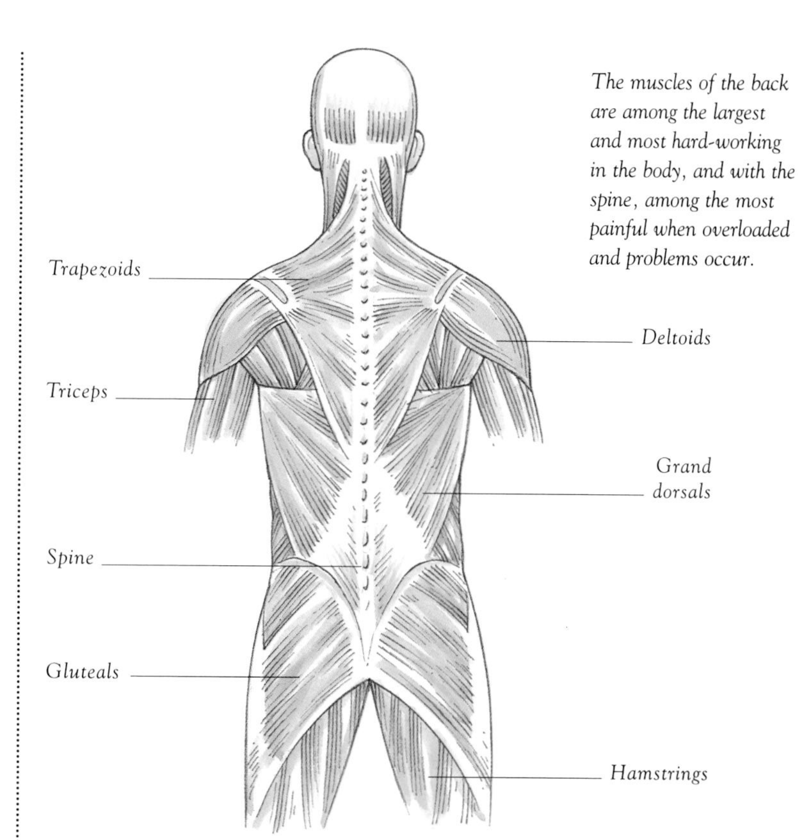

The muscles of the back are among the largest and most hard-working in the body, and with the spine, among the most painful when overloaded and problems occur.

SPINE

The spine has four natural curves—but they should be gentle and upright curves. A good spine should have the right balance of curves for best performance and to avoid strain on muscles and joints. When they are neither gentle nor upright, a variety of problems can occur. The most common abnormalities are kyphosis, lordosis, flat back, sway back, and scoliosis.

Figuring out whether you have a postural problem and deciding on treatment is best done with help. Consult a specialist, such as a qualified osteopath, chiropractor, physiotherapist, or a teacher of yoga or the Alexander technique.

KYPHOSIS

Kyphosis describes a spine with exaggerated outward and inward curves: the upper (thoracic) spine curves out too much—usually producing round shoulders, a flat chest, and an extended neck with the head coming too far forward; and the lower (lumbar) spine curves in too much, producing a hollow back. This is the most common postural problem, and it is often seen in people confined to a wheelchair, or who spend most of their time sitting.

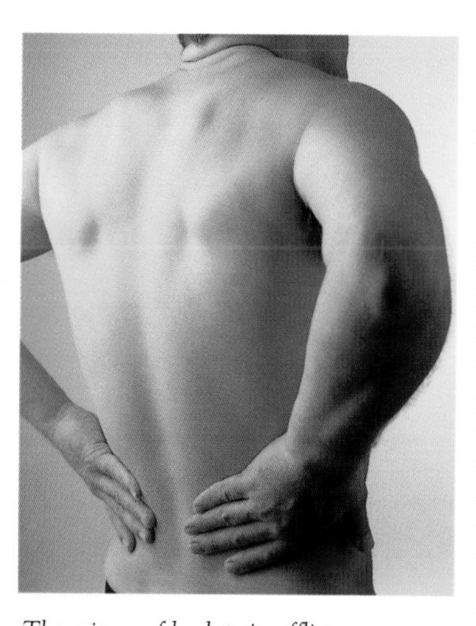

The misery of back pain afflicts most people at some time. Natural therapies can help prevent and reduce pain. If the problem is postural, it is best to seek advice from a specialist.

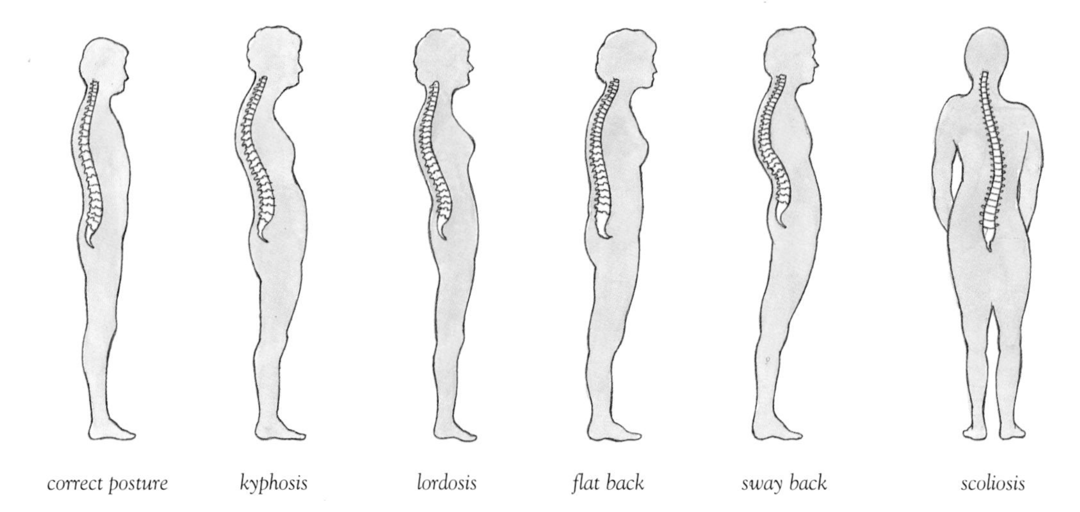

correct posture — kyphosis — lordosis — flat back — sway back — scoliosis

Kyphosis puts pressure on the lungs and compresses the digestive system. This can affect a person's breathing capacity, sometimes leading to tingling and numbness in fingers from the shortage of oxygen to the tissues, asthma and other respiratory problems, and constipation, incontinence, and depression. Treatment for kyphosis should concentrate on deep-breathing and posture-correcting exercises, such as those shown opposite.

LORDOSIS

Lordosis is a posture in which the lower spine is curved excessively inward, and can be due to sitting too much or standing too long with the knees locked backward. It is associated with weak stomach muscles and tight back muscles.

To correct lordosis, stand "tall" but relax the knees—do not force them back. Stand with the pelvis tilted slightly forward, and the stomach muscles gently pulled in. Tuck the chin in. This will lengthen the back of the neck and help reduce the "poked forward" look. Exercises for strengthening stomach muscles will also help.

FLAT BACK

Flat back means largely what it says: the pelvis is tilted too far forward, there is no curve of the lower spine, and the muscles of the bottom are wasted, producing the characteristic flat look. It is also common for people with flat backs to have round shoulders.

To correct a flat back posture, whenever you sit down, straighten your legs out in front of you. This will not only stretch your hamstrings, which are usually tight in this condition, but help accentuate the curve of the lower back. Also clench the muscles of your bottom as often as you can to help strengthen them. A lumbar support cushion or roll is also beneficial. These are available from a variety of sources, including mail order.

SWAY BACK

In a sway back posture, the entire lower back, including the pelvis and upper thighs, is held forward, so that the upper body appears to lean backward. The shoulders are usually rounded and the chin stuck out. It is a posture common in people who are very flexible, and the cause is mainly weak hips. It is sometimes mistaken for lordosis, though it is quite different.

To correct sway back, transfer your body weight onto the balls of the feet rather than the heels when standing, and pull your chin in. This lengthens the neck and lifts some of the weight off the hips. You will also need to do hip and buttock muscle-strengthening exercises.

SCOLIOSIS

Scoliosis is a sideways curvature or twist of the spine, and is usually the result of habitually poor posture, though it can be inherited. The

Posture training

The following therapies can be effective in treating and improving posture.

- *Yoga and tai chi*
- *Alexander technique*
- *Feldenkrais method ("awareness through movement" and "functional integration")*
- *Rolfing (or "structural reintegration")*
- *Hellerwork (a combination of manipulation and movement)*

Specialists in these therapies will be able to offer the detailed individual training and guidance needed. Once learned properly, the exercises taught can usually be carried out safely and successfully at home.

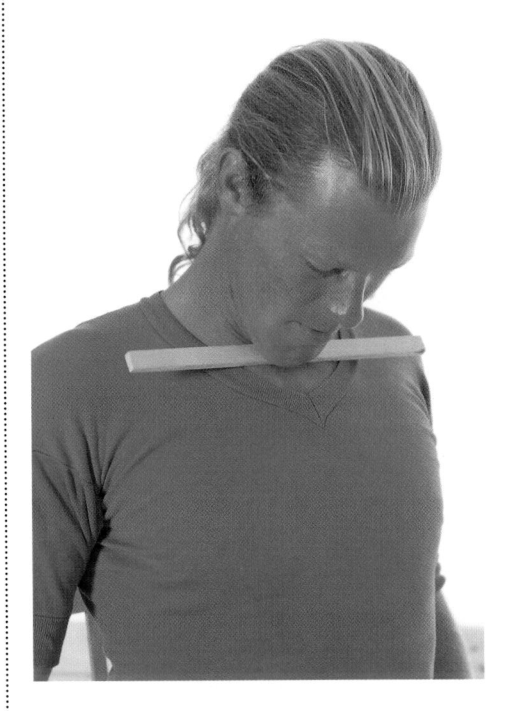

one

Place a stick under your chin and straighten your shoulders, pulling them back slowly but firmly. Your neck muscles will feel pulled and stretched, but persevere without straining. Do only as much as feels comfortable (overtaxing the neck muscles can make the problem worse).

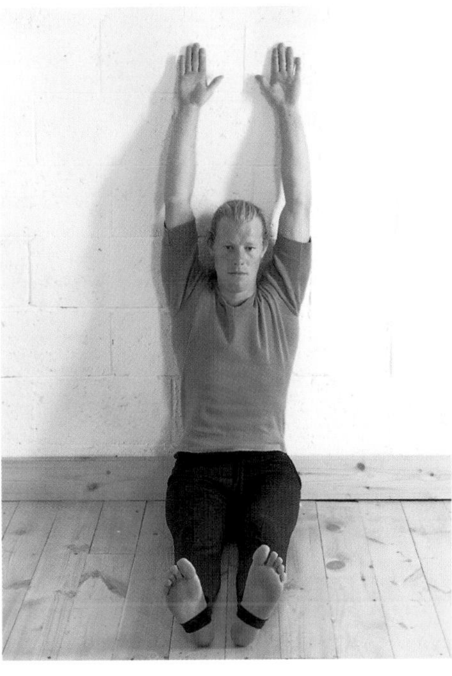

two

Stand or sit against a wall with your shoulders and upper back touching the wall. Stretch your arms above your head and touch the wall. If you can touch the wall easily, your posture is good; if not, it is a lot less good! Keep doing this as often as possible, wherever possible. It will strengthen your back and shoulders muscles as well as helping to straighten your spine.

effect is the same as if you stand with your full weight on one foot and force your shoulders in that direction without actually turning. It is common in varying degrees in many people and characteristically produces different leg lengths.

In severe cases, a special lift fitted into a shoe will help the problem (though it should be done by a qualified person, such as an osteopath), but most people are not badly enough affected to need this sort of artificial aid, and can help themselves easily by regularly stretching the muscles of the hips and trunk. Try this before resorting to artificial aids, if possible. Cranial osteopathy can also help, but must be done by a specialist.

NECK

Neckache can be as mild as a passing discomfort from sitting or lying too long in one position to a more serious and chronic condition, requiring patience and care to correct. Because the neck is one of the most sensitive parts of the body—it is the conduit for all the blood supply and nerve signals to the brain—a problem with the neck can produce symptoms in the head, such as headaches, dizziness, aching eyes, blurred vision, and jaw ache. A mild ache in the neck can be put right simply by massaging the area with your hand until the pain goes. A more severe ache, such as a "crick" or stiff neck (where the head has become "stuck" at an uncomfortable angle and is painful to move), or neck spasm (torticolli) need more complex treatment. But natural therapies have a particularly good success rate whatever the severity.

CAUTION A stiff neck for no obvious reason, with a worsening headache, high temperature, and sensitivity to light, is one of the first symptoms of meningitis: an extremely dangerous infection of the meninges, the thin protective coating of the brain and spinal cord containing cerebrospinal fluid. If these symptoms are experienced, seek immediate medical help.

Massage and aromatherapy

Stroke down the side of the neck and across the shoulders, keeping the muscles relaxed and your hands molded to the contours of your body. Follow a few strokes of this by kneading the muscles and tissues of the neck and shoulders with the palms and fingers of one hand. Start gently and feel for "knots," or

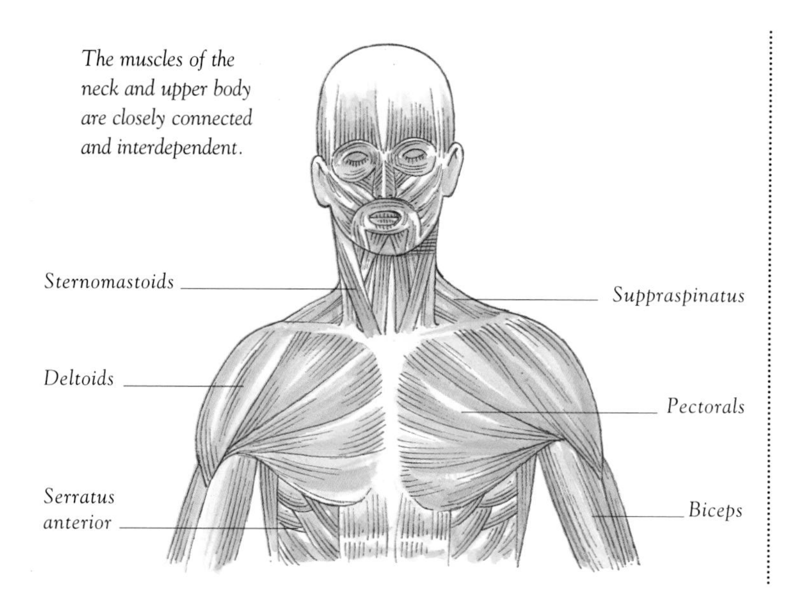

The muscles of the neck and upper body are closely connected and interdependent.

WHIPLASH

Whiplash is pain in the neck (and sometimes the back as a whole) as a result of having the head jolted severely backward—for example, when the car you are in is hit hard in the rear by the car behind. The pain is the result of the muscles, tendons, and ligaments in the neck being strained and attempting to heal. Symptoms, which can also include headaches, disturbed vision, fatigue, pins and needles, anxiety, and depression, can arise immediately or some time after the accident occurred.

areas that are hard and tender, working them until the knottiness goes. Hold any tender area firmly and stretch the now warm muscle by slowly circling your shoulders or head, effectively getting them to massage themselves. Using a few drops of the essential oils of marjoram and/or rosemary, diluted in carrier oil, adds to the benefit. Getting a friend to massage your neck and shoulders is even more effective. Do not massage the throat area.

Physical therapy

Stretching exercises involving the neck and shoulder area can be beneficial. A good physiotherapist or physical therapist should be able to demonstrate them. The example shown here (right) is just one possibility. Posture-correcting exercises (see page 69) aim to improve the position of the neck in relation to the head, and so can aid recovery from neck pain and help prevent further problems.

Reflexology and aromatherapy

Massage where the toes join the sole, especially that of the big toe (which corresponds to the neck). Do it for 2–3 minutes, using marjoram or rosemary essential oils.

Neck-stretching exercise

one

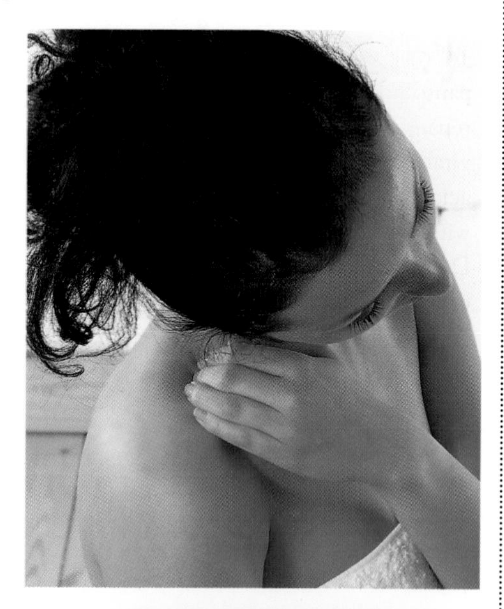

Move your head as far over to one side as you can and press down firmly with your fingers on the shoulder, trapping the muscle under them. Keeping the muscle under pressure, slowly move your head back up from the shoulder. You should feel the muscle stretch. Move your hand a little higher up toward the neck and do it again.

two

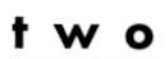

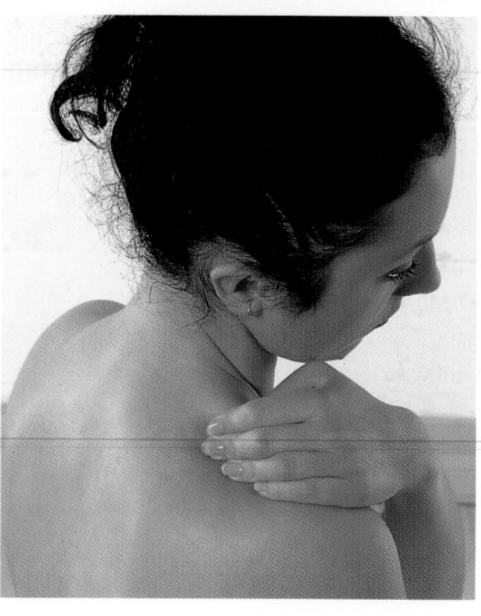

The closer you get to the neck, the harder it gets to move your head back up, but that is normal. The important thing is to feel the stretch. Once you have moved up to the base of the neck in about six steps, repeat the entire procedure on the other shoulder. Cover all of the neck and shoulder area in this way. It should take about 10 minutes.

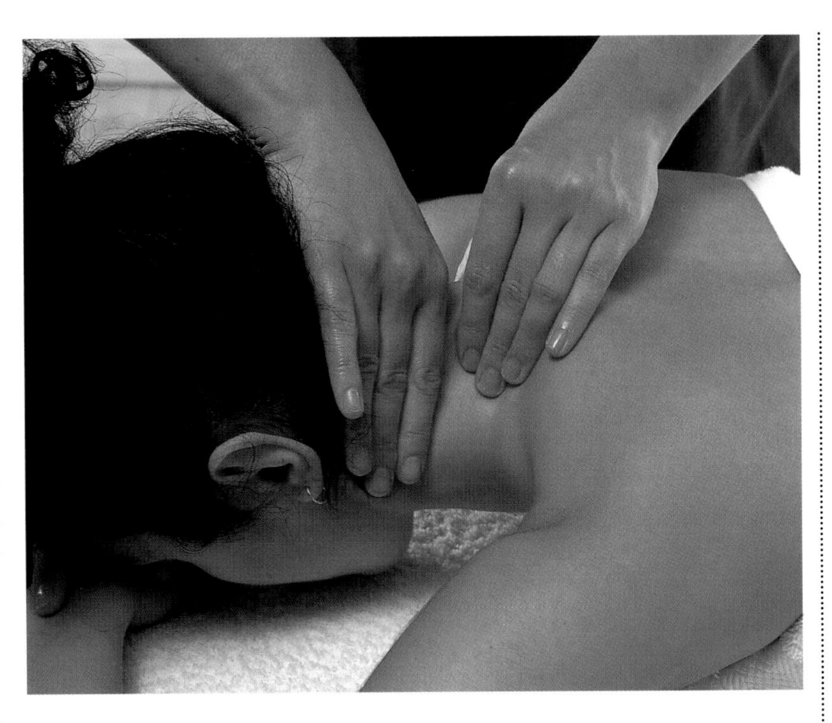

Gentle massaging can relieve neck pain quickly and effectively by encouraging blood into the area.

Herbal medicine and homeopathy

Arnica tincture or ointment on the affected area will help ease any bruising, provided it is applied within an hour of the accident or jolt. The homeopathic remedy arnica 30c can also be taken for the first half hour after the incident (one every five minutes), followed by hypericum 6c (every four hours for up to three days).

Nutritional and dietary therapy

To relieve stiffness, take calcium pantothenate, and to help tissue repair take a good daily multivitamin (with minerals and amino acids) and a fish oil capsule (EPA) with gammalinolenic acid (GLA). Daily doses of vitamin C (3–5 g), calcium (1 g), and magnesium (500 mg) help acute pain, and the freshwater algae spirulina, available in powder form from health food stores, is also recommended.

Hydrotherapy

Alternating hot and cold compresses can bring immediate relief.

TORTICOLLIS

Torticollis (or "wry neck") is the result of spasm of the sternomastoid muscles on either side of the neck, and can be long-term as well as acute. In its chronic state it is more often a genetic problem than due to injury or illness, but in the short term it can be caused by an inflamed gland or rheumatism in the area. Congenital wry neck is hard to correct after childhood without surgery, but the approaches beneficial for neck pain generally can also help alleviate discomfort from short-term spasm.

BACK

Backache, or back pain, is, with headache, one of the commonest and also one of the most serious types of pain experienced. More working days are lost in the western world through back problems than from any other illness except flu. There is little surprise in this, given that the back (and neck), consisting of the spine and a broad swathe of interconnecting muscles and tissues, is almost exclusively responsible for holding us upright and keeping most organs in their correct position. This puts the back (and neck) under constant strain and is the factor that makes back problems difficult to treat.

The record of natural therapies is second to none in both alleviating and curing back pain, and natural approaches are increasingly being incorporated into the treatment being offered at pain clinics around the world. Though pain can happen anywhere in the back, the majority of back pain occurs in the lower part of the back, where it is better known as lumbago.

Massage and aromatherapy

Massage carefully over the entire back, concentrating on "hot spots," or areas of particular pain, *but making sure not to apply pressure to the spine itself.* If unable to reach your back, get a friend to help. A good alternative is to put two tennis balls into a sock and gently roll on them (keeping them away from the spine itself). A mixture of 12 drops of ginger, 5 drops of juniper, and 8 drops of either rosemary or lavender (rosemary is stimulating, and lavender calming), added to a carrier oil, will make massage more effective. Other oils effective for acute pain are black pepper, cypress, eucalyptus, and birch, and for general muscle ache marjoram, chamomile, and clary sage.

Homeopathy and flower remedies

Arnica 6c (every half hour for up to three hours, then every four hours for up to five days) is effective. Alternatives are rhus tox 3c (for muscular strain), and ruta 3c (for bruised bones and tendons). Bach Rescue Remedy may also help.

Yoga exercises for a healthy back

one

The Cat posture can be beneficial. Kneel on all fours, arms straight down, knees under hips, and head up. Breathe in, and slowly raise and lower your head several times. Breathe out.

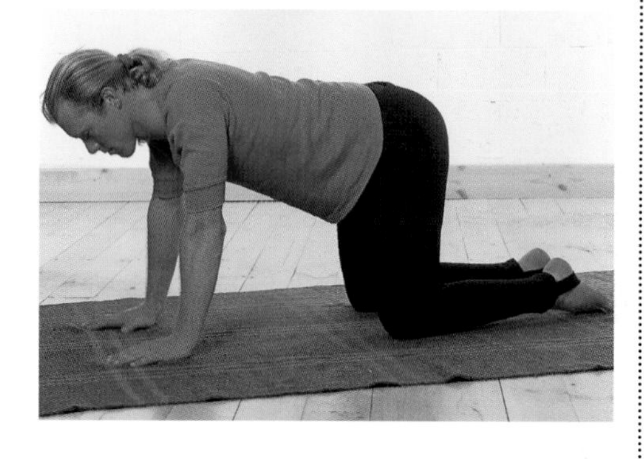

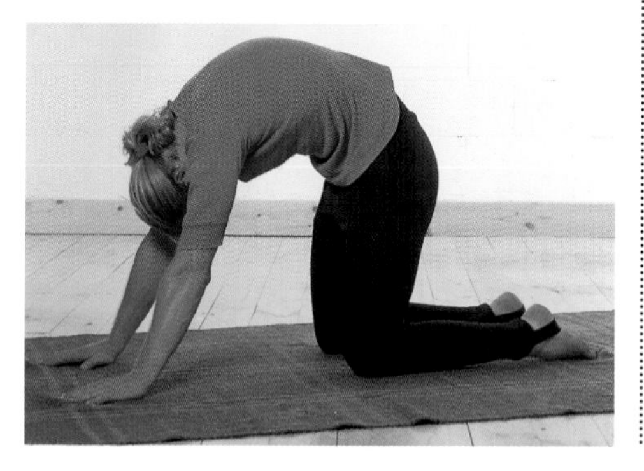

two

Breathe in, lifting your chin right up, and at the same time press down on your hands, dropping your back so that it is curved toward the floor. Hold for a few seconds and breathe out.

three

Breathing out, arch your back upward and pull your chin into your chest. Hold for a few seconds and relax. Repeat three times at first, building up to ten as you gain stamina.

Movement therapy and hydrotherapy

Lie down on a firm flat surface with knees bent, and apply alternate hot and cold compresses. Apply the ice pack for 10 minutes and the hot pack for 5, alternating for as long and as often as helps. Using a large bag of frozen peas and a covered hot-water bottle is the easiest way of doing this at home.

Slowly drawing both knees up toward your shoulders helps gets muscles over spasm by stretching them. But do not force it: stop if it hurts, and let the muscle get used to the stretch before continuing.

Exercise

Gentle exercise is now widely accepted as being much better for treating back problems than rest. Swimming—particularly if combined with a sauna or steam bathing—is excellent, and walking is also good (but not jogging). A wide range of exercises that can help is now on offer in both the western and eastern traditions. Some specialists in back pain offer the best of both, and an initial visit to a therapist could help you find out what is most suitable for your needs and preferences.

The pelvic tilt

Lie flat on your back, arms straight by your side, hands flat on the ground, knees bent. Breathe normally. Pushing down on your hands and arms, and clenching the muscles of your buttocks, raise your pelvis up. Hold for a few seconds and relax. Repeat three times, increasing the number and duration of the tilts as you gain stamina.

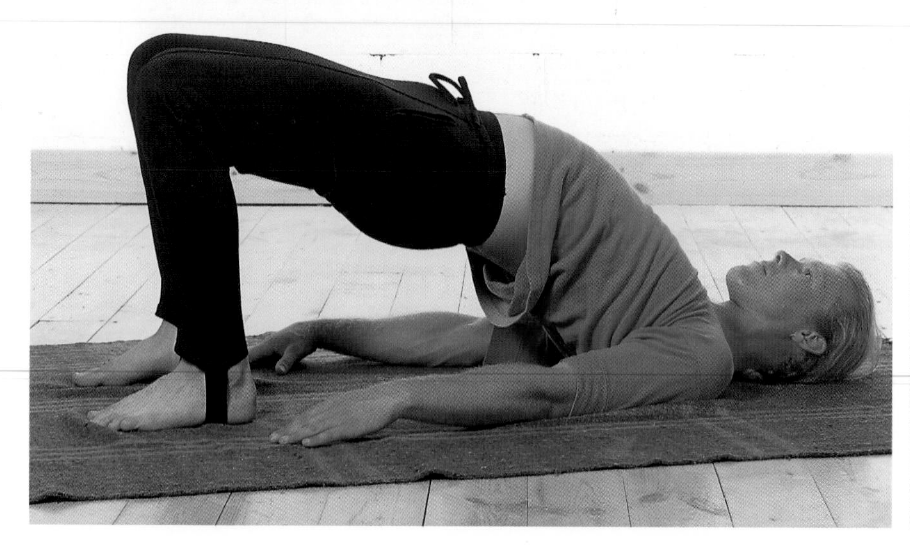

Herbal medicine

If the pain or ache is from a strain or injury, arnica tincture or ointment rubbed gently into the affected area will help ease any bruising, provided it is applied within an hour of the incident. Bromelain (pineapple enzyme) is a powerful anti-inflammatory (2–3 g daily at first, 1–2 g as the pain eases). Other anti-inflammatories, effective drunk as teas, are valerian, hypericum, and Jamaican dogwood. Natural "aspirin" tablets made from willow bark and meadowsweet can help relieve pain, while ginger, cayenne, horseradish, lobelia, and crampbark help recovery if rubbed into the painful area, by stimulating local blood flow.

Electronic devices

TENS provide powerful pain relief, as do devices that encourage blood into the area, such as intasound and vibrating massagers. High-frequency massagers (100 Hz) are best, applied for at least 45 minutes.

Nutritional and dietary therapy

Eat a healthy diet with plenty of fresh fruit and vegetables and as little as possible of animal fats, sugar, salt, alcohol, tea, and coffee. Supplements of fish oils (EPA), evening primrose oil (GLA), and a good multivitamin and mineral supplement will help.

Aromatherapy

Regular hot baths containing a few drops each of chamomile, lavender, juniper, eucalyptus, and rosemary are an effective pain-reliever.

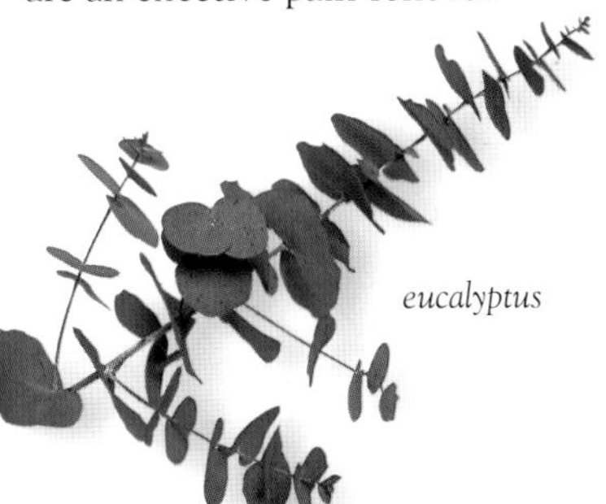

eucalyptus

Relaxation

Encourage relaxation of the back muscles by avoiding stress. Therapies such as meditation, visualization, biofeedback, and self-hypnosis can all help promote mental and emotional relaxation.

Reflexology

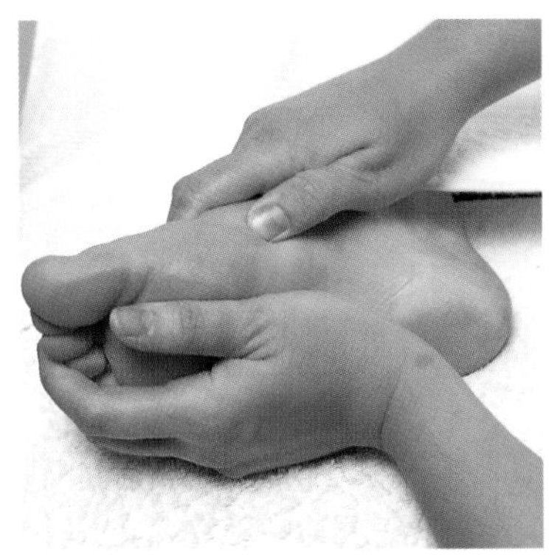

Manipulating the length of each foot along the line of the instep (said to correspond to the spine), can benefit back problems if done regularly. Use a thumb or knuckle to knead along the line of the foot, moving in small circles from the heel to the toe.

Postural therapies

The Alexander technique teaches correct postural habits and is particularly effective for neck and back pain if practiced on a regular basis. Some of the exercises are extremely simple: a classic relaxation exercise good for the back involves lying face up on the floor with knees bent, hands resting on the stomach and head on a book 1½ in (3–4 cm) thick. Other techniques that work along roughly the same lines are Rolfing, the Feldenkrais method, and Hellerwork—but these need even more guidance from a teacher than the Alexander technique.

SLIPPED DISK

Between each of the bones in the spine (vertebrae) is a flat piece, or disk, of springy cartilage that acts as a "shock-absorber." Its jelly-like center can sometimes slip through a crack in the outer ring of the disk—as the result of an awkward movement, for example—and press against the nerves in the spinal column. Pain is sudden, severe, and often accompanied by spasm of the back muscles, a pins and needles feeling, and numbness in one or both legs or feet. *DO NOT MANIPULATE or attempt self-help beyond immediate pain relief, and seek medical attention.*

Electronic devices and hydrotherapy

For immediate pain relief, a TENS device is best, if available, but if not, apply alternating hot and cold compresses. Failing either, a covered hot-water bottle held to the area of pain can help.

Homeopathy and flower remedies

The homeopathic remedy arnica 6c (every half hour for up to three hours, and then one every four hours for up to five days) is effective. Bach Rescue Remedy may also be of benefit.

Other therapies

From a qualified therapist only

The following therapies can give both immediate and long-term relief from back and neck pain, or even a complete cure.

Acupuncture • pages 150–151
Chiropractic • pages 152
Osteopathy and cranial osteopathy • pages 152–153
Hypnotherapy • page 153

NERVE, MUSCLE, AND JOINT PAIN

Aches and pains of the nerves, muscles, and joints are as common as headache and back pain (although back pain is effectively an example of problems in all three of these areas). The source of such pain is not always clear, especially in conditions of the nervous system, such as sciatica, when the site of the pain is often not where the real problem lies. The back is, in fact, the origin of many aches and pains in the nerves, muscles, and joints—even when the pain occurs in the hands, arms, legs, and feet.

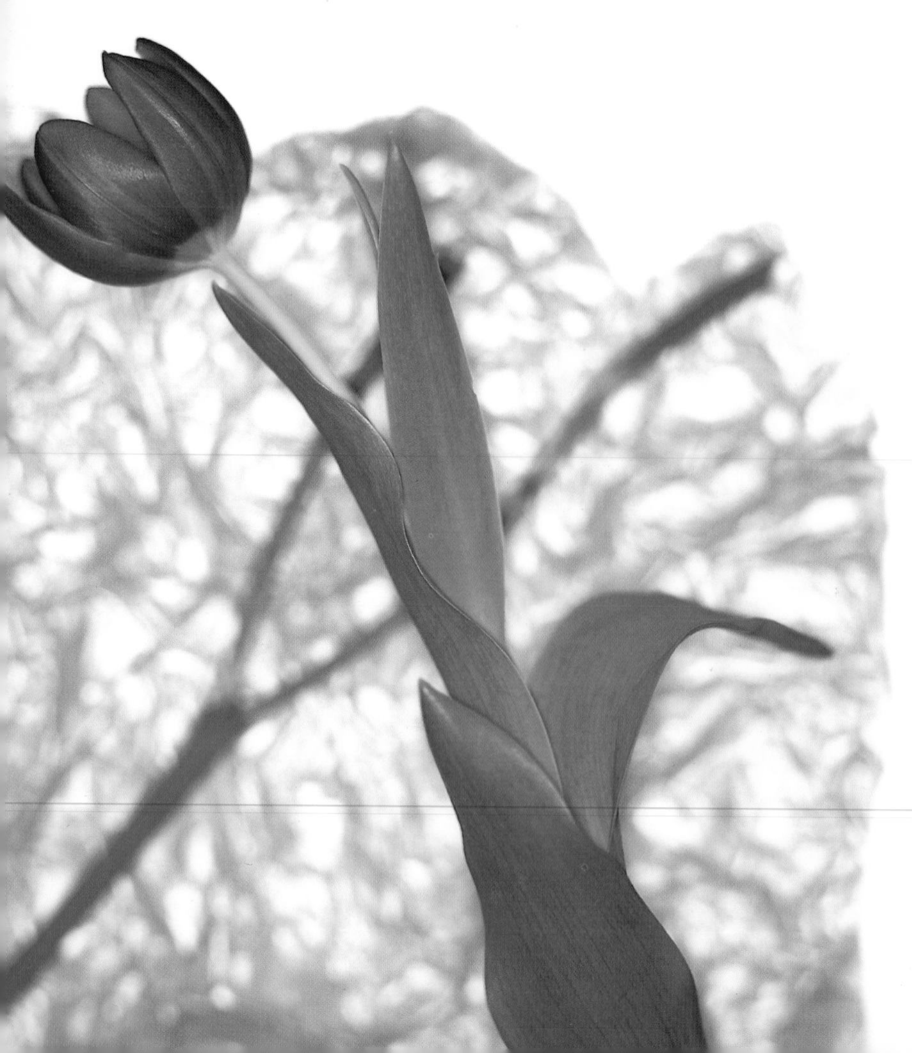

Natural self-help is largely a matter of applying immediate pain-relieving therapy where possible, and then trying to identify the source of the problem to start effective long-term treatment. Most effective immediate natural pain-relief is provided by massage with essential oils, by devices such as TENS, intasound, massagers, and electromagnetic pulsers, by hydrotherapy, by acupressure, and by pain-relieving herbs. Long-term help is often best provided by exercise, by postural and stretching movements, by dietary changes and food supplementation, and by psychological relaxation therapies.

NOTE Though this chapter divides nerves, muscles, and joints into separate sections, the three are in reality so interdependent that often treatment for one will inevitably help the others. The division was adopted to make it easier for readers to identify treatment by their most obvious presenting symptom or symptoms.

NERVE PAIN

A number of different terms are commonly used to describe the various types of nerve pain encountered. The main terms used are neuralgia (meaning pain resulting from injury to a nerve, particularly in the face), sciatica (pain mediated by the sciatic nerve, running from the lower part of the spine down each leg), and neuritis (inflammation in any nerve).

Nerve pain—aching, tingling, pins and needles, and a stabbing or burning sensation are the most common—can be caused by a number of factors, both physical and psychological, but the main ones are circulatory insufficiency, poor posture, wrong diet, stress, and over-exertion. Natural therapies can ease discomfort and accelerate the recovery process.

Nutritional and dietary therapy

Eat plenty of green vegetables and fresh fruit. If a reaction is suspected to something that has been eaten (food "allergy" or intolerance), a fruit (e.g. apples and pears) or vegetable juice (beet and carrot) 48-hour "cleansing" diet can help. Supplementation is recommended as follows: vitamins A, C, E, B-complex, the minerals magnesium, calcium, and selenium, and both omega-3 and omega-6 fatty acids (e.g. fish oils, flaxseed/linseed oil, and starflower/borage oil). Bromelain, an enzyme extracted from pineapples, is a natural nerve anti-inflammatory agent. Take up to 3 g a day *between* meals. A good quality multi-nutrient, available from good drugstores and health food stores, contains most of the supplements needed.

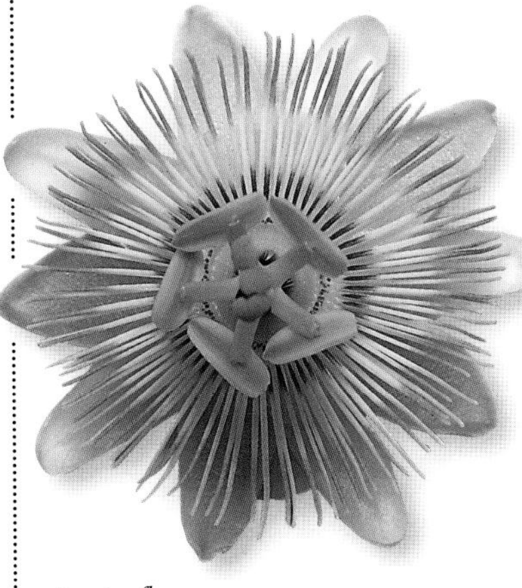

passionflower

Herbal medicine

Regular teas of ginseng, hops, Jamaican dogwood, Pasque flower, passion flower, hypericum, skullcap, and valerian are recommended for nerve pain. "Garlic milk"—that is, two crushed garlic cloves in half a pint of milk (cold or heated, as preferred)—drunk daily, can help sciatic pain.

Homeopathy

Neuralgia can be helped by belladonna 6c and aconite 6c, and nerve injuries by hypericum 6c.

Massage and aromatherapy

Massaging painful areas with two drops each of the essential oils of wintergreen, peppermint, or myrrh can help relieve symptoms (or use a proprietary mixture such as Olbas Oil). Alternatives are rosemary and lavender, or clove, basil, and eucalyptus oils. Hypericum oil can also ease pain if rubbed into the affected area.

Electronic devices

TENS or GigaTENS is highly effective at treating most nerve pain although it does not seem to be quite as good at treating post-herpes neuralgia. Hand-held devices such as massagers/vibrators and intasound are also effective if applied firmly enough for long enough—at least 45 minutes. A frequency of 100 Hz works best.

Relaxation and yoga

Stress management techniques such as meditation (especially autogenics training) and biofeedback can be helpful, together with postures that concentrate on stretching, especially those that tone the spine and back muscles, coupled with breathing exercises. Advice from a trained teacher is best in both cases.

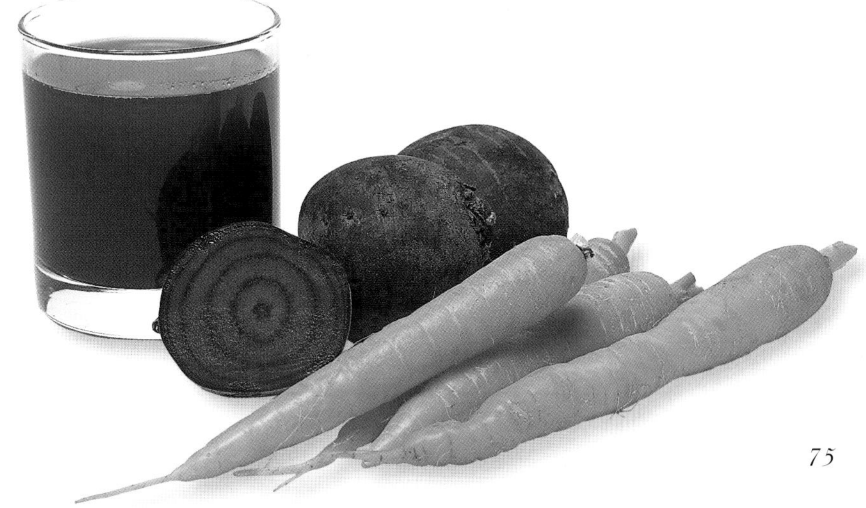

A 48-hour diet of carrot and beet juice mixture can help with mild nerve pain.

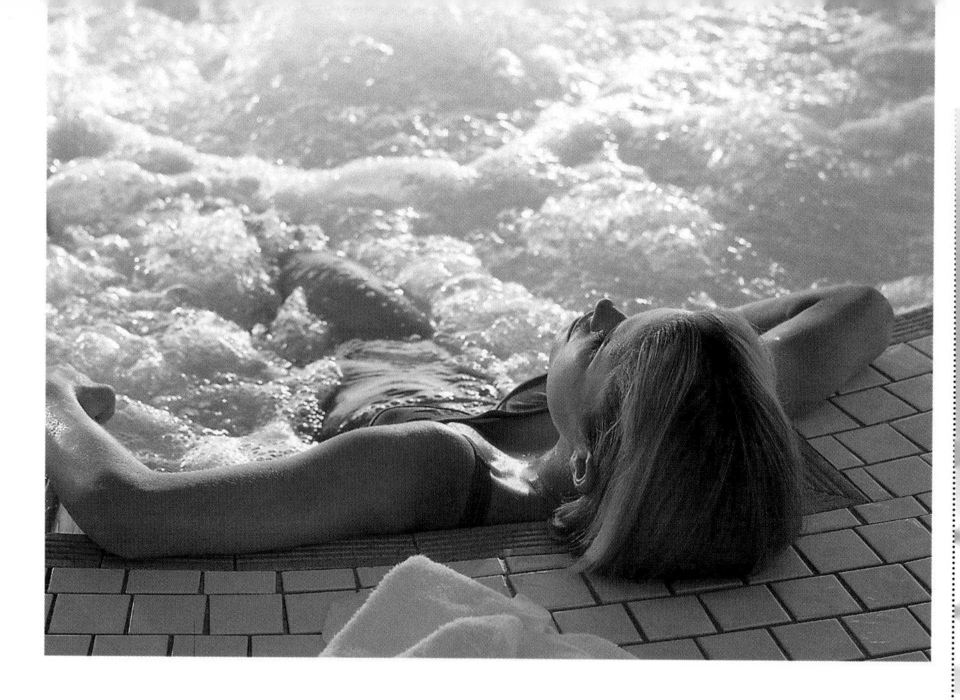

Relaxing in hot water, especially a spa bath with mineral salts added, is particularly beneficial for joint, nerve, and muscle pain.

Acupressure

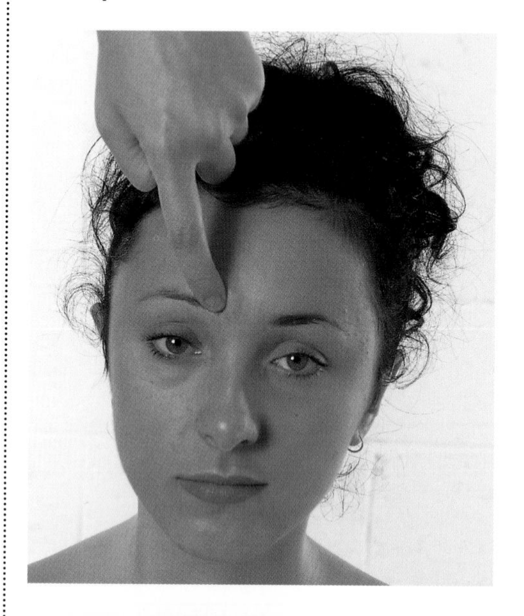

face pain

Press a point on the inner end of the eyebrow on the side of the pain. Alternatively, press points on either side of the mouth.

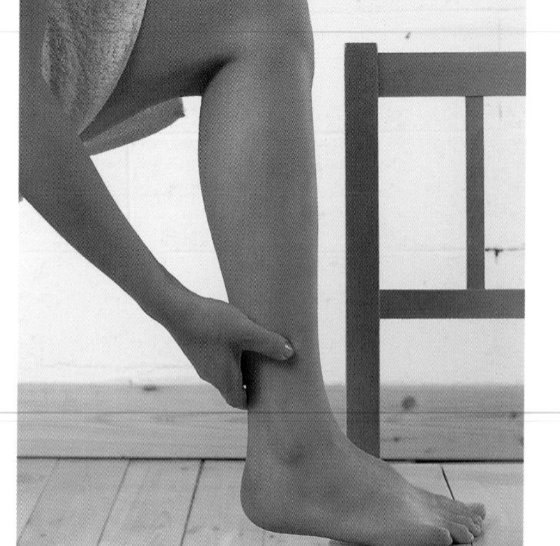

sciatica

Press a point on the outside of the leg a hand's width (including the thumb) from the center of the ankle bone, between the shin bone and the small leg bone. Maintain the pressure for up to 10 minutes and repeat as needed every 30 minutes.

Hydrotherapy

Alternating ice and hot packs helps to relieve pain and promote recovery. A "neutral bath"—that is, bathing in water at body temperature—is soothing. Gentle exercise such as swimming, combined with sauna or steam bathing, is also helpful.

CARPAL TUNNEL SYNDROME

This is inflammation of the carpal tunnel, a tube of sinew through which the nerves and tendons of the arm travel to the hand. The inflammation leads to swelling, which pinches the nerves and produces tingling, numbness, and pain in the hand. It affects particularly the first and index fingers and the thumb. It is most common in pregnant and elderly women. Surgery is the option normally offered by conventional medicine.

Acupressure

Pressing points on either side of the wrist firmly for two minutes three times daily can relieve pain. The point on the underside of the wrist is the "motion sickness" point (see "Nausea and Vomiting," page 25); the other is directly opposite it, on the top center of the wrist.

Hydrotherapy and nutritional therapy

Alternating hot and cold compresses can alleviate symptoms. A daily vitamin B-complex supplement can also help, especially B6 (1 g a day) with magnesium.

MULTIPLE SCLEROSIS

Multiple sclerosis (meaning "multiple hardening") is a disease of the central nervous system as a result of inflammation of and subsequent damage to the myelin sheath, the fatty coating surrounding nerve fibers. This leads to a wide variety of symptoms as a result of interference with nerve signals to the brain, including tingling or pins and needles in the limbs, blurred vision, numbness, difficulty walking, loss of coordination, fatigue, depression, and muscular aches and pains. MS is a degenerative and presently incurable condition of still unknown origin. For reasons still unclear it is much commoner in colder climates than hotter climates and affects women more than men. Depending on the severity of symptoms and how longstanding the problem is, the condition can be considerably helped by various natural therapies.

Movement therapy

Muscular aches and pains are often felt as a result of muscle spasticity due to the right nerve signals not getting through from the brain. A regular routine of muscle-stretching, coordination, and strengthening exercises (stretching being the most important) is therefore one of the single most positive actions anyone with MS can take. *It is important to realise that MS is not a muscle-wasting disease*: there is nothing wrong with the muscles in people with MS—it is lack of use that causes problems. The watchword is "use them or lose them."

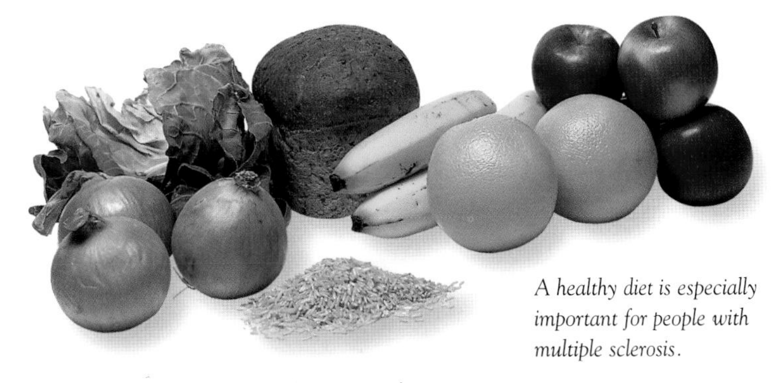

A healthy diet is especially important for people with multiple sclerosis.

Nutritional and dietary therapy

Evidence shows that MS symptoms can be made worse by eating too much animal fat, dairy products, sugar, and salt. At the same time there is evidence that people with MS lack certain important nutrients or their bodies do not use nutrients efficiently. Apart from regularly eating a wholefood diet (fresh fruit and vegetables, brown rice, and wholegrains), the following food supplements can be particularly helpful: polyunsaturated omega-3 and omega-6 EFAs, taken as capsules; vitamin A, preferably as beta-carotene; the B-vitamins, especially B1, B2 (riboflavin), B3 (niacin), B6 (pyridoxine), biotin, B12; vitamin C; vitamin E; zinc; magnesium; manganese; molybdenum; selenium; vanadium. It is advisable to take advice on dose levels from a qualified nutritionalist as individual needs vary.

How to take essential fatty acids

It is important to take omega-3 and omega-6 EFAs in combination and most experts these days agree that the right ratio is two omega-3s to one omega-6 (the so-called "Eskimo diet"). This combination is now available in a single capsule from most drugstores and health food stores.

Type of EFA	*Omega-3*	*Omega-6*
Chemical name	*Alphalinolenic acid*	*Linoleic acid*
Key ingredients	*Eicosapentaenoic acid (EPA)*	*Gammalinolenic acid (GLA)*
Best supplement sources	• *Marine or fish oils* • *Flaxseed (linseed) oil*	• *Blackcurrant seed oil* • *Evening primrose oil* • *Starflower (borage) oil*
Best food sources	• *Oily fish (tuna, mackerel, herring)* • *Dark green leafy vegetables* • *Pumpkin seeds*	• *Sunflower seeds* • *Safflower and sesame seeds* • *Oats, wheat, rice* • *Peas and beans*

NOTE *EFAs are vitamins, not fats, and are more important to healthy body function than any other essential nutrients. The required daily quantities are much higher than for other vitamins and minerals. In the words of one American expert, our intake should be measured "in tablespoons rather than milligrams." Individual needs vary but generally we need more in winter than summer. Care with packaging and storage is essential with EFAs. Unlike powdered nutrients, oils degenerate rapidly if not packaged or stored correctly.*

Sports injuries are one of the most common reasons for damage to the muscles and joints of the body.

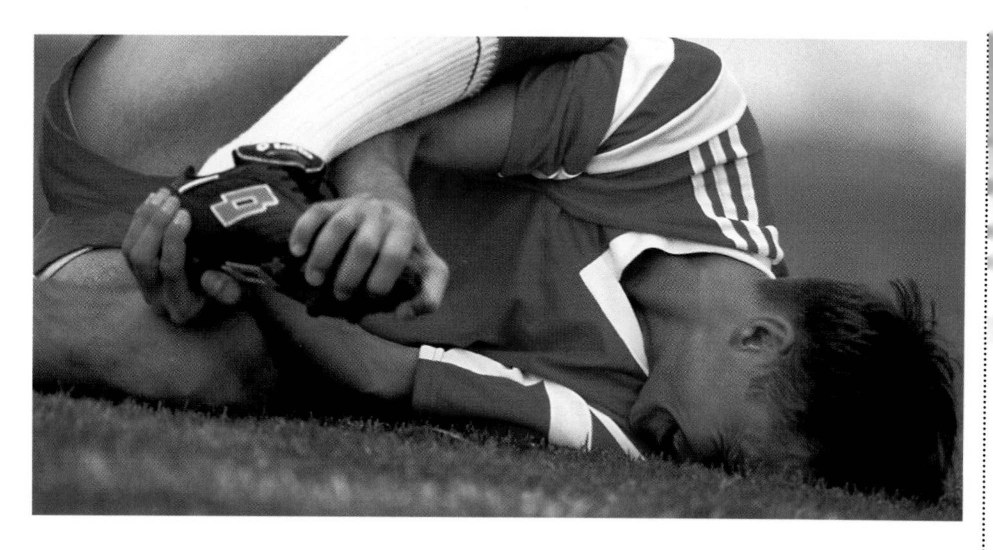

Massage and aromatherapy

Massaging aching and painful muscles and limbs with essential oils is as useful in MS as in any other condition. Many oils can be used—for example, chamomile for bladder and bowels; juniper, rosemary, and black pepper for muscle tone; clary sage and jasmine to relax tension; and basil, rosemary, nutmeg, thyme, geranium, and marjoram for fatigue—so help is best sought from a qualified clinical aromatherapist in the first place. Once they have advised on the right oil or combination of oils for individual symptoms it is then possible to apply self-help or ask a friend to help.

Reflexology

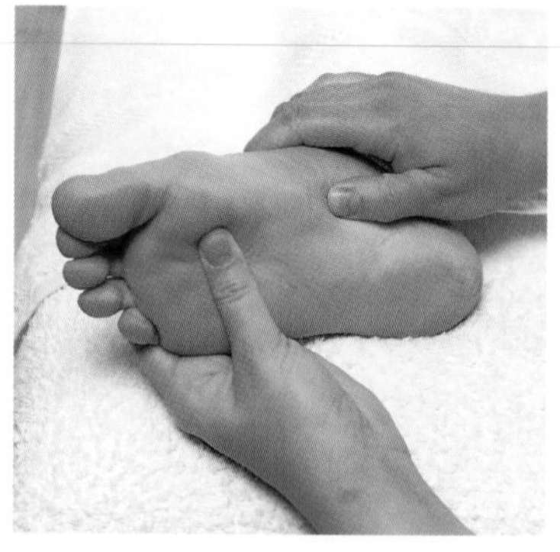

Manipulating the feet can help many of the symptoms of MS, including bladder and bowel problems, fatigue, depression, and sexual problems. The reflex point being pressed here relates to the bladder.

MUSCLE AND TENDON PAIN

Fibromyalgia, also known as fibrositis, is inflammation and pain in the soft tissues or "fibers" of the body, especially the tendons and muscles. Conditions include tendonitis (inflammation of the tendons), tenosynovitis (inflammation of the tendon covering), Repetitive Strain Injury (RSI), frozen shoulder, tennis elbow, and housewives' knee—though frozen shoulder, tennis elbow, and housewives' knee are usually the result of a condition called bursitis or inflammation of the bursa (the soft tissue covering joints that allow them movement.) Fibromyalgic conditions are always painful and incapacitating, but they are usually curable.

Hydrotherapy and exercise

Rest the affected limb if possible and apply regular ice packs (a package of frozen peas is the easiest option), three times on and off every five minutes. Once improvement starts, change to alternating hot and cold compresses and begin very gentle exercise to keep the joints mobile. Elasticated or neoprene sports supports are beneficial at this stage too.

Nutritional and dietary therapy

A wholefood diet (fresh fruit and vegetables, particularly celery) promotes recovery as does supplementing with a range of nutrients, especially essential fatty acids (EPA and GLA), vitamins A, C, E, and B-complex, minerals magnesium and calcium, and the enzymes bromelain and papain. Avoid tea, coffee, alcohol, sugar, and acid fruits, such as and berries.

Herbal medicine

Regular hot teas of valerian, bogbean, golden seal, willow, and primula are recommended to promote recovery, and chamomile with hops or passionflower at night to aid relaxation and sleep. Hot herbal poultices can also be highly effective, particularly using comfrey, marshmallow, slippery elm, and/or flaxseed (linseed).

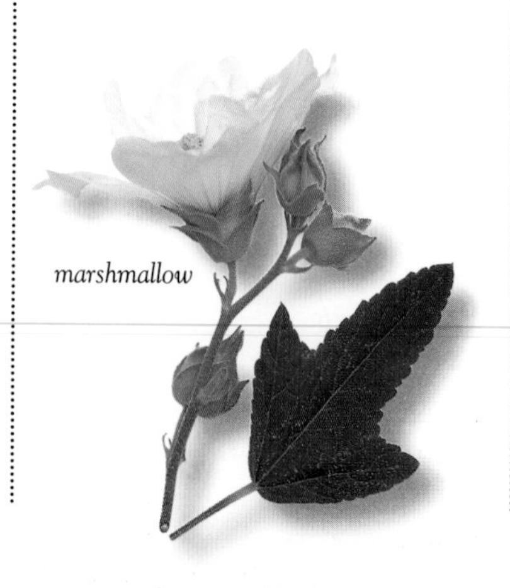

marshmallow

JOINT PAIN

Pain in the legs, feet, and ankles not due to accident, injury, or an inflammatory disease such as arthritis or gout is usually a combination of poor circulation and musculo-skeletal problems, often from poor posture and being overweight. For physical accident or injury see "First Aid for Pain," pages 22–25; for poor circulation see "Heart and Circulation Pain," pages 92–97; for musculo-skeletal pain see "Neck and Back Pain," pages 66–73.

GOUT

Gout is a failure by the body to process uric acid properly (uric acid is a natural by-product of waste elimination), causing crystals to build up around joints, which produces swelling, redness, and pain. It famously affects the big toe but also the knees, elbows, and hands. Attacks come and go, sometimes producing a high temperature. Constant attacks gradually damage the joints so recovery is harder, and less frequent over time, unless corrective action is taken.

Acupressure

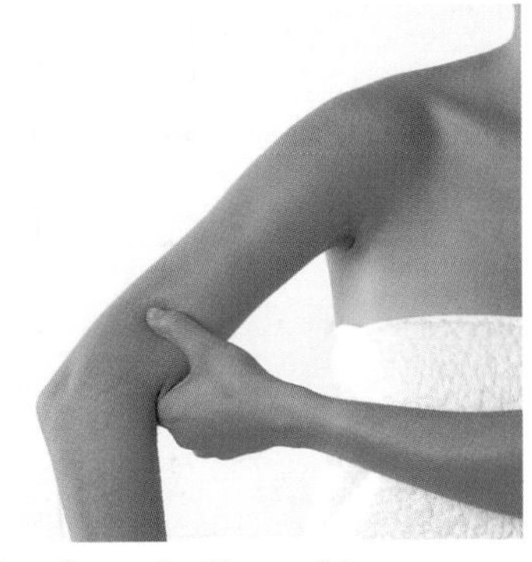

For a frozen shoulder, applying pressure upward to either end of the upper arm bone (humerus) can help but pressure must be strong and held for up to three minutes each time. Repeat daily.

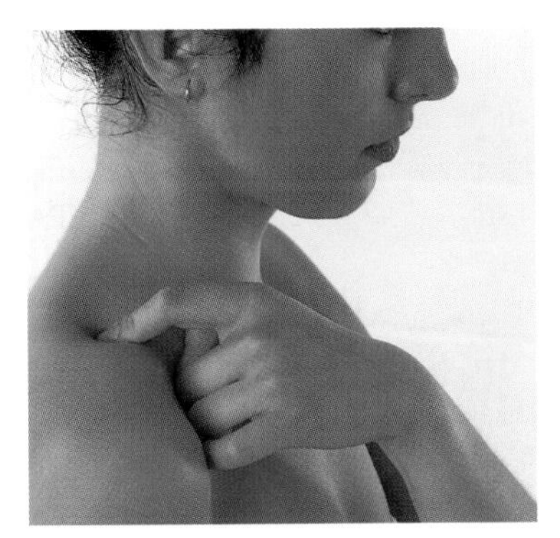

Pressing on a point halfway along the shoulder can also be effective.

Homeopathy

For acute inflammation arnica 6c or apis 6c every two hours; for recurrent attacks rhus tox 6c or bryonia 6c twice daily for two weeks. If inflammation persists, it is advisable to see a qualified therapist for an individual prescription.

Massage and aromatherapy

Massage the affected areas with essential oils of lavender, sandalwood, juniper, eucalyptus, thyme, and/or rosemary (5 drops diluted in a little carrier oil). Knead rather than smooth the affected areas. Alternatively, hot baths with 10 drops of rosemary and/or pine oil added are beneficial.

Hydrotherapy

A simple cold compress can alleviate the pain of a severe attack. A hot Epsom salts bath (a cupful to a bath and soak for 20 minutes) can help the elimination of uric acid.

Herbal medicine

Apply a comfrey and calendula poultice to the affected area as and when necessary. Daily infusions of burdock, nettle, wintergreen, wild carrot, sassafras, juniper, parsley, and/or willow (choose two or three) can clear the problem if taken regularly.

Nutritional and dietary therapy

Drink plenty of pure (not carbonated) water and cut out caffeine and alcohol. Try not to eat shellfish, sardines, beans, kidneys, liver, or "sweetbreads," which aggravate the problem. Eating plenty of garlic, cherries, and other berry fruits dissolves and neutralizes uric acid.

Homeopathy

Arnica and belladonna are remedies that can reduce the severity of an attack. Take a 6c dose every half an hour for up to ten doses (less if the pain subsides) and then 30c three times daily. If attacks recur, see a qualified therapist.

Massage and aromatherapy

Massage the affected area with the essential oils of cypress, peppermint, lavender, chamomile, geranium, eucalyptus, or rosemary (2 drops in a little carrier oil) or add 3–4 drops of your preferred combination to a bath.

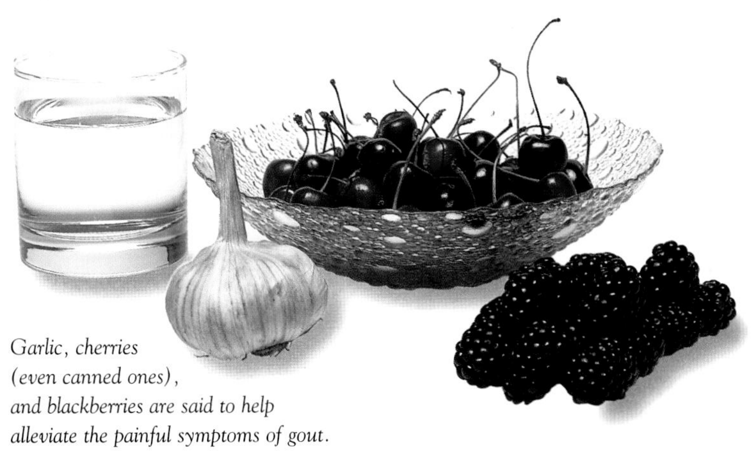

Garlic, cherries (even canned ones), and blackberries are said to help alleviate the painful symptoms of gout.

RHEUMATISM AND ARTHRITIS

Arthritis is a degenerative joint disease and one of the commonest and most severe forms of pain from all causes in the western world, affecting an estimated 10 percent of the population. The two main types are osteoarthritis and rheumatoid arthritis. (Rheumatism is a general term once used to cover all forms of arthritis but it is imprecise and no longer recognized medically.)

Osteoarthritis is "wear-and-tear" arthritis as a result of the gradual wearing down of the protective cartilage between the joints with age. The consequent damage to the bone joints leads to inflammation, reduced movement, and deformity of the joint. Osteoarthritis is the most common form of arthritis worldwide, experienced mainly in the hips, knees, and hands. It affects men and women equally.

Rheumatoid (or poly) arthritis is joint inflammation of varying severity that can affect the whole body, starting usually in the hands and feet and spreading to the rest of the body. It is an auto-immune disease, which means that the body turns against itself and attacks its own tissues. Diet, lifestyle, and inherited predisposition are widely regarded as the main causes, and women are three to four times more likely to suffer than men, especially between the ages of 20 and 40. Apart from swelling, stiffness, and pain in the affected joints, producing a characteristically red and shiny skin, sufferers usually experience fatigue, loss of appetite, and often, a slightly raised temperature.

Natural therapies have an excellent record in the treatment of both forms of arthritis, both for prevention and cure—so much so they are now the treatments of choice of many doctors over conventional drug therapy.

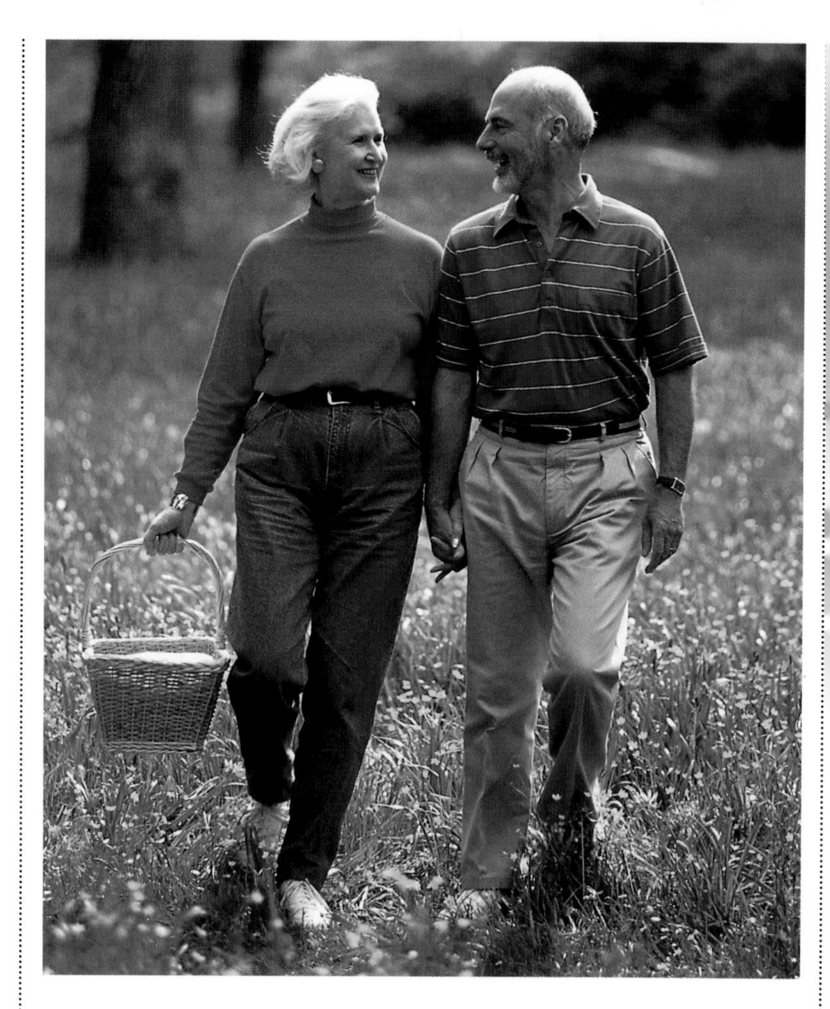

Keeping joints moving is essential in all forms of rheumatism and arthritis. One of the best ways is gentle walking.

Naturopathy

For pain relief both hot and cold compresses are effective as are a variety of baths: choose from seawater, seaweed (bladderwrack), or Epsom salts (3–4 tablespoons in a hot bath). Juice fasts—a combination of celery, carrot, beet, potato, white cabbage, and cucumber—can be safely carried out indefinitely, provided a varied intake is kept up. Contradictory as it may seem, gentle daily exercise is important for both forms of arthritis. It is now recognized that unless joints are kept moving they quickly seize up and the problem gets worse. Swimming is excellent (with a sauna or steam bath), as is gentle walking. Though controversial, wearing a copper bracelet or, the latest development, elastic supports impregnated with copper is claimed to help many with arthritis.

Nutritional and dietary therapy

Adjusting diet is probably the single most important step in the successful treatment of arthritis. Reduce consumption of all animal fats, tea, coffee, and alcohol, and drink 3–4 pints (1.5–2 liters) of pure water every day. Avoid acid-producing foods such as red meats and citrus fruits. Drinking cider vinegar mixed with honey three times a day is also said to help. Recommended daily food supplements include high dose fish oils (such as MaxEPA, but balance with omega-3 oils), vitamins A, C, E, B-complex, the minerals zinc, iron, magnesium, manganese, copper, molybdenum, and selenium, the enzyme superoxide dismutase (SOD), and the amino acid complex glutathione. Results are unlikely to show for between three and six months.

Herbal medicine

Celery seeds, yucca, bogbean, devil's claw, black cohosh, wild yam, willow bark, and feverfew are effective at reducing inflammation. Some may be taken as teas, others as tablets or diluted tinctures.

Homeopathy

Ruta cream rubbed directly into the affected area can help, as can rhus tox, ruta, arnica, and bryonia taken internally.

Massage and aromatherapy

Massage the affected area with capsicum (paprika) cream or the proprietary Asian herbal blend "Tiger Balm." Alternatively, use 2–3 drops of lavender and/or chamomile essential oils combined in a little carrier oil. Cypress, eucalyptus, and rosemary, either massaged in or added to a bath, can also help.

Movement therapy

Yoga and tai chi are excellent for arthritis of all types as they are both gentle and encourage the right mental approach to dealing with pain. Dance offers a less structured, more free-flowing alternative.

Electronic devices

TENS and GigaTENS can help relieve pain very effectively in both the high (70–100 Hz) and low frequency (under 10 Hz) range. Experimentation is needed. Hand-held electronic devices such as massagers/vibrators and intasound are also effective if treatment is applied firmly enough for long enough—at least 45 minutes. High frequency works best.

Acupressure

Apply pressure to the appropriate points for two minutes every morning and evening.

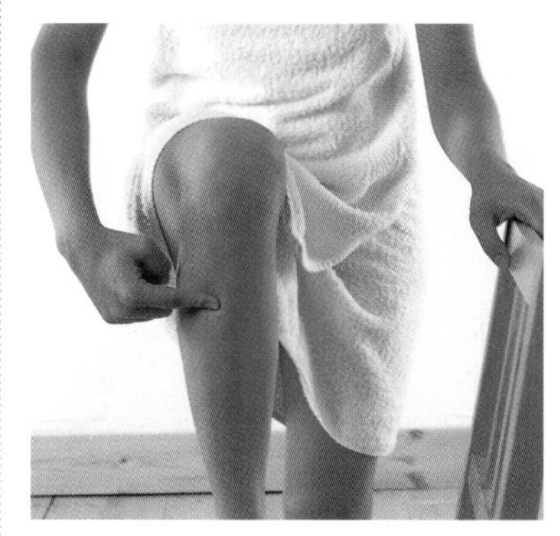

For knee pain, press a point on the front of the leg four fingers' width below the bottom of the kneecap and about a finger's width to the outside of the shin bone.

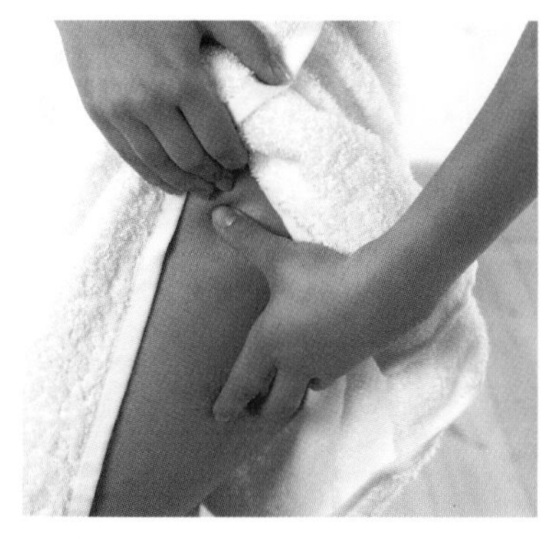

For hip pain, press in firmly at the sides of the hips in the hollow where the leg joins the pelvis.

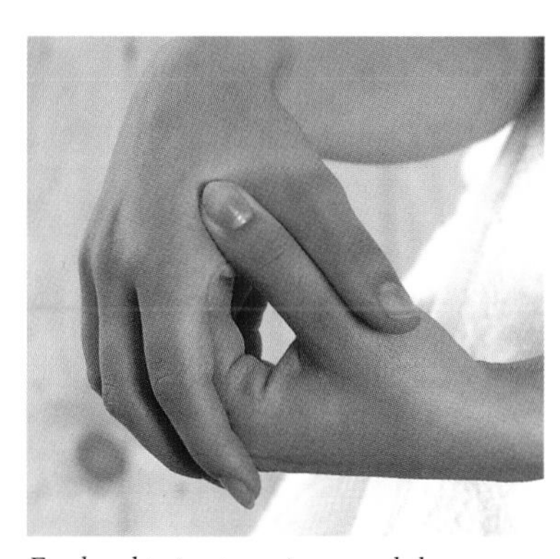

For hand pain, press in toward the forefinger at the end of the crease made between forefinger and thumb. Do NOT use this method during pregnancy.

Relaxation

Visualization, meditation, and biofeedback have a good record of helping to deal with arthritic pain.

ANKYLOSING SPONDYLITIS

Ankylosing spondylitis is a slowly developing degenerative disease in which the joints of the spine become inflamed, stiff, and eventually weld together, affecting other parts of the body, especially the hips, knees, chest, shoulders, and neck. It is most often the consequence of an injury or a disease such as tuberculosis or rheumatoid arthritis and affects mainly young men. As with arthritis, rest usually makes the condition worse and gentle exercise improves it. Treatment is very similar to that for arthritis but the following additional approaches can also help.

Hydrotherapy

Soak in a hot bath of Epsom salts for half an hour to help relieve pain and increase mobility.

Herbal medicine and homeopathy

Daily herbal teas of black willow, devil's claw, and bogbean can help, as can the homeopathic remedies arnica, rhus tox, and bryonia.

Massage and aromatherapy

Massage the back with lavender, rosemary, or basil essential oils—*but never massage the spine itself.*

Other therapies

From a qualified therapist only

Acupuncture and traditional Chinese herbal medicine
• pages 150–151
Osteopathy, cranial osteopathy, and chiropractic
• page 152–153
Counseling and psychotherapy
• page 154
Hypnotherapy • page 153

DIGESTIVE AND URINARY TRACT PAIN

The digestive and urinary tracts are concerned with nutrition and elimination. Food enters through the mouth, is swallowed, and digested; nutrients are extracted and passed into the bloodstream to feed the body (together with oxygen from lungs), and the leftover waste is eliminated through the intestines (solid) and urinary system (liquid). Because these are complex processes, and waste products are often poisonous, the digestive and urinary systems are a common source of aches and pains, which are sometimes removed from the source of the problem.

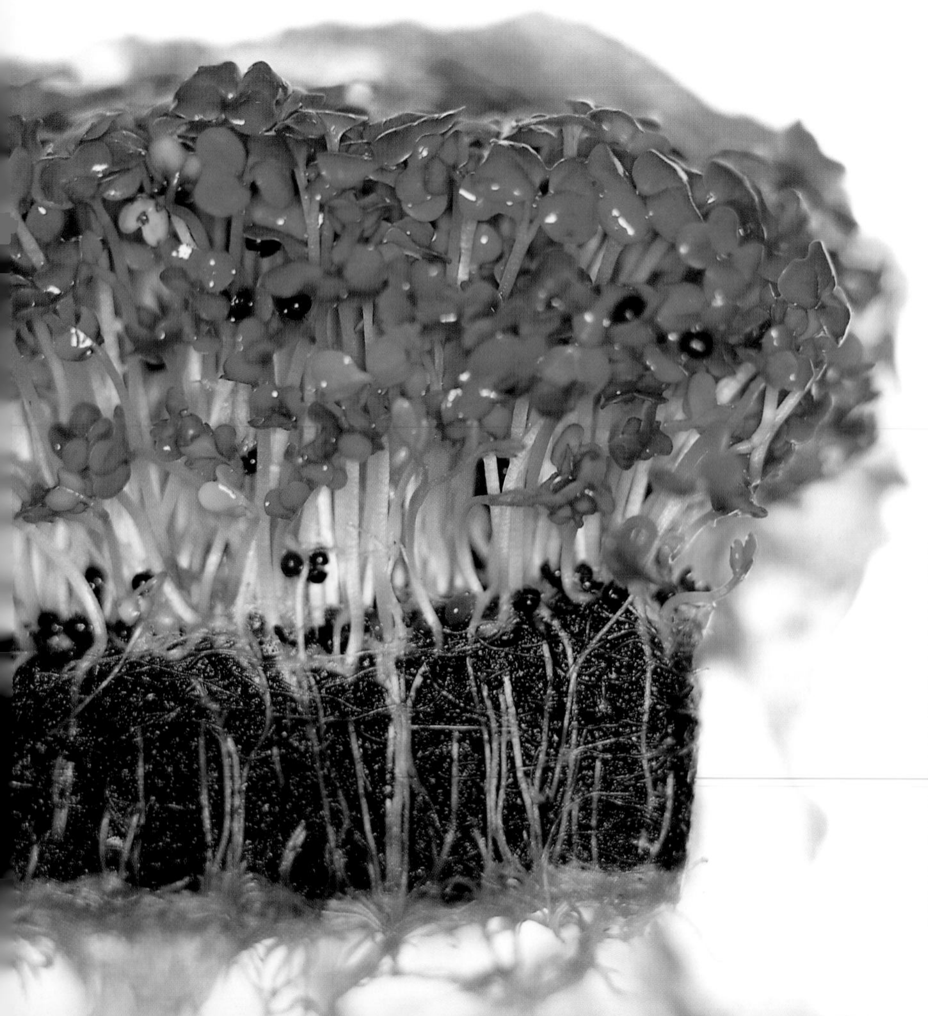

Some natural therapists consider the digestive and elimination systems to be the main source of referred pain, which would put them behind many of the aches and pains felt in areas such as the head, back, chest, and legs. Even without referred pain, however, the two systems are still a major source of discomfort. Problems directly related to them range from stomachaches and ulcers to potentially life-threatening kidney infection and cirrhosis of the liver.

Warning

Seek immediate medical help if your symptoms are:

- *severe or prolonged pain in the stomach, liver, kidneys, intestines, or genitals*
- *if there is blood in the urine or stools.*

STOMACH PAIN

Stomach pain can be extremely debilitating but natural remedies are particularly effective in bringing quick relief.

STOMACHACHE

One of the body's commonest pains, stomachache is most often the result of unlucky or unwise eating—in other words, from eating the wrong food or too much food. Anxiety and stress are also causes. Cases of severe stomach pain that is prolonged or recurring for no obvious reason should be reported to a doctor as soon as possible.

Naturopathy and dietary therapy

Resting with a hot-water bottle on the stomach can bring immediate relief, but for pain from overeating and drinking, or eating the wrong food, a mini-fast—not eating for 12 hours—is most effective. Make sure you drink plenty of pure, non-sparkling water throughout. Do not drink coffee, tea, or alcohol.

For prevention of stomachache, eat little and often rather than a lot of food all at once, and eat healthily (wholefoods, and fresh fruit and vegetables), reducing the intake of fatty foods as much as possible. Do not exercise too soon after eating (wait at least 30 minutes, and preferably an hour), and wear loose, comfortable clothes.

Acupressure

Pressing a point on the cheek, on either side of and below the nose, in line with the eyes, can relieve stomachache caused by stress. For a general "tonic," lie flat on a firm surface and press down vertically in two parallel lines from the breastbone to about halfway toward the navel.

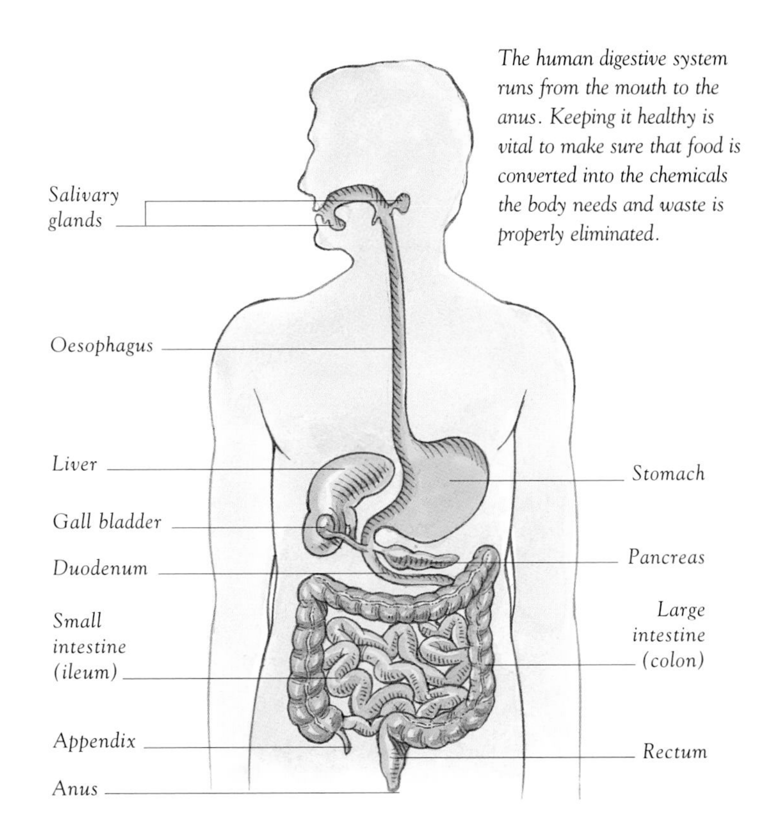

The human digestive system runs from the mouth to the anus. Keeping it healthy is vital to make sure that food is converted into the chemicals the body needs and waste is properly eliminated.

Herbal medicine

Infusions of chamomile, peppermint, lemon balm, marshmallow, or comfrey are soothing and relaxing. Slippery elm is also effective, taken either as a tablet or powder dissolved in hot water.

Yoga and tai chi

A variety of routines can help pain caused by both physical and psychological causes.

Homeopathy

Take the remedies arsenicum album 6c and bryonia 6c, or nux vomica (6c or 30c): one tablet every hour for three hours.

Relaxation

Progressive muscular relaxation (see "Depression," page 28), followed by visualization and meditation, can help stomachache brought on by tension and anxiety.

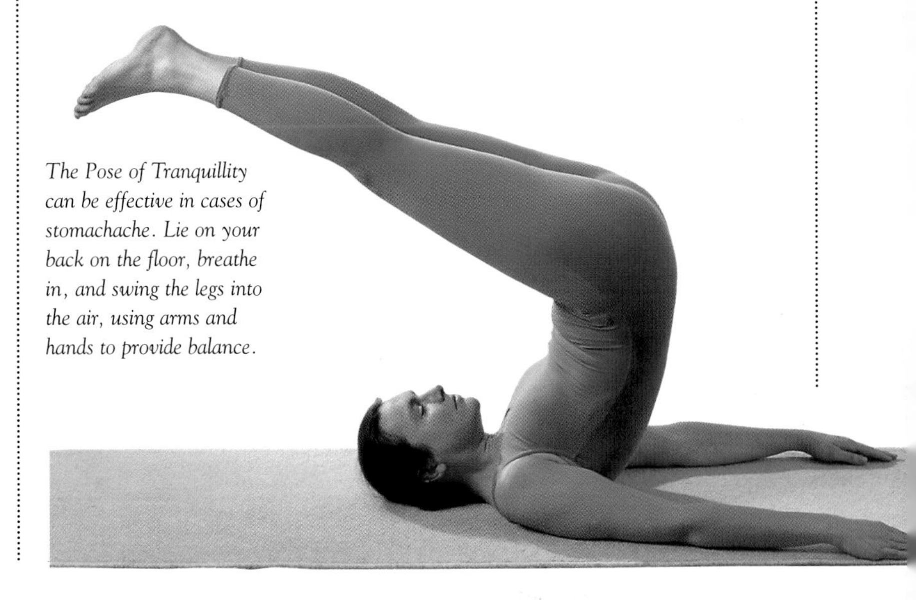

The Pose of Tranquillity can be effective in cases of stomachache. Lie on your back on the floor, breathe in, and swing the legs into the air, using arms and hands to provide balance.

NAUSEA

Nausea is usually a result of eating and drinking too much or unwisely, but it can also be a symptom of food-poisoning, motion sickness, pregnancy, and migraine. It is often accompanied by the urge to vomit.

Naturopathy

Vomiting can clear the problem, and if it does not happen naturally it can be triggered by putting a finger down the throat. After vomiting, eat "neutral" foods, such as rice and boiled vegetables, for 24 hours to let the system recover.

Herbal medicine

Teas of ginger and peppermint (together), chamomile, and black horehound are effective.

Acupressure

Firmly press a point halfway between the breast bone and the navel. An alternative is the point on the wrist for motion sickness (see page 25).

Homeopathy

Arsenicum album 6c (for vomiting after eating), ipecacuanha 6c (for recurring vomiting after meals), and pulsatilla 6c (for vomiting after rich foods) are recommended.

INDIGESTION

A burning pain in the center of the chest is usually a symptom of indigestion or dyspepsia (heartburn). It is a result of acid in the stomach "backing up" into the gullet, usually from eating and drinking too much too quickly. Its symptoms are similar to those of an ulcer, hiatus hernia, or heart attack, so they must taken seriously even though indigestion is the more likely cause.

Naturopathy, and nutritional and dietary therapy

Sipping cider vinegar or lemon juice in hot water and applying a hot-water bottle to the area can bring quick relief. If the indigestion is severe, follow this with a 12-hour fast, drinking only herb teas or crushed apple or carrot juice. Taking a tablespoonful of whey concentrate (milk "serum") with meals is said to be the best regulator of stomach acids in the long term, but natural therapists stress prevention as the main aim. This means always eating in a relaxed manner, eating little and often, spacing meals out, and eating a balanced, nutritious diet. Regular acidophilus and pectin supplements can also help prevent indigestion.

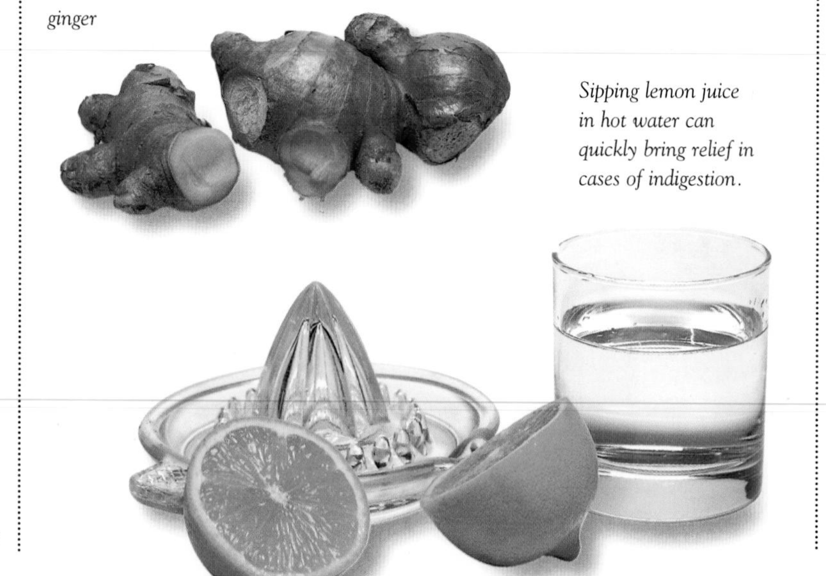

ginger

Sipping lemon juice in hot water can quickly bring relief in cases of indigestion.

Reflexology

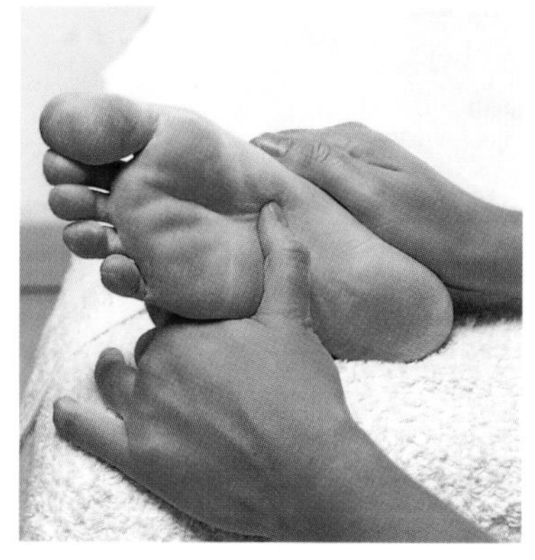

Work across the middle part of the sole of each foot, pressing firmly on any points of tenderness until they disperse. This is the area corresponding to the digestive and elimination organs, including the stomach, pancreas, duodenum, liver, gall bladder, adrenal gland, kidneys, and colon (gut).

Herbal medicine

Meadowsweet, coriander, and slippery elm tablets (or powders) taken with warm water, aid indigestion pain, and so do teas of ginger, peppermint, chamomile, parsley, fennel, lemon balm, raspberry leaf, and/or cinnamon. Ginger and parsley eaten raw can also help.

HIATUS HERNIA

In a hiatus (or diaphragmatic) hernia, part of the stomach slips up through the opening in the diaphragm, where the gullet comes in, entering the area occupied by the lungs. The most frequent cause is being overweight. Often there are no symptoms, but when they are felt, the sharp pain experienced behind the breastbone can feel much like an ulcer, often with the complication of further heartburn pain. Except in extreme cases, surgery is rarely carried out to correct the problem these days.

Naturopathy

The problem can be self-correcting, especially if surplus weight is shed and a healthy and moderate diet is eaten. Sleeping with the head higher than the feet, or even sleeping in an armchair, can bring relief. Other effective treatments are the same as for ulcers.

Movement therapy
Many of the breathing techniques and postures in yoga can help, as can the postural re-education taught in the Alexander technique.

ULCERS/GASTRITIS

Ulcers in the stomach and duodenum are known as peptic ulcers, but are named more specifically for the organ where they appear: so ulcers in the stomach are gastric ulcers, and in the duodenum, they are duodenal ulcers. They are the most likely cause of severe, recurring pain in the stomach, but are usually preceded by inflammation (gastritis), so there is some warning in most cases. Peptic ulcers are far commoner in men than women, and are classically caused by stress and anxiety combined with poor eating and drinking habits. This can penetrate any weakness in the protective mucus lining the two organs and form a painful cavity in the walls. The pain and tenderness is greater in the case of gastric ulcers than duodenal. Gastric pain can cover an area on the stomach about the size of a hand, and normally comes after eating. Duodenal pain is not so closely linked to eating, and is only "finger-point" size.

CAUTION See your family doctor as soon as possible if peptic ulcer is suspected. Untreated stomach ulcers can lead to cancer, particularly in older people.

Naturopathy and dietary therapy
Successful treatment involves fairly severe dietary and lifestyle changes—including fasting—but it is possible, if hard, to cure the problem with these alone. Drinks such as tea, coffee, and alcohol, and all spicy food should be eliminated entirely, as should smoking. Never take aspirin or aspirin-equivalents, which irritate the stomach lining. Eat brown rice, millet, buckwheat, rye, and wholewheat, along with whey concentrate and fresh-pressed juice drinks. Among a range of recommended juices, raw potato, carrot, celery, cabbage, and banana are beneficial. Exercise helps, and stress management is essential.

Herbal medicine
A teaspoon of oil of hypericum, taken every morning and night, is effective against gastritis, while aloe vera juice extract helps ulcers. Take a tablespoonful in a glass of warm water three times a day. Licorice and bilberry juice drunk daily is also said to be effective, and so are teas of marshmallow, coriander, and lemon balm.

Relaxation and movement therapy
The leading role of stress in ulcer formation means that stress management is important. Practice progressive muscular relaxation (see "Depression," page 28), followed by visualization, biofeedback, and meditation. Biofeedback has been shown to be particularly effective at helping the pain of duodenal ulcers. Regular practice of appropriate yoga and tai chi exercises is also a powerful antidote to stress.

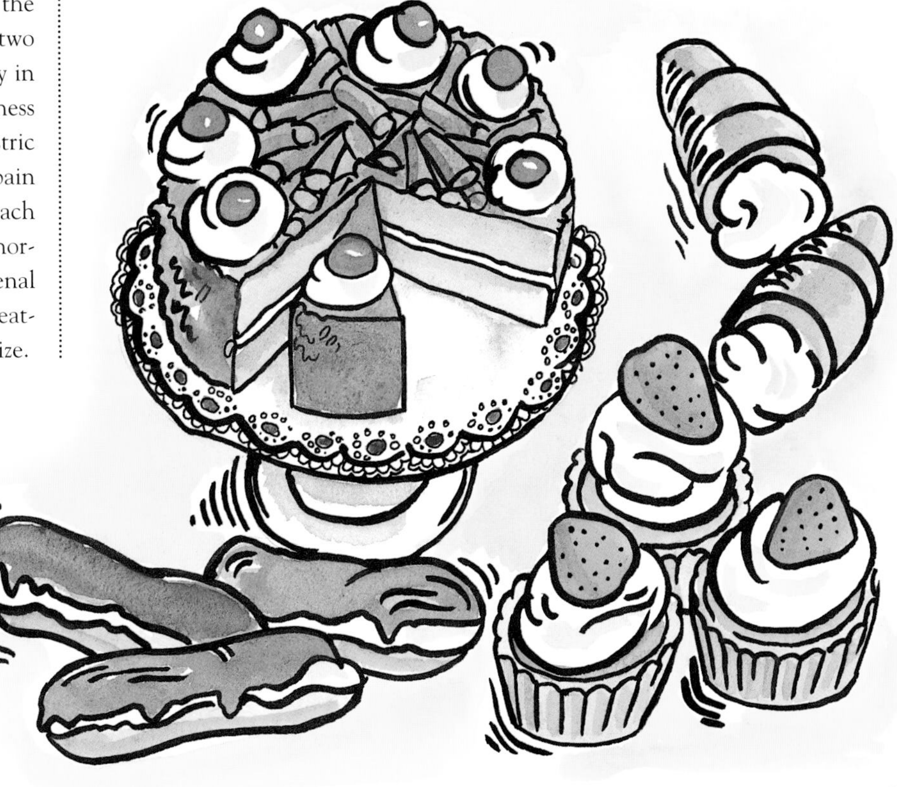

Sugary, sweet foods may taste nice but they are nutritionally worthless and can harm the digestive system as well as lead to problems of overweight.

GALLSTONES

Gallstones are mineral deposits in the gall bladder as a result of a high-fat, low-fiber diet. They are most commonly suffered by diabetics, obese people, and pregnant women, but there also appears to be an inherited tendency. They can become serious, and intervention may be necessary if the stones block the flow of bile for use by the digestive system in breaking down food. Apart from pain, felt usually in the right shoulder or hip, symptoms are jaundice (a yellowing of the whites of the eyes, skin, and urine), heartburn, and fever.

NOTE See a doctor if symptoms are severe. If surgery is advised, ask for ultrasound treatment, which disintegrates the stones and allows them to flush away naturally.

Naturopathy, and nutritional and dietary therapy

Relieve pain by applying a hot pack on the abdomen and lower back for 10–15 minutes. Sipping peppermint oil diluted in water during eating can also help relieve pain. A "liver flush" is the favored treatment to remove gallstones: for six days, eat and drink nothing but wholefoods and apples with plenty of raw apple juice. On the morning of the seventh day, drink a cup of an olive oil and lemon juice mix (half a cup of each). This is claimed to flush the stones out by stimulating bile from the liver. Foods that are good for the liver, and therefore the gallbladder, include globe artichoke, chicory, radish, and dandelion leaves. Drink still water, cut out animal fats and dairy products, and supplement with vitamin C.

Aromatherapy

Vaporizing Scots pine essential oil in a burner can help in pain relief.

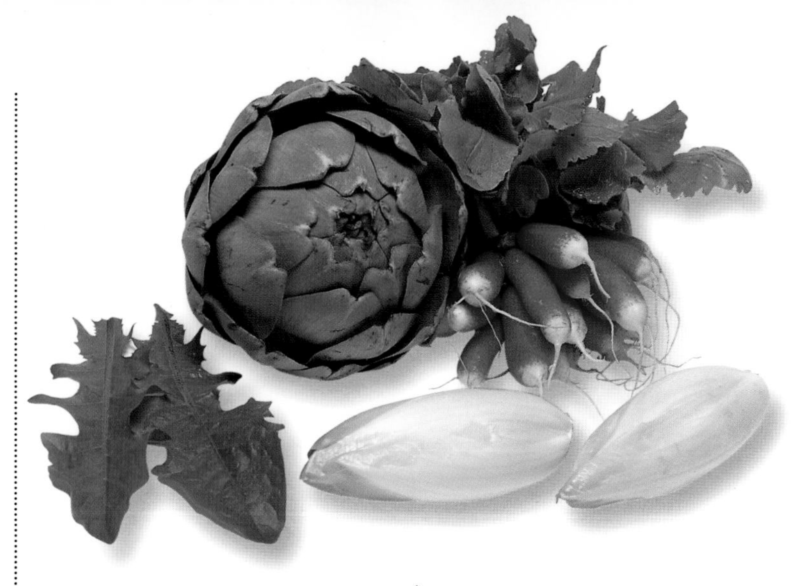

Globe artichoke, chicory, radishes, and dandelion leaves are liver "tonics" said to help with gallstones.

Herbal medicine

The right mix of herbs can clear stones, but time and patience is needed. For example, 2–3 cups of centaury tea every day for 4 weeks can be effective. An alternative is a mix of two parts marshmallow to one part each of balmony, boldo, fringetree bark, and golden seal, drunk as a tea three times a day. Other helpful herbs are stone root, gentian, rosemary, and dandelion.

CAUTION Do not take herbs for gallstones during pregnancy.

Reflexology

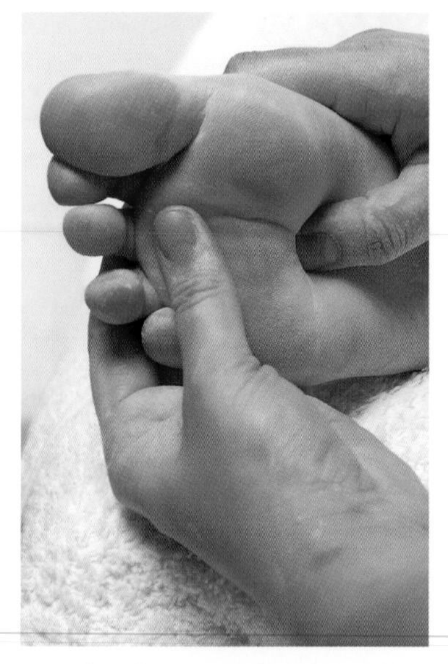

Press the reflex point in the center of the arch on the sole of the right foot (corresponding to the gall bladder) for 10–15 seconds each day.

INTESTINAL AND BOWEL PAIN

The intestinal system is extremely important, and variations in the operation of this system can produce many painful symptoms.

CONSTIPATION

Constipation is having bowels in which waste matter has become stuck in the colon and will not pass through. It is most often caused by a poor diet, lack of exercise, anxiety, and stress. Regular bowel movements are important to bodily health. Fecal waste is of no value to the body, and has the potential to do great harm by allowing the buildup of poisons. These can seep into the bloodstream, from where they spread throughout the body and cause symptoms such as headache, fatigue, joint and muscle pain, and even allergic reactions.

Naturopathy

A heating pad or hot-water bottle placed on the abdomen can help alleviate pain, and flaxseed (linseed) oil taken with psyllium husks can help clean out a sluggish colon. Regular exercise is essential.

Nutritional and dietary therapy

Prunes are an excellent natural laxative, but only in the short term. Never take laxatives long-term. The best method is to increase fiber intake (bran, grains, fresh fruit and raw vegetables, brown rice) and avoid refined foods, especially sugar and white flour. Drink plenty: at least 6–8 glasses daily of clean, preferably filtered, water. Apple juice with fiber is also good, and make sure your diet contains potassium (in most good multivitamin tablets). Juices of carrot or celery with garlic and onion can help.

Herbal medicine

Senna pods and cascara bark made into teas are powerful laxatives, but can cause stomach pain in the process. Chamomile, hops, and fennel help counteract this, but a gentler alternative is flaxseed (linseed) oil (a tablespoonful morning and evening), or dandelion. Eat the leaves or root with salad, or make a tea, and drink three times daily. Cape aloes and slippery elm (tablets or powder) are also effective.

Massage and aromatherapy

Massage the essential oils of marjoram, rosemary (10 drops each), and black pepper (5 drops) into the abdomen and lower back.

Colonic irrigation

Some naturopaths advocate a special treatment for washing out the large intestine, known as colonic irrigation. This involves inserting a small hose-like device with two tubes into the rectum. One of the tubes pumps water in and the other draws it out again, hopefully with any impacted feces that may be blocking the system. It is a far more drastic procedure than a simple enema, which most people can perform on themselves fairly easily—and it is not without risk. It needs special equipment, practitioners must be skilled as well as knowledgeable, and a high degree of hygiene is vital.

DIARRHEA

Diarrhea is waste matter that is too liquid—usually as a result of infection, food-poisoning, or anxiety and stress. It is normally self-correcting after about a day, but it can lead to fecal incontinence—a temporary loss of bowel control.

CAUTION See a doctor if diarrhea lasts longer than 48 hours (24 hours in children), and especially if there is blood or mucus in the stools and it is accompanied by vomiting.

Herbal medicine

Peppermint tea helps, as can an infusion of agrimony, plantain, and geranium, or golden seal.

Homeopathy

Arsenicum album 6c, pulsatilla 6c, and causticum 6c are among many remedies that may be beneficial.

Nutritional and dietary therapy

Excess fiber can cause diarrhea—an example of the importance of moderation in all things being the watchword. Drink lots of pure water, or water from boiled rice, avoid solid food, but eat plenty of live yogurt and/or take acidophilus capsules three times a day.

Massage and aromatherapy

A bath containing 4–5 drops each of juniper, peppermint, and geranium oils can help, or try gently massaging a blend of peppermint, tea tree, sandalwood, and geranium into the abdomen and lower back (5 drops each in a little carrier oil).

Acupressure

Press in the abdomen very firmly at a point three fingers' width on either side of the navel.

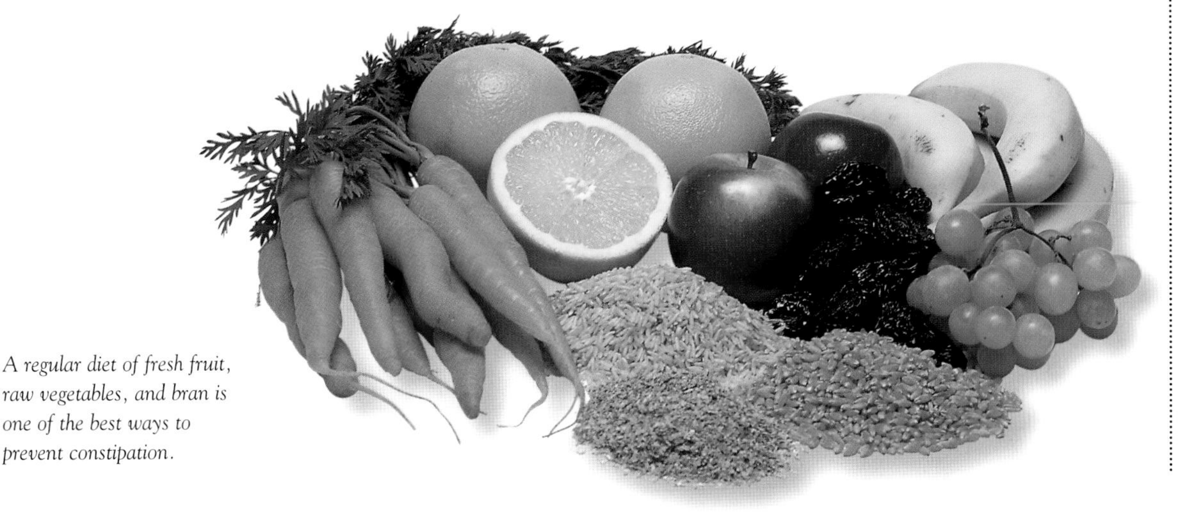

A regular diet of fresh fruit, raw vegetables, and bran is one of the best ways to prevent constipation.

GASTROENTERITIS

Severe inflammation of the stomach and intestines—usually as the result of a bacterial infection from contaminated food or water—gastroenteritis causes strong intestinal pain, diarrhea, fever, headache, and fatigue. "Delhi belly" and "Gippy tummy" are just two of its many colorful nicknames, but the condition is serious if symptoms are powerful and/or persistent, especially in the young or elderly.

CAUTION An adult should see a doctor if the symptoms last more than 48 hours, but consult a doctor immediately if symptoms appear in anyone under 12, or the elderly. Severe cases may need antibiotics.

Naturopathy

An immediate fast is recommended, but it is important to keep taking liquids, especially water with added sea-salt and sugar or honey, if diarrhea is severe and prolonged. See also "Diarrhea," page 87.

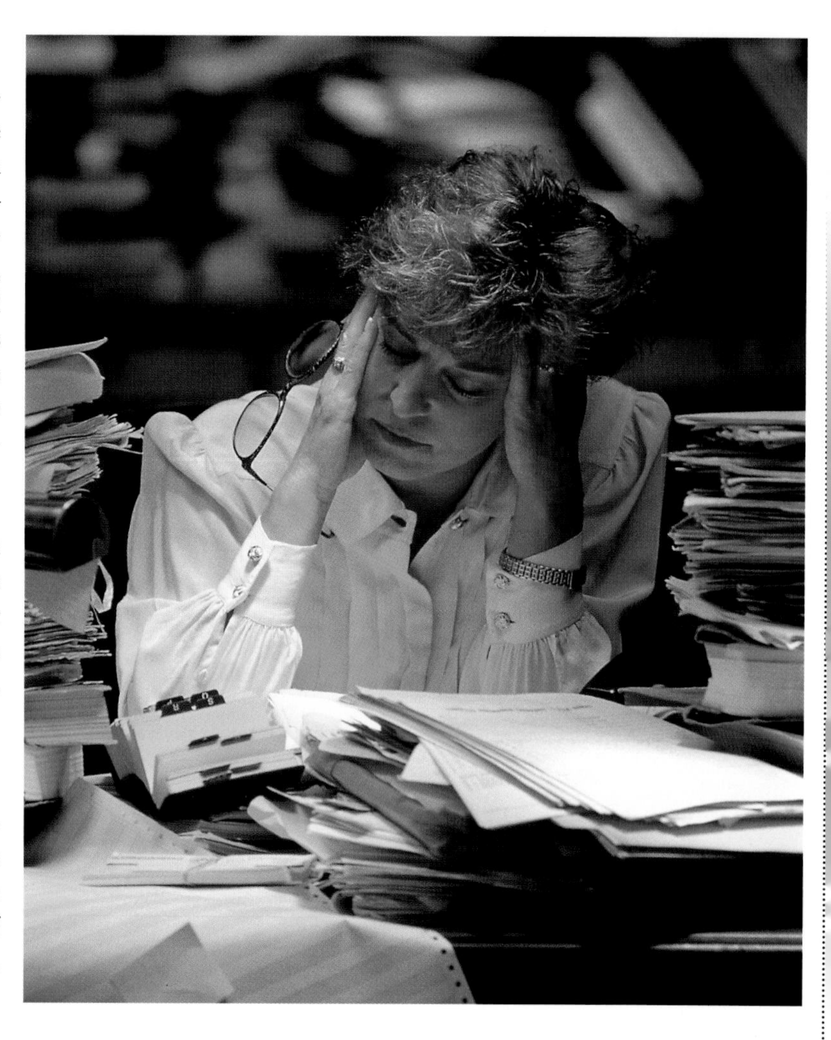

Fatigue is just one of a range of ailments not easy to pinpoint that can be caused by problems with the digestive system.

IRRITABLE BOWEL SYNDROME

Irritable bowel syndrome (IBS) used to be called "spastic colon," and although the term is no longer used, it explains the condition better: the colon muscles go into spasm, causing abdominal pain and cramps, bloating, back pain, flatulence, lethargy, headache, fatigue, and diarrhea alternating with constipation. The problem is common in the western world in both sexes, and increasing. No one is yet sure why, but diet and stress are widely believed to be to blame. The condition can come and go, but once it starts it tends to become long-lasting. The treatments that are useful in constipation and diarrhea (see pages 86–87), such as herbal medicine, aromatherapy, and acupressure, can also help IBS.

Nutritional and dietary therapy

A healthy, wholefood diet is seen as essential for IBS, with regular exercise and stress management. Checking for food intolerances with an experienced therapist is also recommended.

DIVERTICULITIS

Inflammation of the large intestine as a result of "clots" of infected waste lodging in parts of the gut wall, diverticulitis is one result of chronic constipation and irregular bowel movement. The naturopathic and dietary approaches useful for constipation (see pages 86–87) are also appropriate here.

INFLAMMATORY BOWEL DISEASE

A blanket description for a range of uncomfortable and sometimes painful disorders that occur in both the small and large intestine, inflammatory bowel disease (IBD) covers excessive flatulence, ulcerative colitis, and Crohn's disease (enteritis). Colitis occurs in the large intestine, or colon, and Crohn's disease in the small intestine. Crohn's, the result of recurrent inflammation, is the more serious, since it can damage the small intestine's vital role of absorbing nutrients from food, and can cause fever, diarrhea, and weight loss. The cause of colitis is uncertain, but not eating enough fiber may be partly to blame. It can also cause diarrhea, and sometimes mucus and blood in the stools.

Naturopathy and dietary therapy

The same eating advice applies here as in all digestive disorders, but avoid particularly dairy products and refined and processed foods. Check for food intolerances through an experienced therapist. A 24-hour liquid fast followed by a diet of boiled vegetables, rice, and stewed apples is beneficial, and garlic and charcoal tablets can help.

Herbal medicine

Slippery elm taken twice a day, and regular teas of lemon balm and chamomile are said to help.

HEMORRHOIDS (PILES)
See page 97 for suggested natural remedies for hemorrhoids.

> **Appendicitis**
>
> *Appendicitis is inflammation of the appendix. Symptoms are pain in the groin on the right-hand side. It can be life-threatening if untreated, as it can lead to peritonitis—inflammation of the peritoneum, the membranes lining the walls of the abdomen. In severe cases, it may have to be removed by surgery. Always see a doctor immediately if appendicitis is suspected.*

> **How the mind and gut are linked**
>
> *The mind–body link in inflammatory bowel disease is controversial, but evidence is growing, based on the fact that nearly every substance that helps run the brain can also be found in the gut. In the words of one researcher, IBD is a "neurobiopsycho-social phenomenon"—in other words, "a reflection of how aspects of life and living are not working." Conflicts of authority and personal autonomy are cited as classic neurobiopsycho-social causes of IBD. Claims have been made that resolving such conflicts with a skilled counselor or psychotherapist, coupled with natural bodily therapies, have removed the symptoms entirely.*

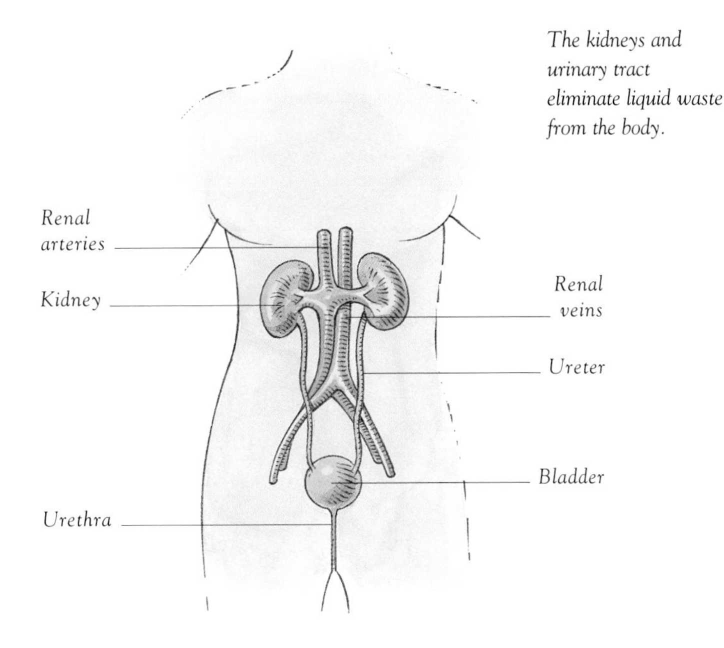

The kidneys and urinary tract eliminate liquid waste from the body.

KIDNEY AND URINARY TRACT PAIN

The urinary system, consisting of the kidneys, ureter, bladder, and urethra, is extremely important for good health. Its job in the cleansing of waste products from the blood and their elimination from the body as urine involves many complex biological processes and chemical balancing acts. All parts of the urinary system can develop infections, causing inflammation and pain, but though serious they can usually be safely and effectively treated by natural means.

CYSTITIS

Cystitis is inflammation of the bladder caused by bacterial infection. These days cystitis is a relatively common condition—especially among adult women (though both men and children can be affected also)—and tends to recur. Symptoms, which can be mild or severe, include pain or a burning sensation on passing urine and, occasionally, blood in the urine. In severe cases, there can be fever and backache also.

Causes are many and varied, but include poor hygiene and diet, certain drugs, having an infection such as a cold or flu, poor posture, anxiety and stress, an allergic reaction to chemicals in toiletries, clothing, and other textiles such as bath towels, and having uncomfortable sex.

Cystitis will usually clear of its own accord in time, with care given to personal hygiene, and abstaining from penetrative sex. But it is such an unpleasant, embarrassing, and uncomfortable condition while it lasts that few are prepared to wait, so it is fortunate that a number of home remedies are highly effective.

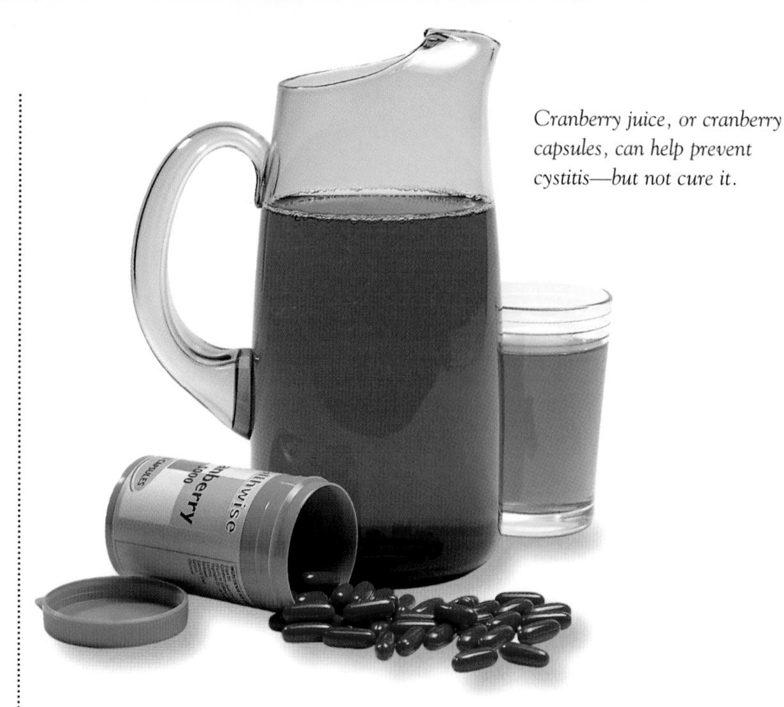

Cranberry juice, or cranberry capsules, can help prevent cystitis—but not cure it.

Acupressure and massage

Massaging and applying pressure to the lower abdomen at a point immediately over the bladder can soothe symptoms.

Aromatherapy

Three or four drops of essential oils of sandalwood, juniper, lavender, or bergamot, mixed with a neutral carrier oil (such as grapeseed), and used in the above massage, or added to the bath, can help ease pain and discomfort.

Reflexology

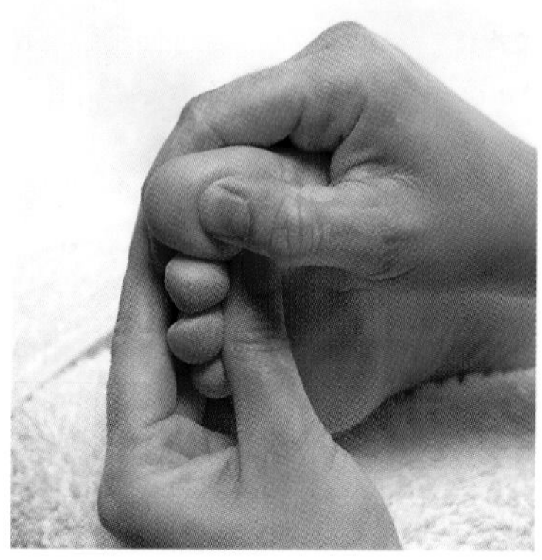

Manipulate the center of the sole of each foot, in a diagonal line to each heel (corresponding to the kidneys and bladder), and also the center of the pad of each toe (the pituitary gland, shown above).

Hydrotherapy

Alternating hot and cold sitz baths—the hot bath at a temperature around 98°F (37°C)—for about half an hour can help, although they are not recommended for those with high blood pressure or a weak heart. Wearing cotton underwear, rather than nylon or other synthetic materials, is also recommended.

Nutritional and dietary therapy

Drinking half a teaspoonful of sodium bicarbonate dissolved in warm water can bring pain relief in 20 minutes. Plain live yogurt applied generously to the genitals also helps. To prevent an attack, eat as nutritious a diet as possible, especially one high in fresh vegetables and fruit—but not acidic fruit, such as oranges and lemons, which can exacerbate the problem. Cranberry juice is said to be an excellent preventive, but do not take cranberry during an attack—it will make it worse. Chamomile and cornsilk tea are reputed to be a helpful safeguard. Drink plenty of pure, clean water (6–8 glasses a day), and cut out coffee and alcohol during an attack.

Herbal medicine

Chamomile tea is effective at the first sign of an attack, and pain can be relieved with teas of cumin, coriander, and fennel (a cup three times a day). Regular infusions of calendula, yarrow, and hypericum are also said to help, as are couch grass and buchu. Echinacea, in a liquid or capsules, is good for any infection.

Homeopathy

Take cantharis 6c and staphysagria 6c hourly while symptoms last.

How the urinary system works

The job of the urinary system is to rid the body of waste liquid known as urine that comes from the kidneys. Kidneys are filters, and their function is to filter out waste from the blood supply and pass it to the bladder down a tube known as the ureter. The bladder is a muscular expanding "bag," which can hold about 1.3 pints (750 ml) of liquid in an adult. From the bladder, urine is expeled via the urethra, which forms part of the genitals in both men and women.

The bladder is controlled by two rings of muscles known as sphincters. The first ring is controlled by the autonomic nervous system—which means that control is involuntary and unconscious, or automatic. But the second set is under our conscious and voluntary control, and this is the set we relax when we urinate. As the urine starts to flow, the muscles that control the bladder (known as detrusor muscles) contract, and this is what forces the urine out in a usually pleasurable rush.

URETHRITIS

Urethritis (also known as urinary tract infection, or UTI) is inflammation of the urethra. It is more common in women than men, but in women it is usually the result of bruising from sex than of infection. In men, it is more likely to be caused by infection from a sexual disease. Symptoms are similar to cystitis, but when the cause is an infection, blood or pus may appear at the opening of the urethra. The infection will usually clear naturally in two or three days, but the treatments effective for cystitis will also work here.

CAUTION Untreated UTI can be dangerous. Medical attention is advisable as soon as possible.

Nutritional and dietary therapy

Drink 3½ pints (2 liters) of water a day. Barley water (5 cups a day) is also effective. Do not drink coffee, tea, alcohol, or acidic fruit juice. Daily supplementation with vitamin C (1 g) helps.

Herbal medicine

Teas of chamomile, yarrow, couch grass, buchu, and cornsilk can be beneficial, and so can two drops of tea tree oil in a glass of warm water.

KIDNEY STONES

Kidney stones are hard deposits of chemical salts that lodge in the kidneys (and sometimes the ureter) as a result of not drinking enough, and of too much calcium and animal protein in the diet. They are more common in some countries than others, which suggests that high mineral deposits in water supplies may be one culprit. The usual symptom is constant, if mild, pain in the lower back on one side. Severe pain (colic) usually means a stone has passed from the kidney but become stuck in the ureter. Natural treatment involves reducing the mineral content of what you eat and drink, and taking remedies that help dissolve the stones.

CAUTION Severe pain usually requires immediate medical intervention, but ask for ultrasound therapy rather than surgery. Ultrasound disintegrates the stones harmlessly and allows them to flush away naturally, without surgery.

Herbal medicine

Regular tinctures of gravel root, stone root, parsley, and wild carrot are said to help dissolve stones over a period of time. An alternative is drinking nettle tea regularly (three times a day).

Hydrotherapy

A hot pack or compress of Epsom salts applied to the back over the kidneys and abdomen can relieve pain. Apply it for 10–15 minutes, then as often as needed. A hot bath with Epsom salts will also help.

Nutritional and dietary therapy

Drink lots of clean water, preferably filtered, and cut down on dairy products and other calcium-rich foods, such as chocolate, strawberries, rhubarb, grapes, spinach, and beet. A daily dose of a little cider vinegar or lemon juice in warm water with honey is said to be effective in dissolving stones.

Acupressure

Three different points around the ankle help kidney and bladder problems: a point under the ankle bone on the inside of the foot; a point midway between the ankle bone and the tendon on the inside of the foot; and a point on the outside of the ankle midway between the ankle bone and the tendon.

Homeopathy

The remedies berberis 6c, sarsaparilla 6c, magnesia phos 6c, and calcarea 6c are said to help relieve pain from a blocked ureter.

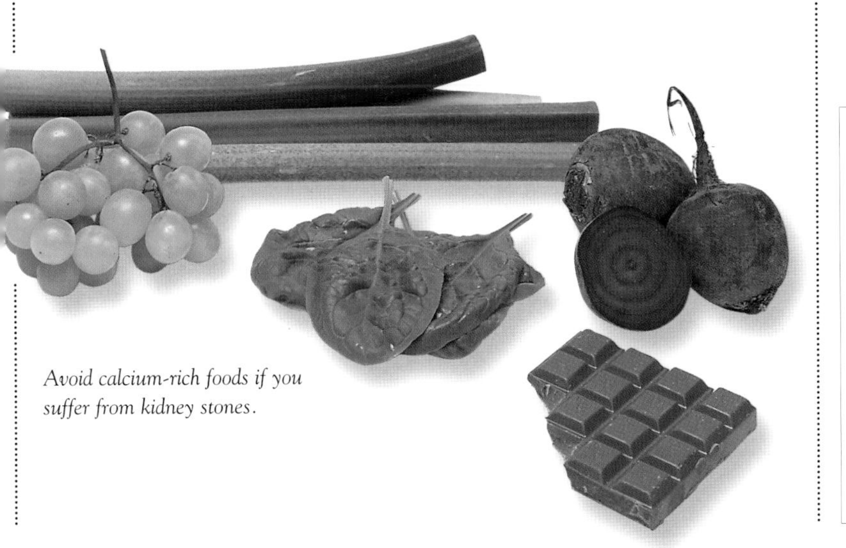

Avoid calcium-rich foods if you suffer from kidney stones.

Other therapies

From a qualified therapist only

Acupuncture and traditional Chinese herbal medicine • pages 150–151
Osteopathy and chiropractic • page 152–153
Hypnotherapy • page 153
Counseling and psychotherapy • page 154

HEART AND CIRCULATION PAIN

Pain in the heart and blood vessels can range from a mild ache to an agonizing cramp, and is usually the result of poor or impaired circulation. Impaired circulation, in turn, usually arises from atherosclerosis or arteriosclerosis (two medical names for hardening and clogging of the arteries), and from tension and stress. Excess weight, smoking, high blood pressure, and heredity are contributing factors. Heart disease results in more deaths in the western world than all other diseases together, usually from heart attack but also from stroke.

Hardening and clogging of arteries, including those around the heart muscle, is widespread in affluent populations throughout the world that consume the so-called "western diet," containing large amounts of animal fat, sugar, and salt. Over time—and the process starts almost from birth—fat deposits (atheroma) from such a diet line the artery walls and turn hard (calcify). This, in turn, prevents the arteries from being able to expand and contract as they should. Tension, for its part, not only causes blood vessels to narrow and tighten—and so circulate blood less efficiently—but, by a complex chemical process, also helps trigger the buildup of unhealthy fats in the bloodstream in the first place. The result of this lethal combination of diet and stress is generally what is meant by "heart disease."

Unconventional (non-drug) treatments concentrate on helping

blood vessels, particularly the all-important arteries, to become less clogged and more flexible to cope with the flow of blood to and from the heart, as well as promoting the health and strength of the heart muscle. The seriousness of circulatory disease means that natural approaches are generally more suitable for prevention than treatment, especially for people with severe and long-standing problems, but a number of non-conventional treatments have been shown to be highly effective in countering poor circulation, particularly that relating to stress.

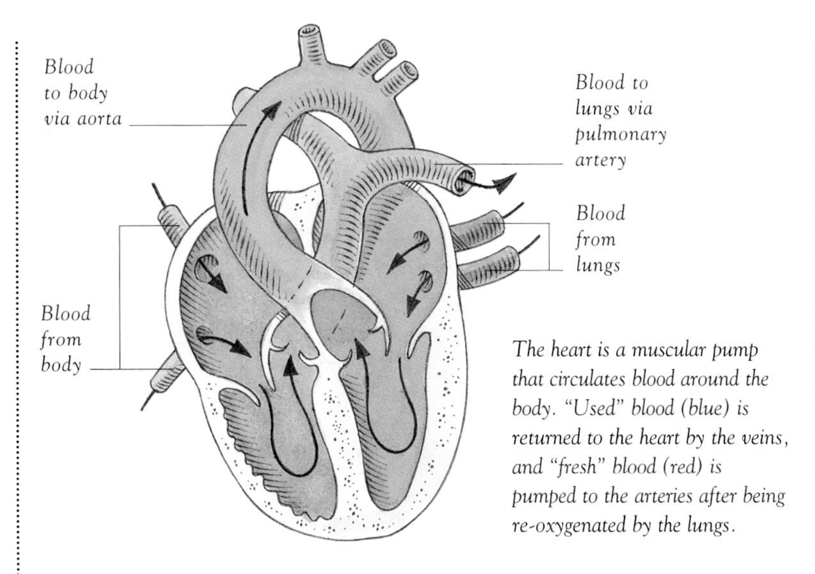

The heart is a muscular pump that circulates blood around the body. "Used" blood (blue) is returned to the heart by the veins, and "fresh" blood (red) is pumped to the arteries after being re-oxygenated by the lungs.

Warning

Seek immediate medical attention if you have any of the following symptoms:

- *a tight, cramp-like pain in the center of your chest*
- *pain down your left arm and up the left side of your neck*
- *extreme breathlessness with sweating and a cold, clammy skin, for no apparent reason.*

HEART PAIN

Whilst heart pain should always be taken extremely seriously, it is worth noting that natural remedies can make a real difference.

PALPITATIONS

Palpitations (rapid and/or irregular heartbeat) are alarming but not unusual. The anxiety they cause can be more serious than the physical problem itself. They can have a psychological cause, such as worry or panic, but are just as likely to be the result of infection or something eaten and drunk: tea, coffee, alcohol, and drugs, for example.

Slow, deep breathing, and biofeedback techniques are effective. Bach Rescue Remedy, or the homeopathic remedy aconite 6c can help, as can massage of the acupressure "heart" point, beneath the pisiform bone on the wrist below the little finger. The herbs valerian and hawthorn berry (as tablets), and a tea of lemon balm, lime blossom, motherwort, and passionflower are also beneficial.

ANGINA

Angina (angina pectoris) is pain in the front of the chest, sometimes with radiation to the neck, jaw, or other areas, usually as a result of poor circulation in the arteries that supply the heart muscle with the blood to keep it working properly. It is a serious sign that action is necessary if a full-scale heart attack is not to follow sometime in the future. The remedy is essentially the same as for all heart and arterial problems: exercise, diet, stress reduction, and emotional support.

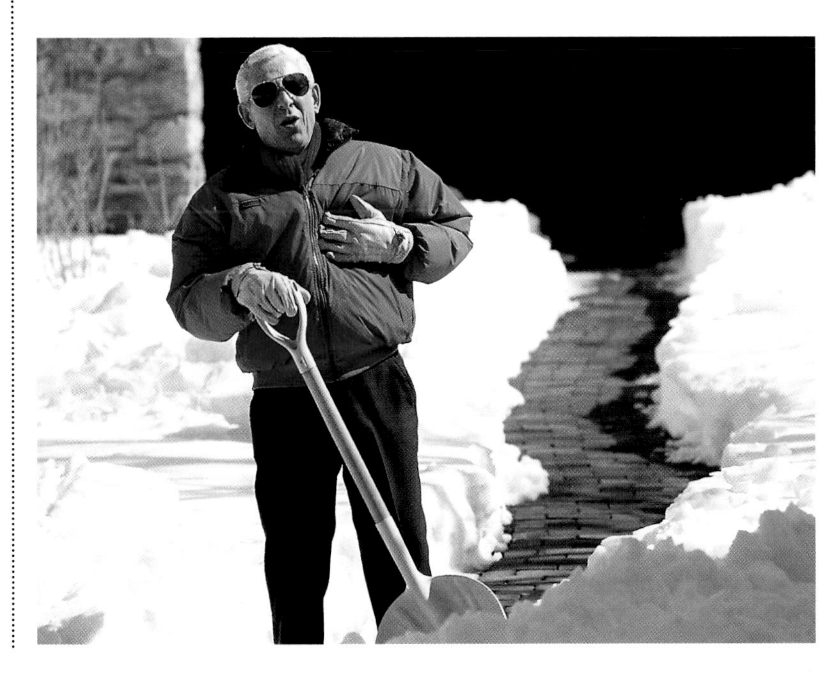

Severe pain in the center of the chest during exercise, particularly in elderly people, is a symptom of heart attack from heart disease.

Nutritional and dietary therapy

Healthy eating applies particularly strongly for every condition involving the heart and arteries. The so-called "Mediterranean diet" of salads, fish, garlic, red wine, vegetables, and fruit is considered ideal, because heart disease rates in Mediterranean countries are a half to one-third those of northern Europe and north America. Taking regular supplements of the "antioxidant" nutrients has now been shown to have outstanding preventive and recuperative benefits. The main ones are the vitamins A, C, E, the minerals selenium, zinc, magnesium, the amino acid lysine, the essential fatty acids EPA (from fish oils), and GLA (from starflower/borage and evening primrose oils), and lecithin.

Herbal medicine

Garlic, bromelain, lime blossom, lily of the valley, motherwort, and hawthorn berries all have a reputation for removing angina symptoms completely over the long haul. Yarrow tea can also be beneficial. Make an infusion of two teaspoonfuls of the dried herb, and drink three times daily.

Self-help stress reduction techniques

Physical

Exercise (but make sure it is gentle exercise and check it out with your doctor first)
Massage • pages 128–129
Aromatherapy (oils of black pepper, orange, lemon, juniper, cypress, and rosemary are recommended) • pages 130–131
Reflexology • pages 144–145

Psychological

Meditation (including autogenics) • pages 138–139
Visualization • page 137
Self-hypnosis • page 136
Biofeedback • page 139

Physical and psychological

Yoga • pages 132–133
Tai chi • page 134

NOTE *Talking to family and friends and enlisting their help and support is an important factor in combating stress and promoting heart health.*

Warning: severe heart pain

Severe heart pain, accompanied by pains in the left arm and neck with breathlessness, pallor, and sweating, may be a heart attack, and is not suitable for self-help or treatment by non-medical means. If symptoms such as these occur, seek immediate medical help.

Stress reduction

There is a wide choice of self-help stress reduction techniques, including physical and psychological approaches. The most important thing is to find out which approach works best for each individual.

CIRCULATION PAIN

Aches and pains in parts of the body other than the heart are often the result of poor circulation of blood in those areas, particularly the hands, legs, and feet. Poor circulation can be helped by the same action that helps pain in the heart muscle, especially exercise, diet, and stress reduction.

Yoga

The Shoulder Stand, followed by the Fish posture, are said to be beneficial for circulatory problems in the hands and feet (see opposite).

This ultrasound picture shows the four chambers of the human heart responsible for blood circulation. The two chambers on the left control the flow of used blood and those on the right refreshed blood.

The shoulder stand

CAUTION These yoga postures are not recommended for those with high blood pressure or a diagnosed heart condition. They are also not advisable during menstruation, or with eye, ear, or brain infection. Check with your doctor before attempting them.

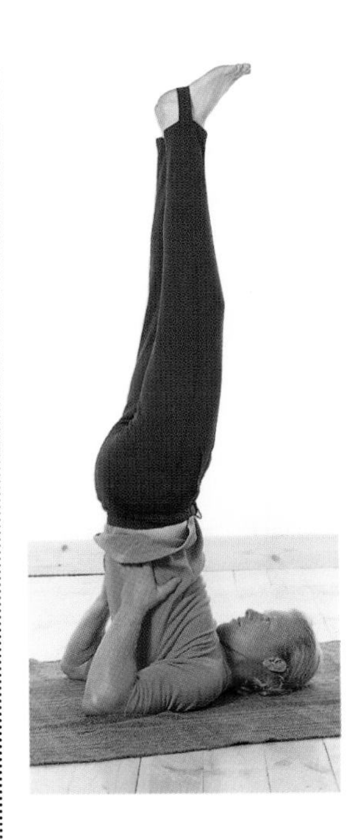

one

Lie on your back, arms by your side, palms face down. Breathing in, raise your entire bottom half so that you are supporting yourself on your shoulders, with your hands and arms supporting your back. Keep your spine straight and breathe normally. Tuck your chin into your chest and relax. Try to hold the posture for a minute, increasing the time as it becomes easier.

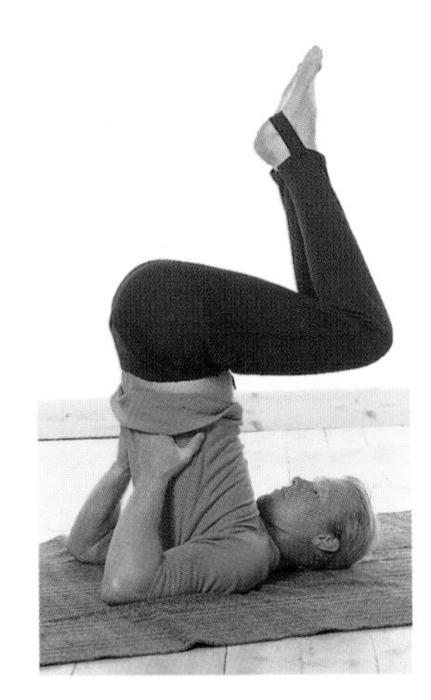

two

To come out of the posture, breathe out, bring your knees to your chest, and slowly let them uncurl back to the ground. Relax in that position for as long as you held the posture.

The half shoulder stand

The easier half shoulder stand can be just as effective as the full one. Raise your legs, but instead of holding them upright, let them fall back at an angle of about 45° over your head, bending the knees if this is easier. Alternatively, use a chair to support your legs.

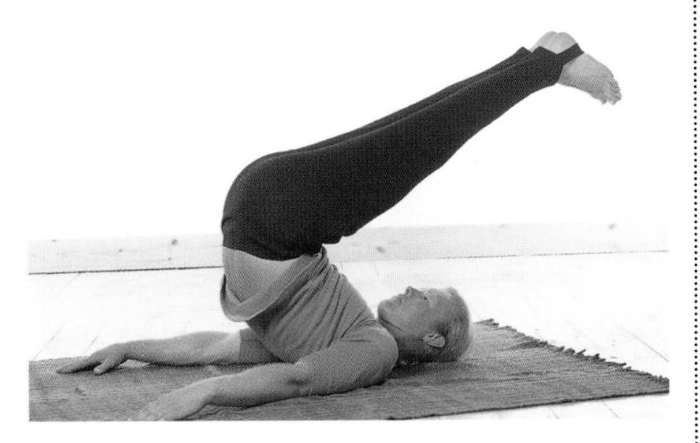

The fish

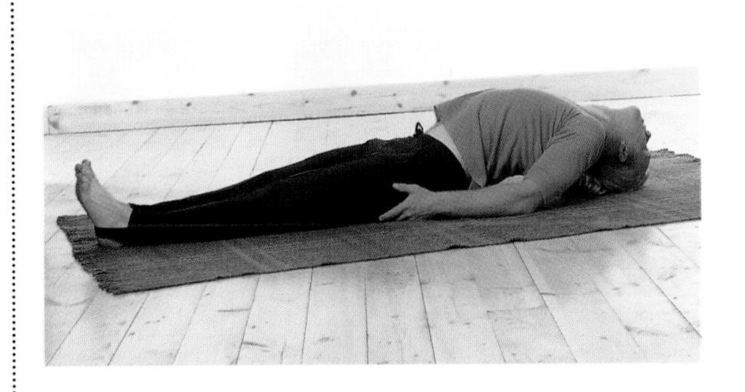

one

Lie on the ground with your arms by your side, breathe in, and arch your back. Holding your stomach in and your chest high, breathe deeply. Hold the position for 30 seconds, then relax by breathing out and lying straight for another 30 seconds. Increase the time as the posture becomes easier.

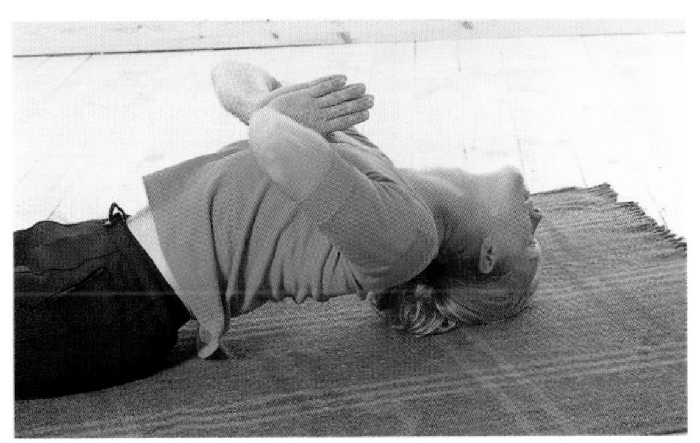

two

A variation is to bring the palms of your hands together across your chest in a prayer position. Again, breathe slowly and deeply and hold the position for approximately 30 seconds, then release.

Herbal medicine

Garlic, onion, ginger, chili peppers, and alfalfa seeds have all been shown to aid circulation by becoming a part of a regular diet. Among many other herbs said to help circulation, especially in the hands and feet, are cayenne pepper, lily of the valley, dandelion, and broom.

CRAMP

See page 25 for natural remedies.

RAYNAUD'S SYNDROME

An unusual but painful condition as a result of spasm of the nerves of the small arteries, especially in the fingers, that makes them go cold, white, and often numb. For reasons as yet unknown, it affects mainly young women.

Nutritional and dietary therapy

Eat iron-rich foods, such as liver, chicken, dark green leafy vegetables, soybeans, and black kidney beans, or a multivitamin supplement containing iron with vitamins C, E, B-complex, copper, and selenium. Avoid caffeine-rich drinks, such as coffee and tea, that both constrict blood vessels (smoking does the same) and reduce the absorption of iron.

Biofeedback

Techniques that can control muscular tension and circulation can be beneficial.

CHILBLAINS

See page 24 for natural remedies.

VARICOSE VEINS

More common in women than men, often as a result of pregnancy, varicose veins are caused by blood not circulating efficiently enough, so that small pockets of congestion occur. Other common causes are not taking enough exercise, standing still for long periods, and being overweight. The veins show as lumps that can be both painful and itchy and may lead to phlebitis.

Hydrotherapy

Alternating hot and cold water compresses on the affected area can alleviate pain and improve circulation. Start with a hot pad.

Nutritional and dietary therapy

Mixing the following combinations and drinking them regularly as juices is claimed to be particularly beneficial: carrot, celery, and parsley; carrot, celery, and spinach; carrot, spinach, and turnip; carrot, beet, and cucumber; watercress. A diet of raw beet is also said to help, and foods such as apricots, cherries, rosehips, blackberries, and buckwheat are recommended. Take vitamin C (500 mg), E (400 iu), rutin, and lecithin.

Herbal medicine

Hawthorn berries, horse chestnut, and the bark or berries of prickly ash may be effective in cases of painful varicose veins, but guidance from a qualified herbalist is advised.

Artery stretching

Artery "stretching," a highly specialized form of acupressure barely known outside Japan, where it is practiced widely, is said to be especially effective for circulation problems resulting from hardening of arteries.

Though effective, the therapy is painful in cases of advanced arterial disease, and can be dangerous in untrained hands.

Aromatherapy

The oils cypress, lemon, lime, and sandalwood are said to help circulation, but massaging over affected veins needs great care; putting the oils into a warm (not hot) bath is a better alternative.

Reflexology

Massaging the web between the second and third toes of both feet is claimed to benefit circulation.

Yoga

Practice the Shoulder Stand and the Fish postures (see page 95).

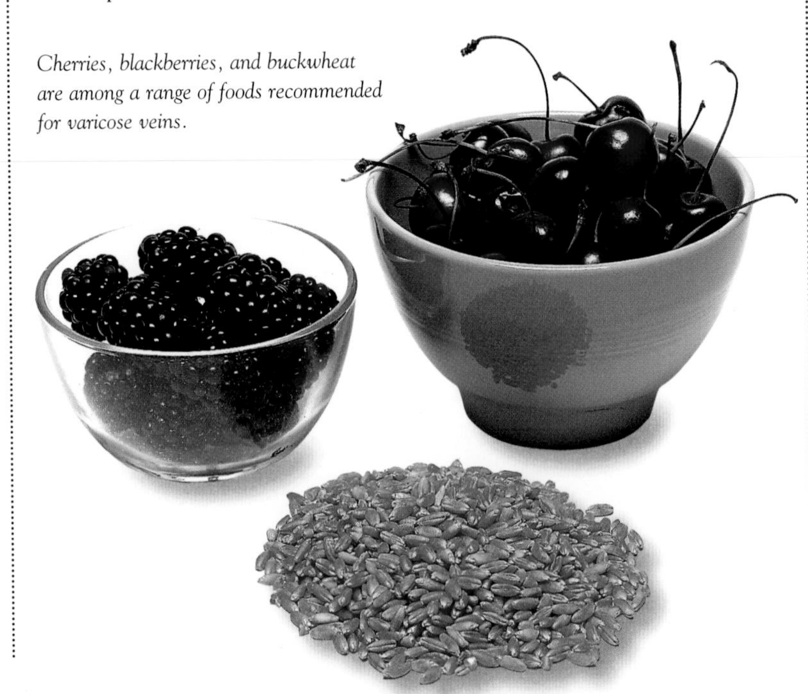

Cherries, blackberries, and buckwheat are among a range of foods recommended for varicose veins.

HEMORRHOIDS (PILES)

Hemorrhoids are a form of varicose vein that forms at the opening of the anus, often as a result of recurring constipation and straining to evacuate. The veins become distended and enlarged and often rupture, causing pain, irritation, and bleeding during bowel movements.

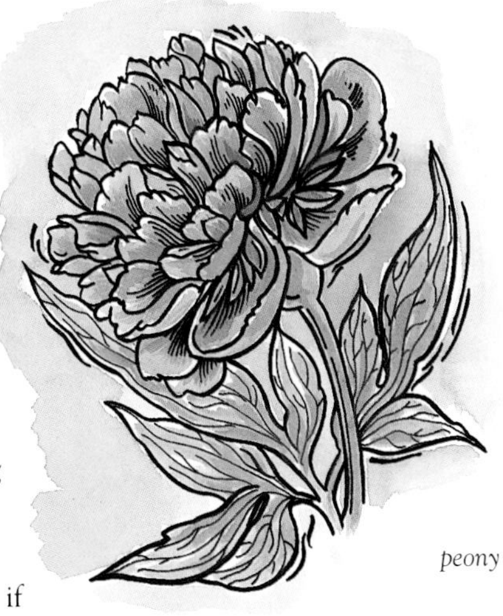

peony

CAUTION See your doctor if bleeding continues for more than 12 hours, or has no obvious cause.

Hydrotherapy

Ice packs can bring immediate relief (packs of frozen peas are ideal), but bathing in alternating hot and cold water is recommended for the longer term. (Sitz bathing, in which the feet are in cold water and the bottom in hot, and vice versa, is the ideal, but this is only really practicable for most people at health spas with such facilities.) An alternative is having a warm bath containing about 1 lb (0.5 kg) of sea salt or 3–4 drops of essential oil of cypress and/or chamomile. Soak for up to 10 minutes.

Yoga

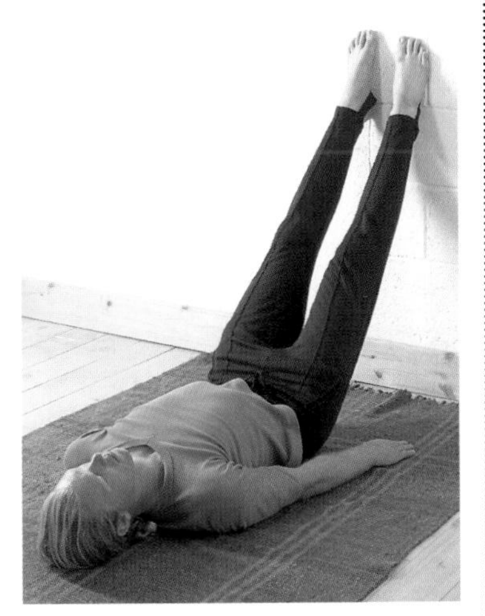

Lie with the legs at a 45° angle to a suitable support for three minutes a day.

Herbal medicine

Apply peony ointment to veins protruding from the anus and peony suppositories to those inside. Use witch hazel if the hemorrhoids are bleeding. Other effective herbal ointments are calendula, hypericum, pilewort, comfrey, horse chestnut, and yarrow. Yarrow can be applied as a compress or drunk as a tea.

Movement therapy

Regular exercise will help the poor circulation that is at the root of the problem. Other forms of movement therapy, such as dance and tai chi, are also beneficial.

Nutritional and dietary therapy

Eat a wholefood diet and drink at least 6–8 glasses of water or diluted fruit juice between meals a day, with a large daily spoonful of flaxseed (linseed) oil. Take the same supplements as for varicose veins (see page 96), and take iron if bleeding is heavy.

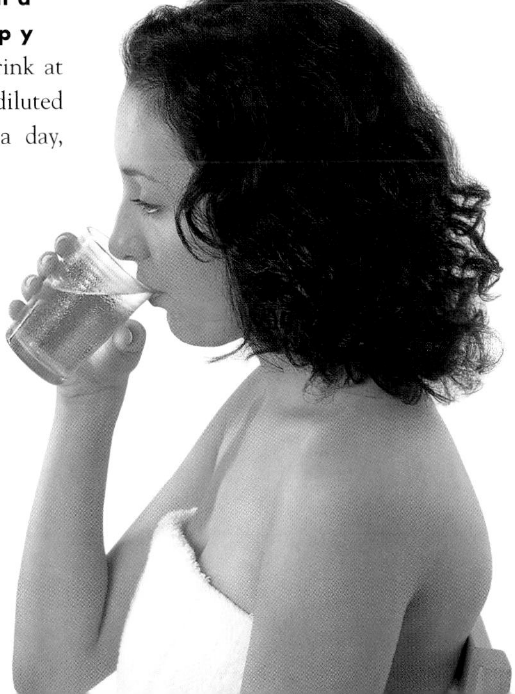

Piles can be helped by drinking plenty of water or diluted fruit juice with flaxseed (linseed) oil.

PHLEBITIS

Phlebitis is inflammation of the veins, most often in the legs and linked to varicose veins. It can sometimes happen at the site of an injection. The condition can lead to complications and should be checked by a doctor.

Naturopathy

The most effective treatment for phlebitis is simply to lift the leg or affected area and rest it. For longer-lasting conditions, elasticated stockings and similar supports can help, as can natural painkillers and anti-inflammatories, such as willow bark and meadowsweet.

Other therapies

From a qualified therapist only

Acupuncture • pages 150–151
Cranial osteopathy • pages 153
Homeopathy • pages 146–147
Counseling and psychotherapy • page 154
Hypnotherapy • page 153
Creative arts therapies • pages 140–141

SEX AND PREGNANCY PAIN

This section deals with pain in the male and female reproductive organs, pain as a result of physical and psychological problems in sex, and pain in pregnancy and childbirth. There is a close and complex relationship between the mind and emotions and the body in sex that affects both men and women and can give rise to psychological as well as physical pain: for example, in problems of impotence (the inability to get or maintain an erection), or vaginismus (an involuntary tightening of the vagina).

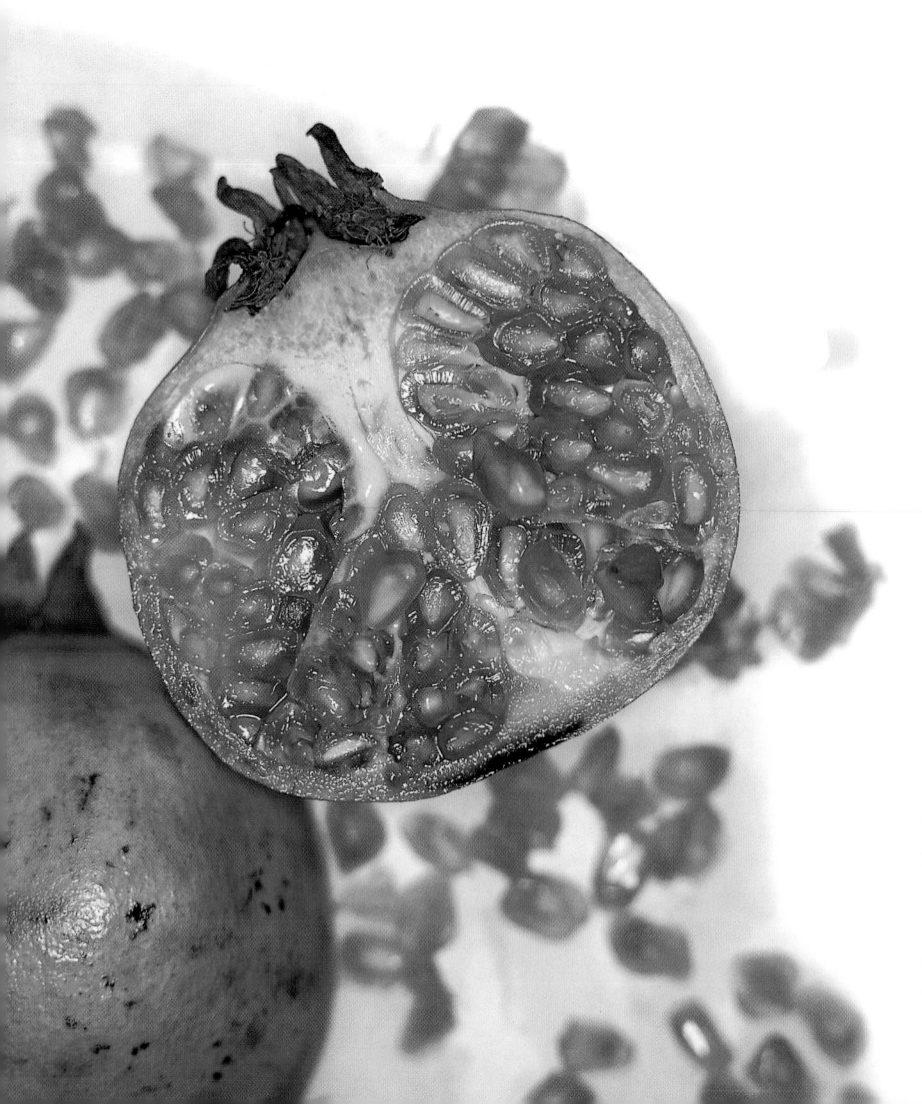

SEX AND GENITAL PAIN IN MEN

The lower pelvic area is one of considerable local trauma, and there are several conditions that can be helped by natural therapies.

HERNIA

A hernia is usually taken to mean a rupture in the groin area, but it actually applies to any part of the abdomen, where the contents —mainly the intestines—push through a weakness in the abdominal wall and cause a swelling that is often painful. Straining to lift heavy weights or make bowel movements are the most common causes. Men are more prone than women to hernia in the groin, but women can also suffer. It should not be confused with hiatus hernia (see pages 84–85).

Attempt to return the contents of the hernia back where they came from by gentle but firm inward

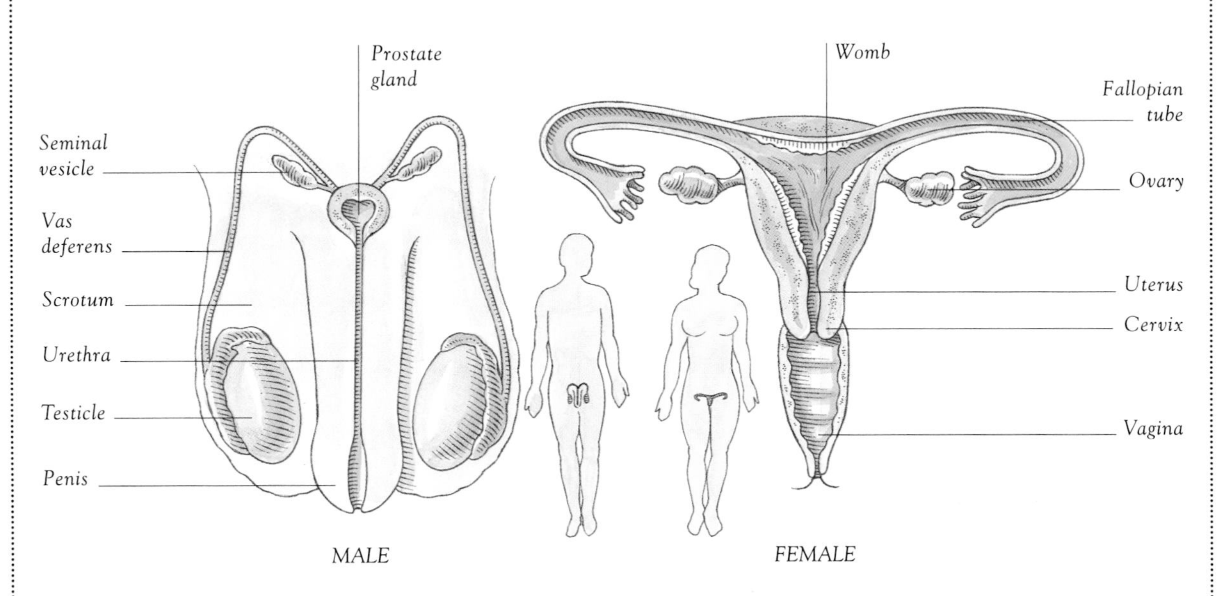

Male and female reproductive organs.

pressure and the use of a support or truss to hold them in place. But do not truss a hernia you cannot return manually and that is trapped. A trapped, or strangulated, hernia can be dangerous and requires surgery to correct, and surgery is almost always necessary if the problem is recurrent.

PROSTATITIS

Inflammation of the prostate gland: the gland is the size of a walnut that lies immediately below the bladder and is involved in the manufacture of semen (not sperm). The inflammation is due to infection, which may be elsewhere in the body. Symptoms are pain in the lower back, abdomen, behind the scrotum and between the legs, and fever. Untreated prostatitis can lead to inflammation of other parts of the genito-urinary system, especially the testicles (orchitis), epididymis (epididymitis), and more seriously, the kidneys. The natural enlargement of the prostate with age (especially over 50) does not produce prostatitis, but can benefit from the treatments outlined here.

Naturopathy

Drink large amounts of liquids, preferably water (but not tea, coffee, or alcohol), and urinate as often as possible, making sure the bladder is as empty as possible before stopping. Sit in a waist-deep hot bath for about 10 minutes, knees bent, and with a cold washcloth on your forehead. Afterward, rub your lower half down with a cold towel, and hold the towel between your legs for a few seconds to cool that area. Some therapists recommend regular ejaculation and massage of the prostate to relieve pressure from enlargement. Walking also helps.

Nutritional and dietary therapy

Avoid spicy and fatty foods, and take daily supplements of vitamins C, E, B-complex, zinc, and magnesium. Regular supplementation with fish oils, olive oil, and evening primrose oil can also help. Juice mixes that are said to be effective are carrot, celery, watercress, and horseradish; carrot, cucumber, beet, radish, and garlic; and pumpkin.

Herbal medicine

Teas of dandelion, saw palmetto, fygeum, horsetail, and couch grass are said to be beneficial, particularly the first three herbs. Tinctures of pipsissewa, echinacea, staphysagria, and pulsatilla can also help, but individual prescription is advisable from a qualified therapist.

Massage and aromatherapy

Massaging or inhaling using the essential oils of lavender, cypress, and thyme may be beneficial.

Reflexology

Massage a point midway between the anklebone and the heel on the inside of the foot. The same point benefits the uterus in women.

Other therapies

From aqualified therapist only

Acupuncture and traditional Chinese herbal medicine • pages 150–151
Colonic irrigation • page 87

IMPOTENCE

Impotence (the inability to achieve or maintain an erection) can be physical—as a result of illness or infection—but is often psychological. A physical problem can usually be detected fairly easily by a family doctor, especially if illness is involved (some medicines and drugs can cause impotence, for example). But if there is no obvious physical reason for it, the cause is most likely psychological. A combination of physical and psychological treatments that simultaneously promote relaxation and desire is most effective.

"Partner" therapy

Recruiting your sexual partner is important. Agree to caress and cuddle without any other expectations, to remove any pressure of having to "perform." Encourage your partner to fondle your genitals in the way you like. Using massage oil can help. Do not feel you must have intercourse until you are completely ready by feeling relaxed and confident about it. Also make sure that the circumstances for lovemaking are right: relaxed and unhurried. This and the following approaches can also help with the problem of premature ejaculation ("coming too soon").

Massage and aromatherapy

Massaging, or preferably being massaged, with the essential oils of ylang ylang, jasmine, rose, sandalwood, jojoba, or patchouli—all renowned aphrodisiacs—is both mentally relaxing and physically stimulating. Massaging the neck and head, including the scalp, with rosemary can also help. Having a partner do this while reading erotic literature or looking at erotic pictures can be highly effective.

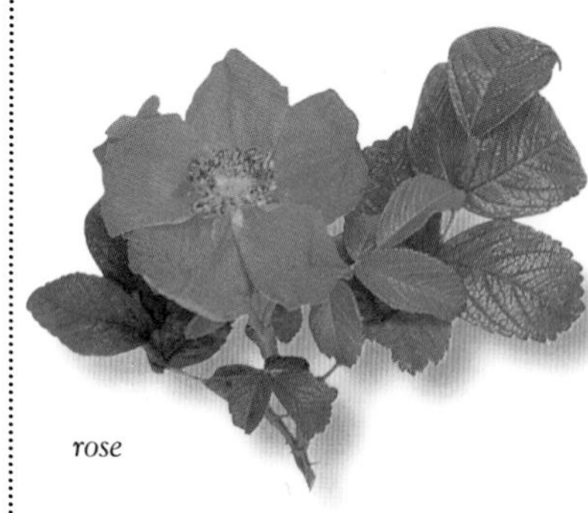

rose

Hydrotherapy and movement

A daily cold bath or a sitz bath, where you sit alternately in hot and cold water, can be extremely effective if done regularly. Regular exercise is always beneficial.

Herbal medicine

Teas of saw palmetto and fygeum are said to help.

Nutritional and dietary therapy

Besides eating and drinking healthily (plenty of fresh fruit and vegetables, and not too much alcohol), foods rich in vitamin C and zinc are beneficial. Examples are (vitamin C) broccoli, red peppers, blackcurrants, and tomatoes, and (zinc) shellfish, sardines, pumpkin seeds, chicken, and brown rice. Taking a regular supplement with vitamin C and zinc can also help.

Relaxation

Muscle relaxation exercises, visualization, meditation, and biofeedback can all help overcome the psychological strain that can lie behind impotence, and reassert a more positive frame of mind.

Other therapies
From a qualified therapist only

Counseling and psychotherapy (including sex therapy) • *page 154*
Hypnotherapy • *page 153*

Foods containing large amounts of vitamin C and zinc, such as broccoli, tomatoes, red peppers, and prawns, can help overcome the problems of impotence.

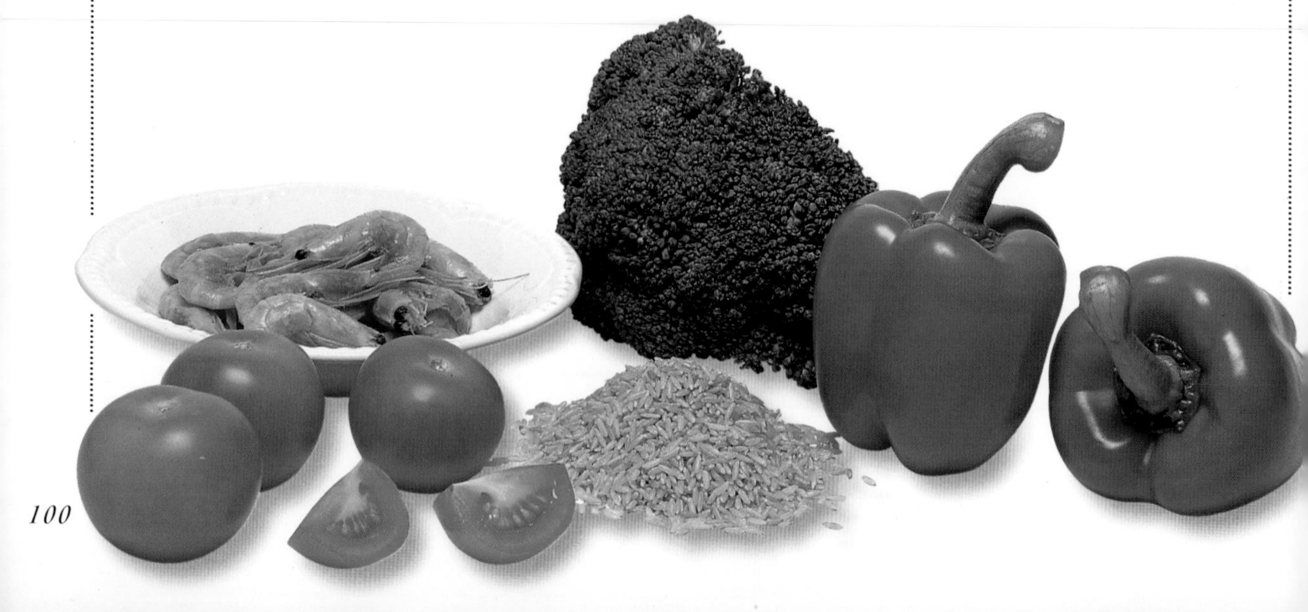

SEX AND GENITAL PAIN IN WOMEN

Like men, women can experience both psychological and physical pain from sexual and genital causes, both of which can be helped enormously by natural means.

VAGINISMUS

Vaginismus is a psychological condition causing the vagina to tighten and make intercourse difficult, if not impossible, without pain. Often associated with low sexual response ("frigidity"), vaginismus is, in fact, not the same: a woman can want penetrative sex but be unable to relax her vagina for reasons she is often unaware of and cannot control.

As the female equivalent of male impotence, its successful treatment is similar—that is, recruiting the help of a partner and creating the conditions for relaxing and trusting sex. Learning to masturbate to orgasm, and teaching your partner how to do it to you, is often effective by itself, especially with the essential oils recommended for male impotence. A hot waist-deep bath can also help as well as relaxation techniques.

VAGINITIS

Inflammation of the vagina, often as the result of uncomfortable sex, but also from infection, vaginitis results in soreness and itching and sometimes a discharge with blood.

NOTE Vaginitis should not be confused with vaginosis, which is a mild and common bacterial condition that causes a vaginal discharge with a fishy smell. Vaginosis is treated simply by inserting natural live yogurt into the vagina and/or taking acidophilus capsules (two a day) until clear. However, you should see a doctor if vaginitis symptoms occur during pregnancy.

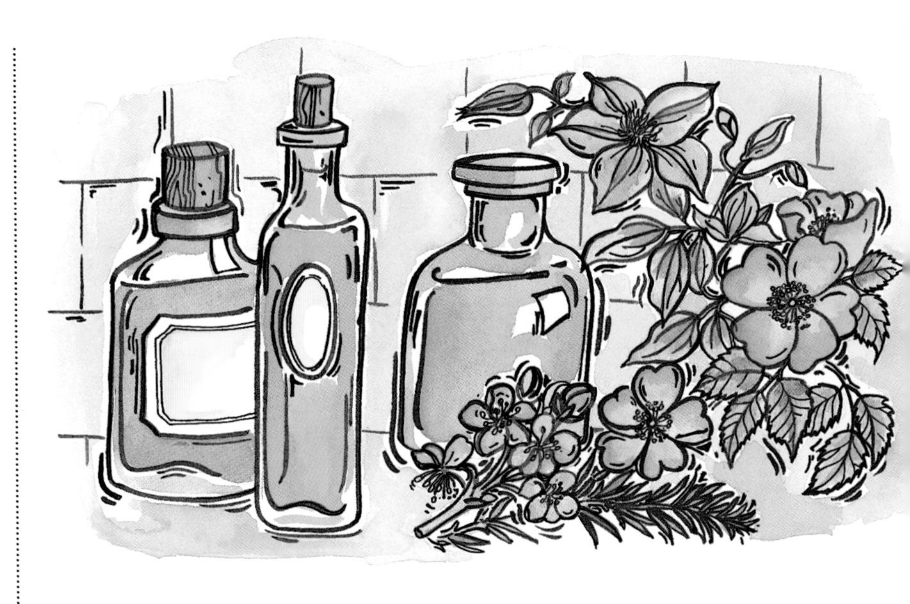

Bathing in or vaporizing your favorite essential oils can aid relaxation if anxiety is causing sexual problems.

Aromatherapy and herbal medicine

Regular herbal douches with hypericum and calendula is an effective treatment (mix 10 drops of each of the mother tinctures in 1 pint/570 ml of boiled warm water). An alternative is a bath with several drops of lavender essential oil in it (avoid chemical soaps and detergents). Aloe vera tincture (diluted) or gel is also effective. If the cause is being too dry for sex—a problem for many women after the menopause—your partner should use a lubricating gel or oil, such as jojoba. If inflammation is already present, a drop or two of tea tree oil with a neutral carrier oil is best.

THRUSH

Thrush is a vaginal infection caused by an overgrowth of the yeast organism candida albicans (the condition is also known as candidiasis). It is characterized by severe itching in the vagina and vulva, and a thick white discharge from the vagina resembling cottage cheese, and it can make having sex and urinating painful.

Naturopathy

To ease itching, insert natural live yogurt into the vagina and leave it there for at least an hour (covering a tampon and inserting it is a good way). Avoid intercourse for the duration of an attack.

Nutritional and dietary therapy

Eat plenty of natural live yogurt (2–3 tubs a day), and supplement with lactobacillus acidophilus capsules (two a day). Avoid sugar, alcohol, and similar refined carbohydrates (yeasts feed on them), and eat plenty of salads, garlic, fresh fruit, and wholegrains.

Aromatherapy

Douche (or bath) with 2–3 drops of tea tree, bergamot, and myrrh, or lavender, bergamot, and rose in 2 pints (1 liter) of warm water. Tea tree oil can also be applied direct as both an antifungal and antiseptic.

Herbal medicine

A warm compress of golden seal, chamomile, or myrrh can relieve the pain and discomfort of symptoms in the vulva.

PREMENSTRUAL SYNDROME

Describing a collection of symptoms that occur as a result of changes in hormone levels just before menstruation, premenstrual syndrome (PMS) is characterized as depression, tension headaches, irritability, mood swings, food cravings, feelings of being bloated, and breast tenderness. Reactions range from mild to severe, and differ between individuals as well as from month to month.

Herbs for PMS

Recommended herbs include the following, but a wide range of herbs is available, so it is best to see a qualified herbalist for individual prescription.

Depression and anxiety:
• starflower (borage), lemon balm
Breast pain and tenderness:
• evening primrose
Water retention:
• dandelion, cleavers
Headache:
• meadowsweet, willow bark
Insomnia: • chamomile

Reflexology

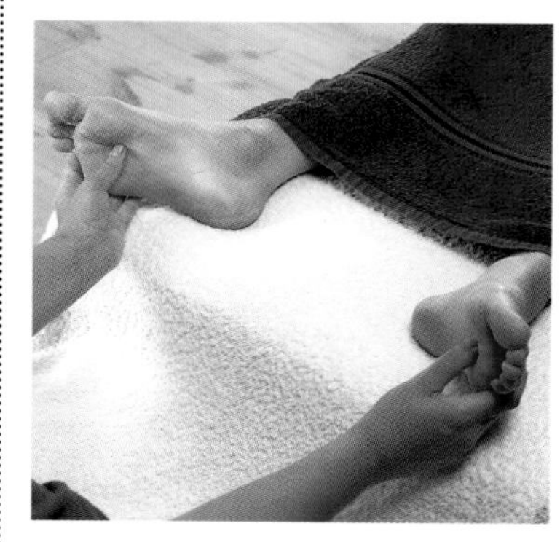

Manipulate the points on the soles of both feet said to be associated with PMS symptoms, especially the big toe, instep, and center of the foot (above).

Hydrotherapy and aromatherapy

Learning to handle stress and relax is an important part of PMS treatment. A warm bath with lemon grass essential oil is calming.

Nutritional and dietary therapy

Eat a healthy diet with plenty of salads and leafy green vegetables, and cut down on dairy products, sugar, salt, caffeine, and alcohol. Supplementing with vitamins C, B-complex, E, the minerals zinc, magnesium, and iron, and a balance of essential fatty acids (2 EPA:1 GLA) can help.

Herbal medicine

A tea blend containing chaste-tree berries, Mexican yam, ginseng, licorice, fennel, kelp, black cohosh, and false unicorn—drunk three times daily during the second half of the menstrual cycle for at least three months—is said to regulate hormone levels.

MENSTRUAL CRAMPS

Menstrual cramps, or painful periods (dysmenorrhea), are the result of too-strong contractions to expel the lining of the womb at menstruation. The reason is usually an over-production of prostaglandins, hormone-like substances that promote contractions. Too many result in contractions so strong they cause pain. This may be no more than a dull ache in the lower part of the back or abdomen, but it can be a cramp-like pain accompanied by nausea and even diarrhea. Stress and tension can be important contributing factors. Dysmenorrhea is different from menorrhagia (heavy bleeding)—usually caused by normally non-painful and harmless fibroids (growths) in the uterus—and PMS. Painful periods can sometimes be caused by inflammation of the uterus.

Other therapies for menstrual pain

From a qualified therapist only

Acupuncture • pages 150–151
Counseling and psychotherapy • page 154
Hypnotherapy • page 153
Creative arts therapy • pages 140–141

Regular, energetic exercise can help female hormonal problems such as premenstrual syndrome (PMS).

Pain in the uterus

Pain in the uterus (womb) is normally the result of two similar-sounding but quite different conditions. Endometritis is a rare but painful condition caused by inflammation of the walls of the uterus (endometrium), usually from bacterial infection after childbirth. Symptoms are pain in the lower part of the back and abdomen, and erratic menstruation. Conventional treatment involves antibiotics and, if the problem recurs, dilatation and curettage (D and C) surgery.

It should not be confused with endometriosis, in which uterine tissue grows outside the uterus and swells in normal response to the monthly hormone cycle, sometimes causing sudden pain. Neither condition is considered suitable for self-help, though many of the treatments for menstrual pain are likely to help pain in the uterus also.

Hydrotherapy and relaxation

Exercise and a hot bath with caraway seed oil in it are beneficial. Learning to relax is beneficial for all forms of period pain. Biofeedback has been shown to be particularly effective.

Nutritional and dietary therapy

Healthy eating and drinking will help, especially reducing animal fats, saturated oils, and salt intake. Try a multivitamin with vitamin B6 and magnesium, and evening primrose oil with vitamin E.

Herbal medicine

The Chinese herb dong quai relieves menstrual pain. Raspberry leaf tea and ginger can also help.

PROLAPSE

Prolapse of the uterus usually results from a combination of age and overweight, often as a result of earlier pregnancy, in which slack muscles allow the pelvic organs to sag, causing aching sensations in the lower back and abdomen, incontinence, and constipation. Surgery is sometimes necessary.

Movement therapy

Taking outdoor exercise and losing weight are the two essentials. A specific exercise to tone up the muscles of the pelvis is the Pelvic Tilt (see page 72).

Herbal medicine

Drink black cohosh, raspberry leaf, and chaste-tree as tinctures diluted in water, or in teas.

PELVIC INFLAMMATORY DISEASE

The female reproductive organs are both complex and vulnerable, and prone to infection from a number of sources. Pelvic inflammatory disease (PID) is when more than one of the many organs involved—for example, the ovaries, fallopian tubes, uterus, and cervix—becomes infected or inflamed. It can be caused by injury through sex, the intrauterine contraceptive device (IUD), endometriosis, sexually transmitted diseases, or abortion, and results in severe pain, backache, fever, vaginal discharge, fatigue, and long-term debility.

CAUTION PID can be extremely serious, and medical assistance should be sought without delay. Antibiotics are likely to be necessary for PID.

Aromatherapy and dietary therapy

Rest, eating a healthy diet, and hot baths—especially with the essential oils of cypress and lavender—are recommended to alleviate symptoms. A good multivitamin and mineral supplement with vitamin A, B-complex, C, E, zinc, magnesium, and selenium can help; so can both the EPA and GLA essential fatty acids, and lactobacillus acidophilus (two capsules daily).

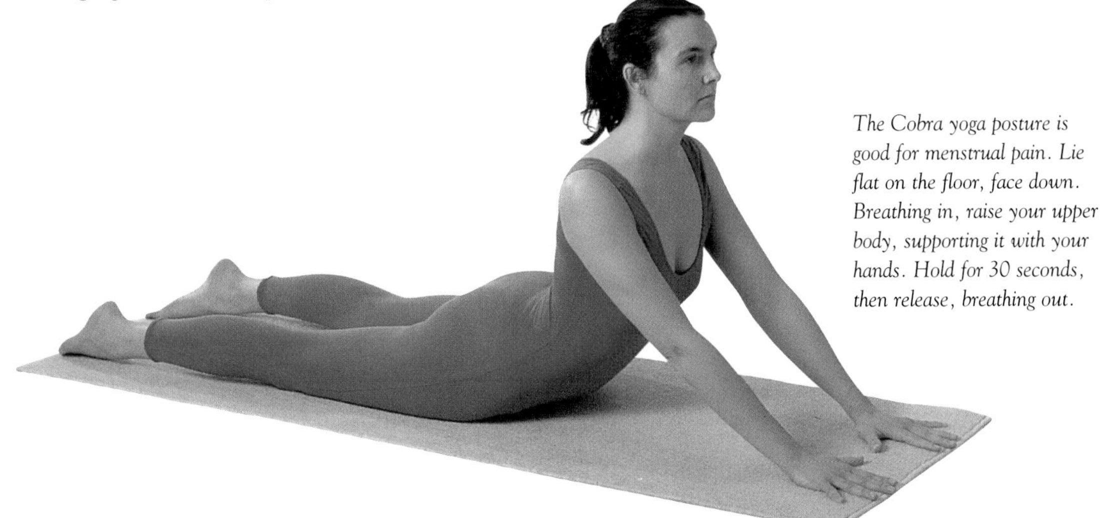

The Cobra yoga posture is good for menstrual pain. Lie flat on the floor, face down. Breathing in, raise your upper body, supporting it with your hands. Hold for 30 seconds, then release, breathing out.

SEXUAL DISEASES

Sexually transmitted diseases (STDs)—once called venereal diseases (VD)—are diseases spread by having sex with an infected person. Symptoms usually show first in the genitals, but disease is not necessarily confined there. A few, such as pubic lice ("crabs"), genital warts, genital herpes, nonspecific urethritis (NSU), and chlamydia, are common and relatively harmless, causing more discomfort and embarrassment than pain—though pain can be associated with herpes, NSU, and chlamydia. But others—particularly gonorrhea, syphilis, and human immunodeficiency virus (HIV)—are serious and, with the exception of HIV, not suitable for self-help. They should be seen and diagnosed by a medical doctor before being treated medically.

HIV and AIDS

The situation surrounding HIV—and the condition Acquired Immune Deficiency Syndrome (AIDS) that it may or may not lead to—is extremely complex and controversial. Emotions on both sides of the conventional versus nonconventional debate currently run so high that we have taken the decision not to include its treatment by self-help in this book on the grounds that the space available is too limited to do justice to the importance of the subject.

GENITAL HERPES

A viral infection caused by the herpes simplex virus (also responsible for cold sores), genital herpes shows as small, painful sores on the penis or in the vagina that form blisters, burst, and dry.

Hydrotherapy and herbal medicine

Wash the affected parts with salt water (use a teaspoonful of salt to 1 pint/570 ml of water), or apply tea tree oil to the sores/blisters, and witch hazel to dry them afterward.

NONSPECIFIC URETHRITIS

Nonspecific urethritis (NSU) is inflammation of the urethra, usually as a result of having sex with a partner with cystitis or urinary tract infection (UTI). It affects women more than men, causing an unpleasant discharge, soreness, and painful sex. The treatment for cystitis is also effective for NSU.

CHLAMYDIA

Chlamydia is an infection caused by the parasite chlamydia trachomatis, which lodges in the urethra and, in women, the vagina. It is extremely common (some say the most common STD in the world today), but symptoms are almost exclusively confined to women: a sore vagina, causing pain during sex, a tender cervix, the urge to urinate, and an intensely irritating discharge. If untreated, it can spread to other parts of the reproductive system, causing pelvic inflammatory disease, infertility, and long-term debility.

Hydrotherapy

Colonic irrigation (see page 87), followed by supplementation with lactobacillus bacteria, is recommended, but treatment must be by an experienced practitioner. Both sexual partners should be treated.

Nutritional and dietary therapy

Eat a healthy diet (increasing fresh fruit and vegetables and decreasing sugars, processed food, and alcohol), and supplement with vitamins A, C, E, and, especially, zinc.

Herbal medicine

A vaginal douche of calendula, golden seal, and echinacea every morning is effective, followed by inserting plain yogurt into the vagina in the evening.

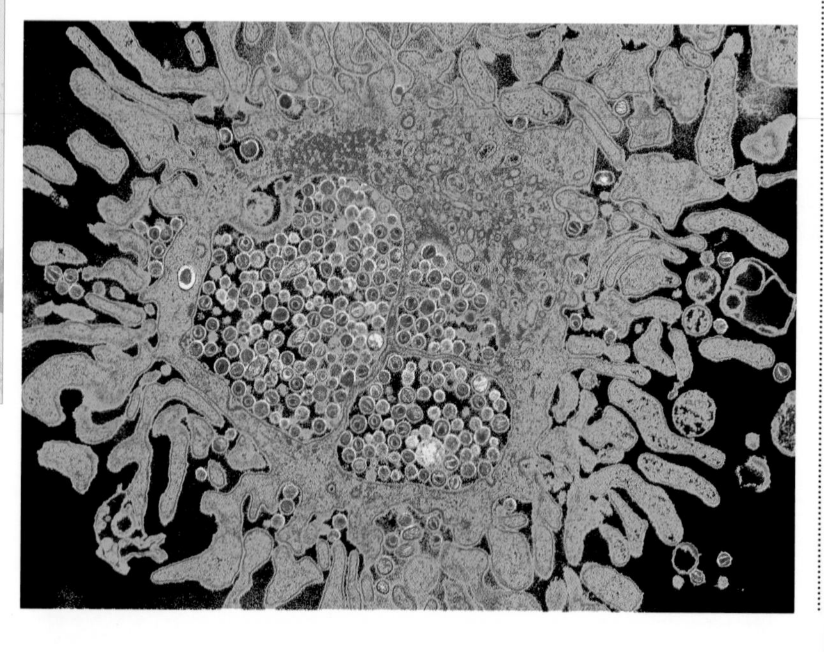

The human immunodeficiency virus (HIV), which may be responsible for AIDS, is shown here developing in a body cell at a magnification of nearly 11,000.

PREGNANCY PAIN

Different women will have different experiences of pregnancy. For example, one may suffer morning sickness for the entire nine months, another may not be affected at all.

MORNING SICKNESS

A feeling of nausea, sometimes causing actual vomiting, as a result of changed hormone levels due to pregnancy. The symptoms are commonest in the morning, but they can happen at any time.

Herbal medicine

Fresh root ginger (either chewed raw, or cut up, simmered for 10–15 minutes, and drunk) can help. Alternatively, a few drops of the essential oil of either chamomile or peppermint in a glass of warm water can be drunk instead of tea.

Acupressure

Pressing the point on the wrist for motion sickness (see page 25) is claimed to help most sufferers. Special wristbands can also work.

acupressure wristband

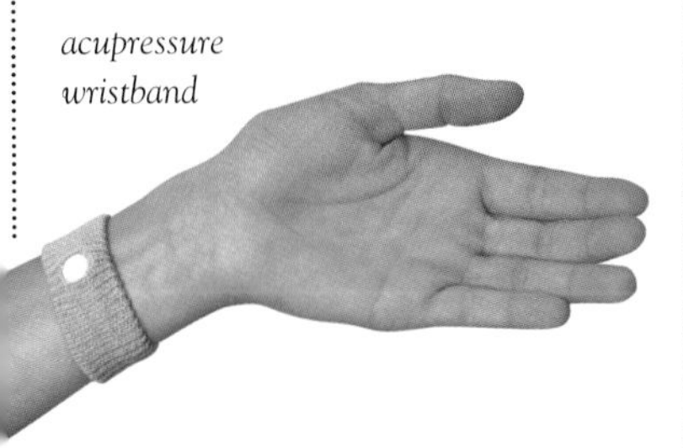

Homeopathy

The remedies nux vomica, pulsatilla, and ipecacuanha may help.

Aromatherapy

One or two drops of essential oil of lemon, vaporized in a burner in the bedroom before going to sleep, is sometimes effective.

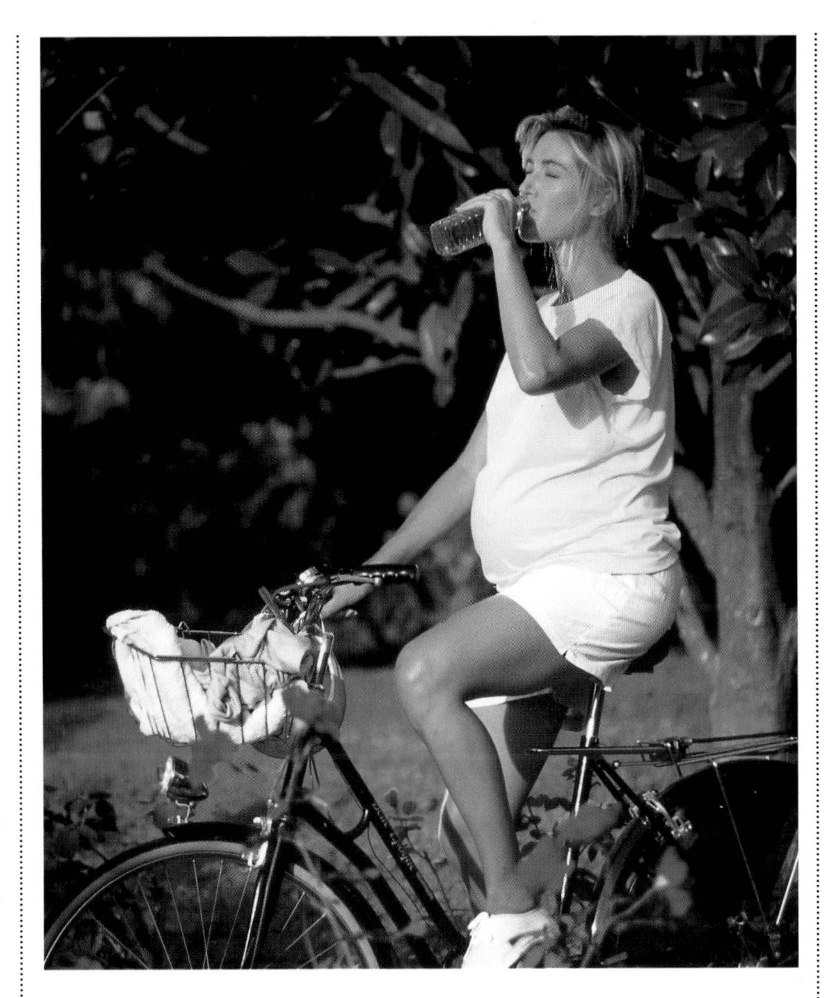

Gentle exercise in fresh air can benefit both mother-to-be and her baby, but always remember to keep up fluid intake, preferably by drinking pure water.

CAUTION The following oils should never be used during pregnancy: angelica, cinnamon bark, clary sage, hyssop, juniper berry, lovage, myrrh, origanum, pennyroyal, rosemary, sage, savory, sweet fennel, sweet marjoram, thyme.

SORE BREASTS

Breasts can often become sore as they enlarge as a normal part of pregnancy. Cracked nipples can develop later from breastfeeding.

Massage and aromatherapy

Gently massaging the breasts with lavender or geranium essential oils, diluted in a little carrier oil, can help. Alternatively put a few drops of the oils into a warm bath and let the water cover your breasts, or soak a washcloth or small towel in the liquid and place it over them.

Homeopathy

The remedies conium and bryonia can help. If the nipples become cracked use castor equi.

HEARTBURN

Heartburn is a common symptom of women in their final months of pregnancy, and is caused by excess acid in the stomach. Treat as for indigestion (see page 84). In addition, a tea or infusion of meadowsweet and marshmallow calms the stomach. Two drops of sandalwood to a large tablespoonful of carrier oil massaged into the solar plexus can help. Alternatively, drink a drop in some water. Peppermint can be used instead.

BACKACHE

Backache is a common problem as pregnancy advances, for the obvious reason of carrying around a large and unaccustomed weight. This places great strain on the musculo-skeletal system generally but has a particular effect on the spine and muscles of the back. The approaches described in "Neck and Back Pain" (pages 66–73) and "Nerve, Muscle, and Joint Pain" (pages 74–81) are applicable.

CHILDBIRTH PAIN

Every woman knows of the pain, none want it, but few realize how much can be done to alleviate and even prevent it—naturally.

BEFORE LABOR

Preparing early in the pregnancy is vital for a "pain-free" birth, and to minimize any after-effects. There are many natural ways to do this.

Nutritional and dietary therapy

Eating a healthy diet and taking a good multivitamin with folic acid and vitamin E daily will help ensure that you and the baby are not missing vital nutrients.

Herbal medicine and relaxation

Drink raspberry leaf tea regularly over the last three months: it helps tone the womb. Learn special breathing and relaxing techniques: yoga and self-hypnosis are useful.

Massage and aromatherapy

Massage jojoba oil into the perineum—the area between the vagina and the anus—everyday during the last two months or so: it makes the skin more supple, and helps prevent tearing during the last stages of labor. Massage the breasts, thighs, and abdomen with generous amounts of lavender and neroli essential oils (20 drops of lavender to 5 of neroli, mixed into almond or wheatgerm carrier oil), every morning and night for the last four or five months of pregnancy: it improves the skin's elasticity and helps prevent stretch marks. Other useful oils are rosewood and frankincense. An alternative is vitamin E cream.

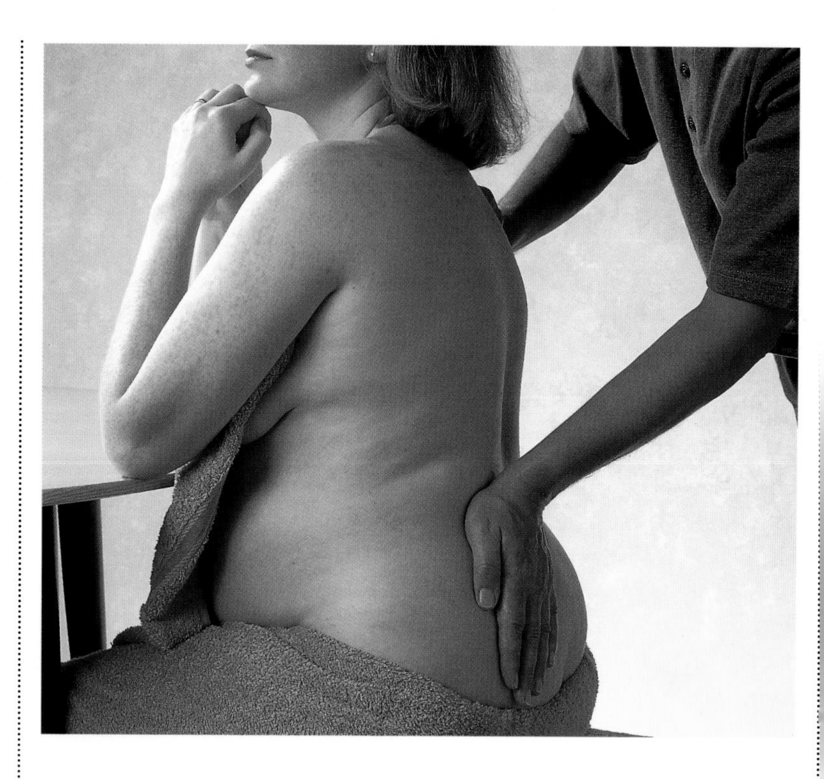

Use firm downward strokes with the heel of the hand to relax the lower back muscles during pregnancy. Work on both sides of the spine simultaneously.

DURING LABOR

Many women prefer not to take drugs during the labor itself, but many have found that the following natural approaches bring welcome relief.

Electronic devices

TENS is only now coming into common usage for all forms of pain—particularly pain of the nerves, muscles, and joints—but it was its help in childbirth pain that was largely responsible for its wider acceptance. Every childbirth clinic or center worthy of the name should now offer TENS to a woman in labor if she wants it. However, it is worth checking in advance that it is available.

Relaxation

Controlled breathing, especially that taught as part of yoga (pranyama), along with meditation and visualization can be used extremely effectively to minimize labor pain, but it is best to be introduced in advance to a method that suits you by an expert.

Massage and aromatherapy

Getting a partner or friend to massage the lower back with a mixture of the oils of lavender (15 drops), rose, and ylang ylang (five drops each) is both relaxing and strengthening, especially if experiencing a long labor. Firm downward strokes should be used.

Rosemary, lavender, or chamomile oil massaged onto the wrists, forehead, or neck is useful for self-help.

Acupressure

Apply firm pressure on a point on the inside of either leg a hand's width above the ankle. Back pain is relieved by pressing a point on either side of the spine immediately below the last rib.

Homeopathy and flower remedies

The remedies caulophyllum 6c (to ease delivery) and gelsemium 3c (to ease pain) are recommended. Bach Rescue Remedy can help if taken during labor.

AFTER LABOR

The aftermath of labor can be painful both physically and psychologically. Again, natural approaches can help enormously.

Psychological therapies

Seek as much help from partner, family, and friends as you need. Do not feel guilty—in most cases they are only too ready to help. Alternatively, your doctor may be able to refer you for help from healthcarers such as counselors.

Water birthing

Many women find that giving birth sitting in a large tub of warm water, supported by others (especially her partner) is both comforting and pain-relieving. Water birthing is more widely available in some countries than others, but it is usually possible to choose this option in modern centers. Failing this, it may be possible to rent your own pool for a home birth, provided you have a qualified midwife in attendance. Inquire well in advance—and be prepared to make a stand if that is your preference.

CAUTION Severe postnatal depression, in which sufferers become manic, experience delusions, and lose touch with reality, is extremely rare, but see a doctor as soon as possible if you feel you may be in this category.

Massage and aromatherapy

Regular warm baths with lavender oil will ease any vaginal pain and promote healing, especially if the vagina tore during labor, or an episiotomy was performed (a cut in the vagina to ease the baby's passage), and stitches inserted. The oils of jasmine or ylang ylang, either in the bath or vaporized, can help ease postnatal depression—a "drop in spirits" that sometimes follows childbirth as a result of hormonal readjustments.

Nutritional and dietary therapy

Regular rest and eating healthily is as important now as before childbirth. However, this can prove difficult during the first few months of caring for a baby, so take a good multivitamin/mineral daily to ensure sufficient nutrient intake.

Flower remedies

Various flower remedies can help a wide variety of problems of mood sometimes arising after childbirth. (Refer to chart on page 149.)

Other therapies

From a qualified therapist only

Acupuncture • pages 150–151
Hypnotherapy • page 153

Massage

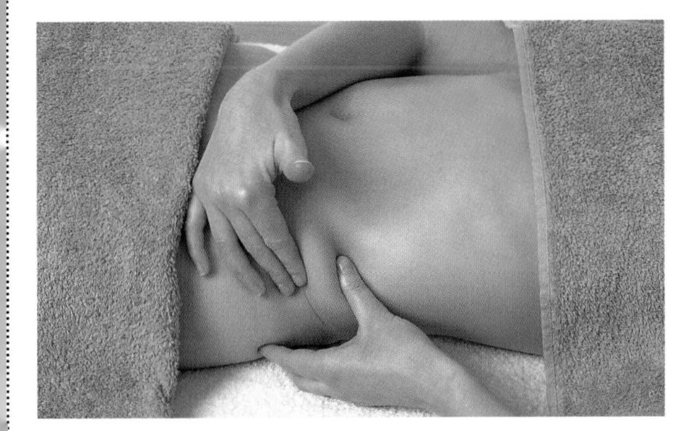

The abdominal muscles are likely to need toning up for some weeks after childbirth. Lie down in a comfortable position and lift and squeeze the tissues on the side of the abdomen between the fingers of one hand and the thumb of the other, then release.

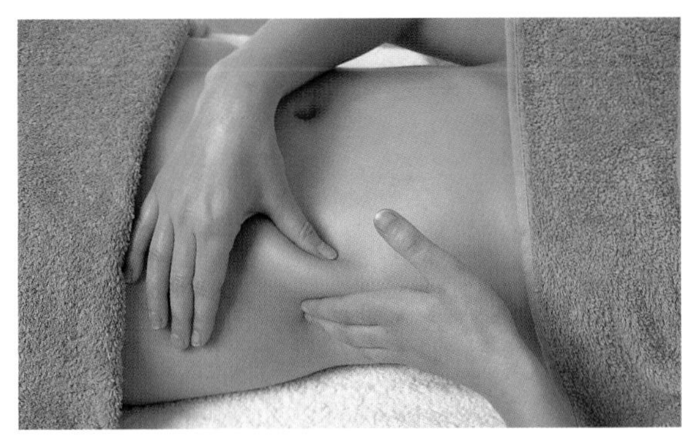

Repeat the lifting and squeezing technique, this time swapping the function of each hand. Continue for a few minutes, alternating hands. Apply the same technique on the other side, then move the hands to the central abdominal muscles and repeat.

BABIES AND CHILDREN IN PAIN

While aches—vague, nonspecific, general discomfort—seem to be almost entirely an adult problem, often associated with aging, pain is common to all age groups. But children, and especially babies, can suffer severe discomfort as a result of illnesses that are confined exclusively to the very young. This section deals with the treatment of pain from illnesses in children (under 12 years old) and babies (under 3 years old).

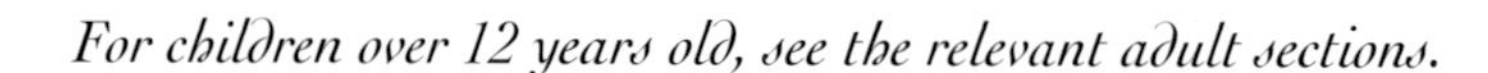

For children over 12 years old, see the relevant adult sections.

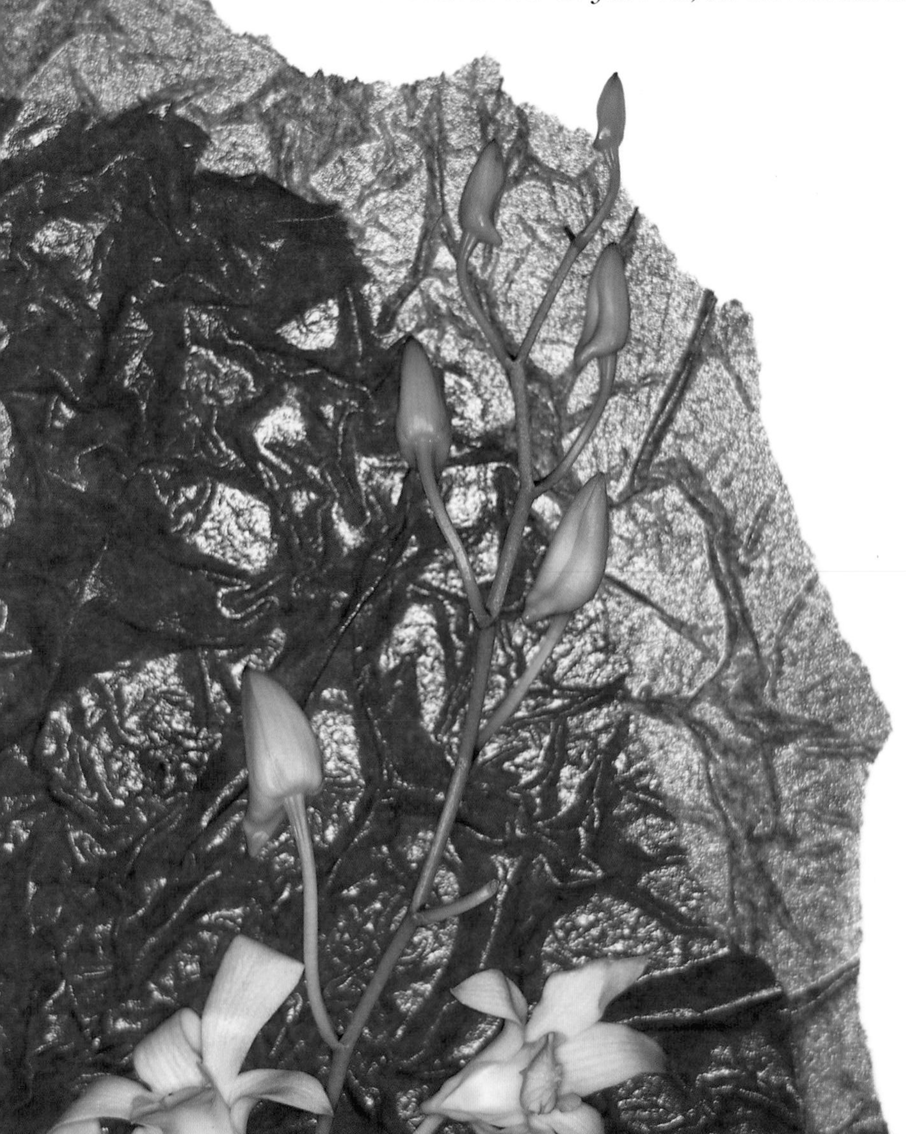

DIAPER (NAPPY) RASH

Keep the area clean with organic (hypoallergenic) cleansing cream and let plenty of fresh air get to it. Chamomile lotion, comfrey, or castor oil ointment, and olive or almond oil, all provide effective relief. The homeopathic remedies sulfur 6c and rhus tox 6c may help.

COLIC AND STOMACHACHE

Colic (pain in the stomach and colon) is caused by a number of factors to do with diet, eating habits, and stress, and is painful enough to lead to chronic episodes of crying and fretfulness.

Herbal medicine

Gripe water (water with dill seed added) is the standard treatment. Add a drop of fennel or chamomile oil to it to make it even more effective. Another method is to make an infusion of fennel or anise (one teaspoonful of dried herb to a cup of water), and give half a teaspoonful every half hour.

Nutritional and dietary therapy
Give half a teaspoonful of apple cider vinegar with water every hour. To strengthen the dose, mix the vinegar half-and-half with water and give two teaspoonfuls. To weaken, mix one teaspoonful of vinegar to 8 fl oz (225 ml) of water.

Massage and aromatherapy
Gently massaging the abdomen can help (see right). Using a drop of fennel or chamomile oil in half a teaspoonful of neutral carrier oil will be soothing.

TEETHING
A zwieback, hard cracker, teething biscuit, or rusk is most effective. Vaporizing chamomile or lavender essential oils can also be beneficial. The homeopathic remedies chamomila or pulsatilla powders applied to the gums can help too.

ORAL THRUSH
A fungal infection caused by the candida albicans organism found in the mouths of very young children (and also the elderly). In adults, it is more usually a problem in the intestines and, in women, the vagina. Symptoms are small, white patches on the lips, tongue, and gums (not to be confused with mouth ulcers). Consult a doctor if it does not clear within a few days.

Nutritional and dietary therapy
Garlic, olive oil, and live yogurt (containing acidophilus or bifidophilus bacteria, but no sugar) prevent the fungus spreading.

Herbal medicine
Mouthwashes containing aloe vera, myrrh, or calendula are useful, but only for children old enough to rinse and spit.

Massage routine for babies

abdomen

Massage can help circulation and enhance body function. Stroke around the abdomen in a clockwise direction (the direction in which the intestines run). This technique is particularly good for colic.

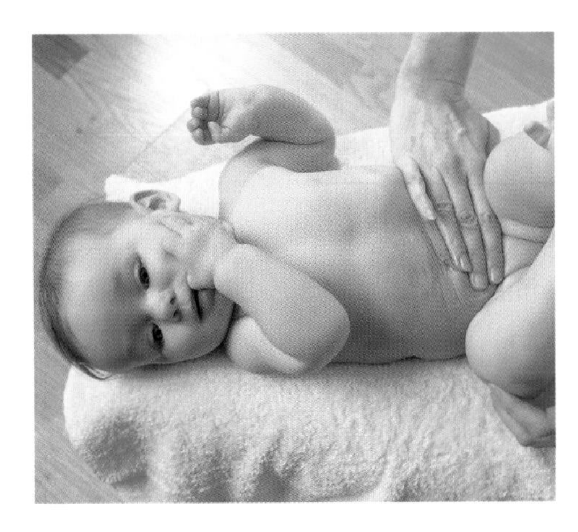

neck

Place the fingers on one side of the neck and the thumb on the other. Gently squeeze, letting the neck slip away from your grip by sliding the hand upward. Combine this stroke with a soothing back massage.

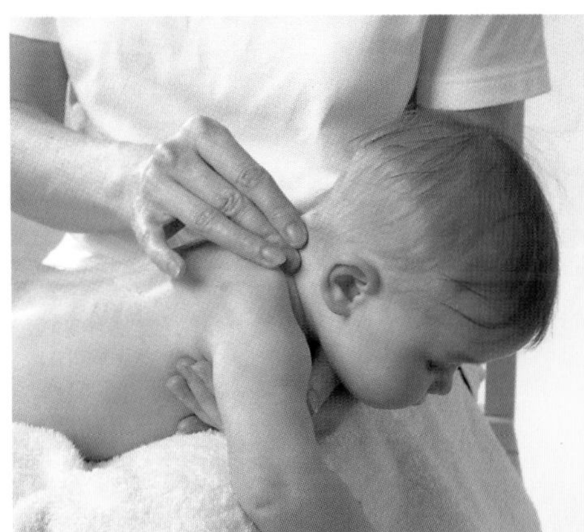

back

Place your hand flat on the small of the baby's back and gently vibrate for a few seconds. Then run your hand up toward the neck, keeping your hand relaxed so as not to crease the baby's skin too much.

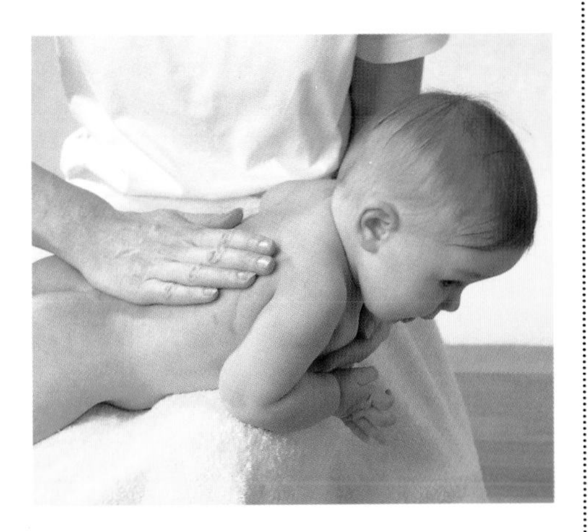

feet

Turn the baby over so that he or she is lying face down and massage the soles of the feet with your thumbs. You can also gently squeeze the whole foot with your hands in this position.

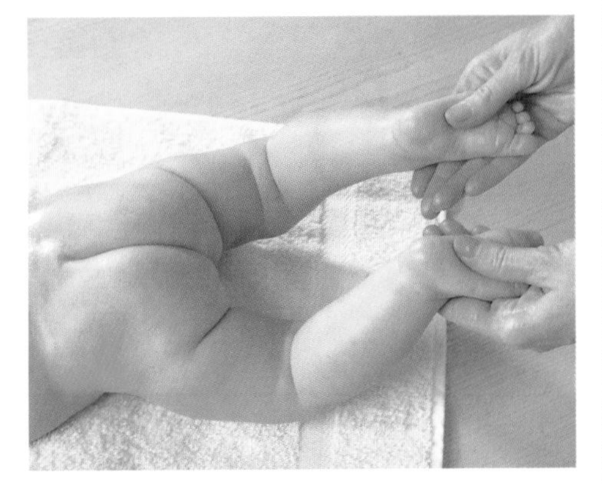

CROUP

A kind of baby version of whooping cough, croup is caused by a bacterial inflammation of the airways, producing a harsh, barking cough and labored breathing with fever, restlessness, and irritability.

Hydrotherapy

Make sure the air for breathing is warm and humid, and the room well ventilated. Humidifiers help or simply boiling a kettle nearby so the child can inhale the steam. However, always stay with the child to avoid accidents occurring.

Herbal medicine

A tea made of equal parts of coltsfoot and vervain will help. Give a teaspoonful to babies and a tablespoonful to children over 3 years, every few hours as required.

Massage and aromatherapy

Gently massage the chest with eucalyptus and sandalwood oil (two drops of each), mixed into a carrier oil (such as grapeseed).

Recommended essential oils for babies and children

Oil	Effective for
Lavender	*All conditions*
Chamomile (Roman, German)	*Earache, colic, teething, vomiting, diarrhea, insomnia*
Mandarin	*Hiccups, upset stomach, insomnia, tearfulness*
Geranium	*Skin problems, throat infections, diarrhea*
Rose	*Headache, eczema, runny nose, tearfulness*
Peppermint	*Toothache, nausea and vomiting, stomachache, itchy skin*
Eucalyptus	*Colds, breathing problems*
Tea tree	*Skin problems (including diaper/nappy rash), thrush, colds, coughs*
Clary sage	*Sleeplessness, tearfulness, excitability*

FEVER

Fever is a raised temperature (in children, a mouth temperature above 99°F/37.5°C, and a rectal temperature over 100°F/38°C). Children suffer from sudden raised temperature much more often than adults, and normally recover from them just as quickly. A fever that continues for more than eight hours, especially if the child is sick and listless, requires medical attention. Herbal teas of elderflower, peppermint, and yarrow can help.

BRUISING AND INJURIES

Ice packs applied immediately, and either arnica tincture or arnica 6c as a homeopathic pill given within the first hour, are effective.

EARACHE

Lying with the head on a covered hot-water bottle can bring relief, especially if the ache is from exposure to cold wind. If due to infection, give vitamin C (1 g) hourly for three hours.

Herbal medicine

Put mullein flower or almond oil drops into the ear (warmed to body temperature and kept in with small swabs of cotton), and give echinacea tincture diluted in water, or garlic capsules.

Homeopathy

Pulsatilla 6c can help earache, but individual prescription from a qualified homeopath is advisable.

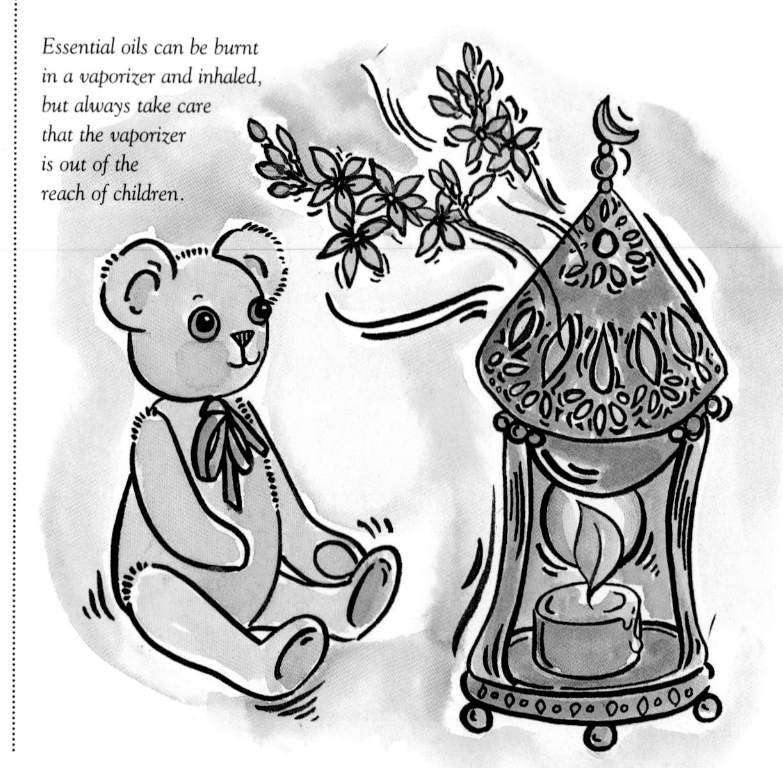

Essential oils can be burnt in a vaporizer and inhaled, but always take care that the vaporizer is out of the reach of children.

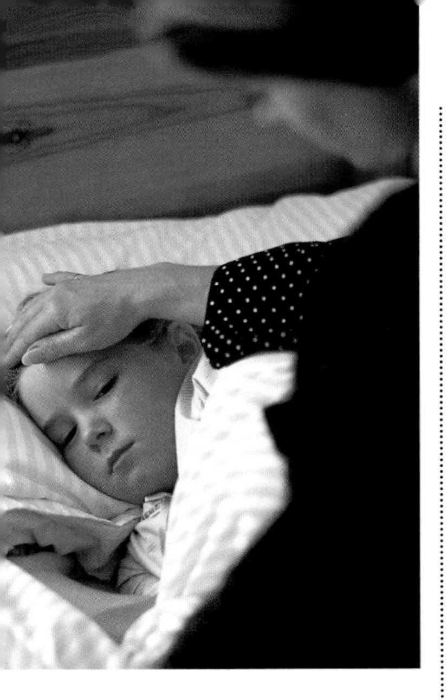

Bed rest, and tender loving care, is all many young children need to recover from minor illnesses.

WHOOPING COUGH

Whooping cough (pertussis) is a bacterial infection of the mucus membranes lining the airways, leading to a cough that ends in a "whoop," accompanied by labored breathing, fever, running nose, and loss of appetite. It can last for weeks and become serious if not treated.

Herbal medicine

Chest compresses made of a hayflower infusion or, in serious cases, onion are highly effective. Alternatives are poultices made of mustard or horseradish, and, if the condition is severe, a mustard bath (but not for too long). White horehound, mullein flowers, thyme, and lavender can also be beneficial.

Nutritional and dietary therapy

Give plenty of liquid, especially fruit juices high in vitamin C.

Homeopathy

Ipecacuanha 3c, coccus cacti 3c, drosera 3c, or aconitum 3c can help (the last two especially at nighttime), but the advice of a qualified therapist is advisable.

Congestion-clearing cocktail for children

Simmer a few slices of ginger root in a cup of water for 15 minutes. Add the juice of ½ lemon and sweeten with honey. Drink while hot.

COUGH

For coughs due to chest infection, wild cherry bark or white horehound "tea" is best (give half a teaspoonful three times daily). A mixture of hot lemon juice, honey, and glycerin can be drunk regularly to ease symptoms. Inhalation of 3–4 drops of eucalyptus oil in hot water for about 10 minutes will also help. Children over eight can have thyme, cypress, or sandalwood inhalations as alternatives.

SORE THROAT

Children are particularly prone to "strep" throat, an acute sore throat caused by streptococcus bacteria. Severe cases may need antibiotics, but try gentler methods first.

Herbal medicine

A gargle or sips of sage, thyme, or lemon tea—sweetened with honey, if necessary—will alleviate the discomfort. For very young children, use just pure lemon juice.

MUMPS

Swollen neck glands, headache, sore throat, and high temperature characterize this illness, caused by a virus and caught by contact with an infected person. It is not serious in children, but can be in adolescent and adult males, often leading to inflamed testicles. Symptoms usually pass after a week to 10 days.

Herbal medicine and hydrotherapy

Saturate a cloth with heated oil of hypericum, wring it out, apply to the swollen glands, and cover with a hot-water bottle. Alternatively, mix the oil with potter's clay, spread on a cloth, and apply in the same way. Another treatment is to apply a warm compress of arnica or calendula extract to the swollen area (add a few drops of either herb to the water the compress is soaked in). Older children can benefit from gargling with diluted tincture of sage.

SKIN IRRITATION

Rubbing on lavender oil is effective against spots; peppermint or rose is good for itchy skin; and tea tree for infected cuts and scratches. With the exception of lavender, oils should be diluted in a little neutral carrier oil before being applied.

CAUTION Major skin irritation resulting from illnesses such as measles, chickenpox, and parasites (worms and head lice) should be treated only after reference to a doctor. If the doctor is agreeable, the oils above, particularly lavender, can help alleviate irritation.

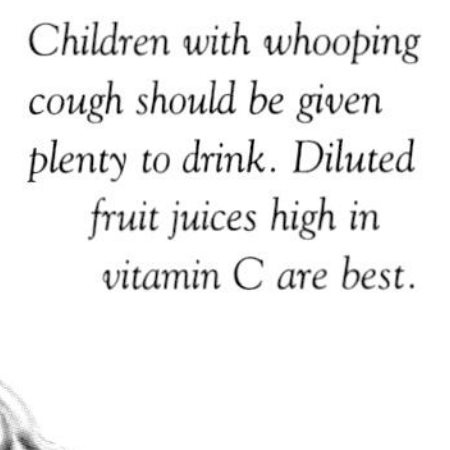

Children with whooping cough should be given plenty to drink. Diluted fruit juices high in vitamin C are best.

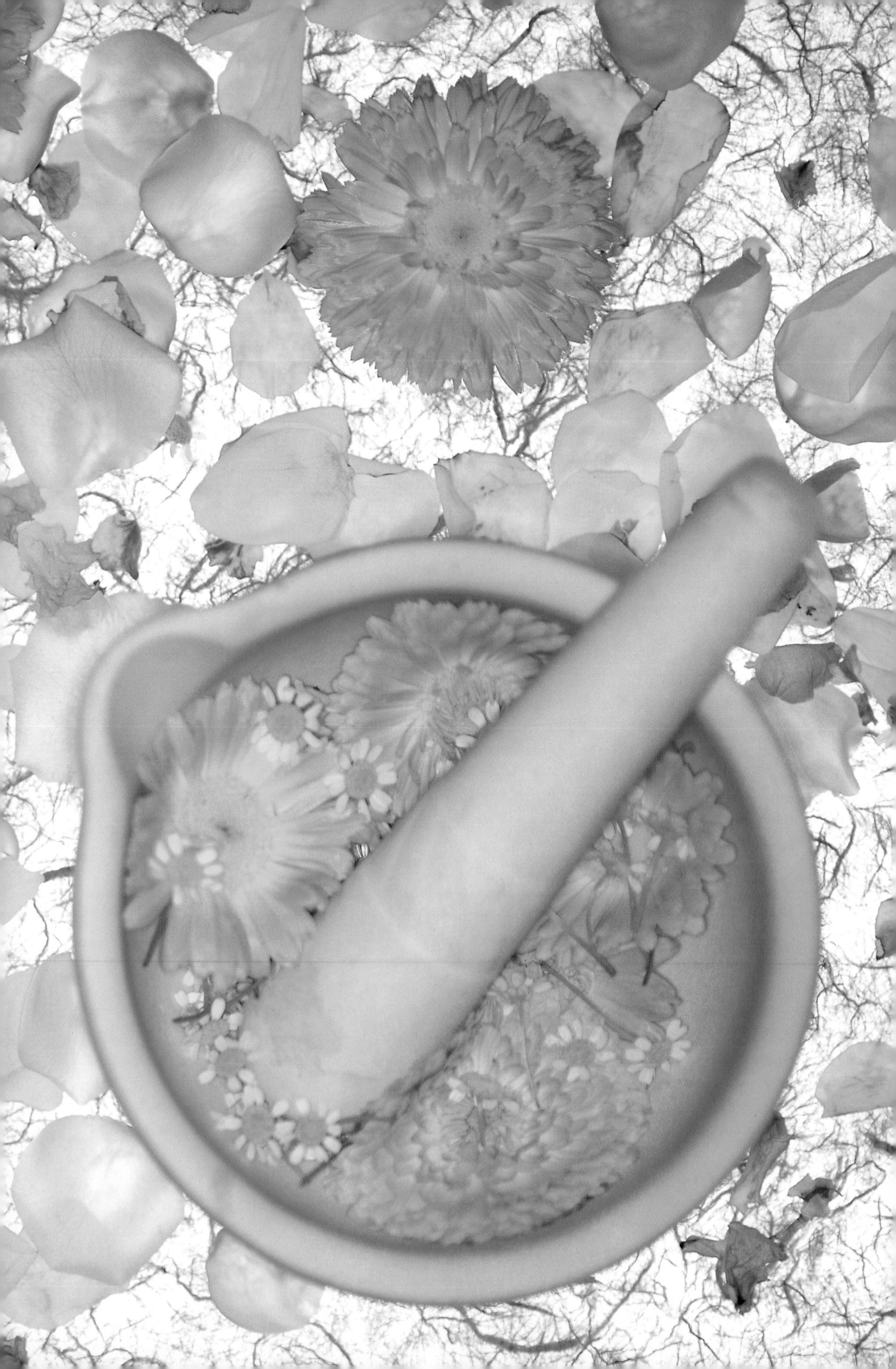

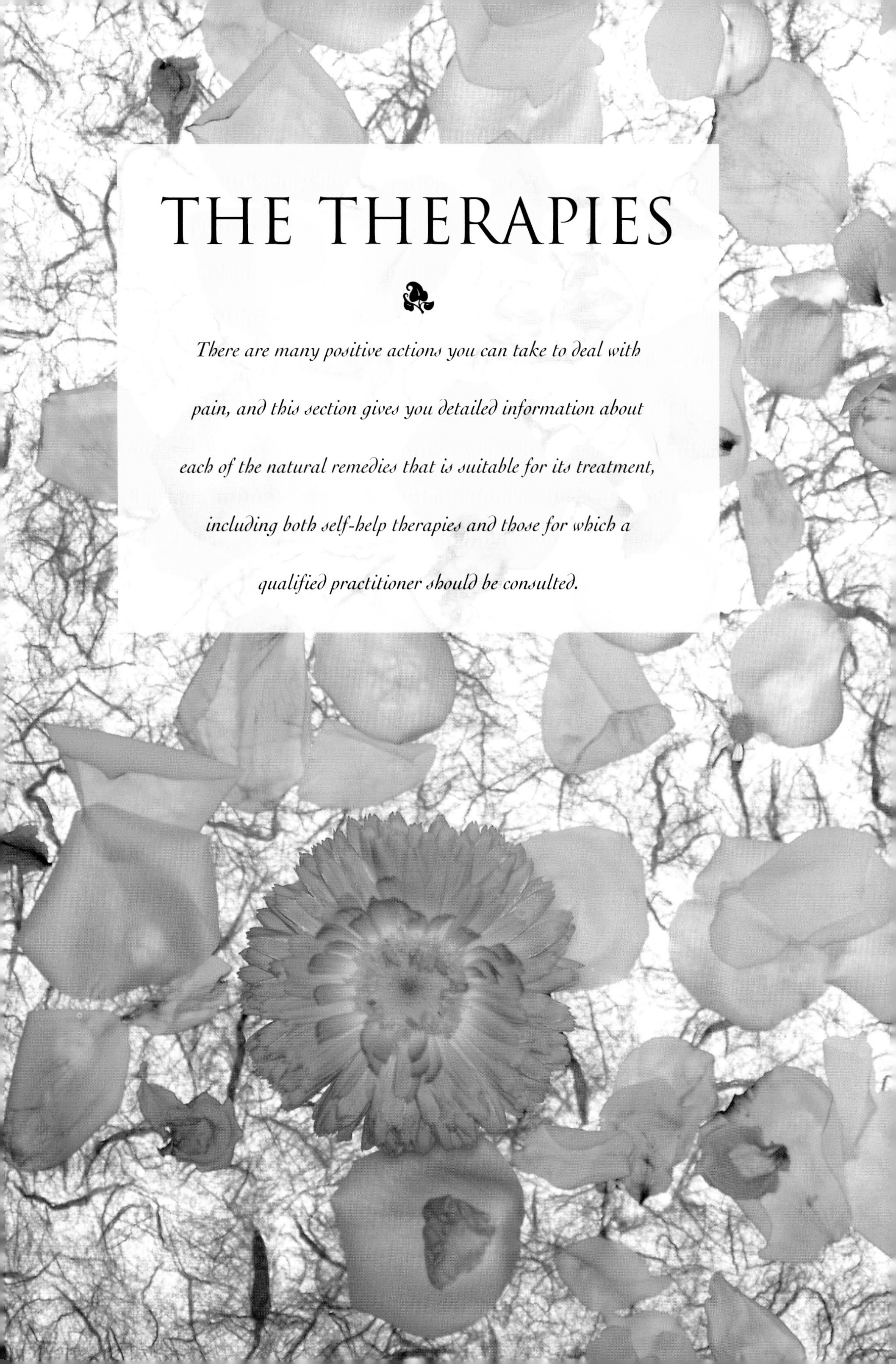

THE THERAPIES

There are many positive actions you can take to deal with pain, and this section gives you detailed information about each of the natural remedies that is suitable for its treatment, including both self-help therapies and those for which a qualified practitioner should be consulted.

AT-A-GLANCE GUIDE TO THERAPIES

SELF-HELP

PHYSICAL

Naturopathy and hydrotherapy
All pain, including headaches, migraines, eyestrain, earache, sinusitis, tooth and jaw ache, sore throats, neck strain, low back pain, coughs, bronchitis, asthma, pleurisy, circulation problems, stomachache, constipation, diarrhea, cystitis, hemorrhoids, nerve pain, fibromyalgia, bursitis, carpal tunnel syndrome, arthritis, heat rash, eczema, psoriasis, chlamydia, vaginitis, pregnancy, childbirth, cancer

Dietary and nutritional therapies
Migraines, depression, angina, circulation problems, hayfever, cold sores, asthma, pneumonia, tuberculosis, stomachache, indigestion/heartburn, nausea, ulcers, gallstones, constipation, diarrhea, irritable bowel syndrome, diverticulitis, appendicitis, inflammatory bowel disorder, hemorrhoids, gallstones, urinary tract infection, cystitis, kidney stones, nerve inflammation, fibromyalgia, carpal tunnel syndrome, gout, arthritis, osteoporosis, ankylosing spondylitis, eczema/dermatitis, psoriasis, pelvic inflammatory disorder, premenstrual syndrome, painful periods, thrush

Electronic devices
Migraines, sinusitis, arthritis, low back pain, slipped disk, sciatica, fibromyalgia, bursitis, cramp, post-herpes infection, sports injuries, breaks and sprains, cancer

Herbal medicine
Headaches, migraines, depression, eyestrain, earache, tinnitus, sinusitis, toothache and sore gums, mouth ulcers, sore throat, neckache, coughs, colds and flu, bronchitis, asthma, pleurisy, pneumonia, tuberculosis, angina, circulation problems, stomachache, indigestion/heartburn, nausea, ulcers, gallstones, constipation, diarrhea, irritable bowel syndrome, diverticulitis, appendicitis, inflammatory bowel disorder, hemorrhoids, urinary tract infection, cystitis, kidney stones, fibromyalgia, bursitis, gout, arthritis, ankylosing spondylitis, heat rash, boils, blisters, tinea/ringworm, eczema/dermatitis, psoriasis, prostatitis, herpes, prolapse, premenstrual syndrome, painful periods, vaginitis, cancer

Massage
Headaches, migraines, depression, eyestrain, sinusitis, neck strain, backache,

MOVEMENT

Yoga and tai chi
Headaches, migraines, depression, neck and back pain, asthma, angina, high blood pressure, constipation, irritable bowel syndrome, nerve pain, arthritis, ankylosing spondylitis, osteoporosis, sexual problems, pregnancy, childbirth

Alexander technique
Headaches, migraines, neck and back problems, fibromyalgia, circulation and breathing problems, including asthma

PSYCHOLOGICAL

Self-hypnosis
Aches and pains due to mental, emotional, and physical problems

Relaxation therapies
Headaches, migraines, depression, back strain, breathing problems, asthma, angina, circulation problems, high blood

SUBTLE ENERGY

Acupressure
Headaches, migraines, sinusitis, hayfever, whiplash injury, back pain, coughs, asthma, angina, palpitations, circulation problems, stomachache, nausea, gallstones, diarrhea, irritable bowel syndrome, urinary tract infection, cystitis, kidney stones, nerve pain, fibromyalgia, bursitis, carpal tunnel syndrome, feet and ankle problems, gout, arthritis, pelvic inflammatory disease, premenstrual syndrome, painful periods, childbirth, cancer

Reflexology
Headaches, migraines, depression, pneumonia, emphysema, stomachache, indigestion/heartburn, nausea, constipation, irritable bowel syndrome, nerve pain, feet and ankle pain, cancer

Homeopathy
Psychological pain, eyestrain, infections, migraines, sore throat, hayfever, coughs, asthma, stomachache, indigestion, colitis, Crohn's disease, flatulence, urinary tract infection, cystitis, kidney stones,

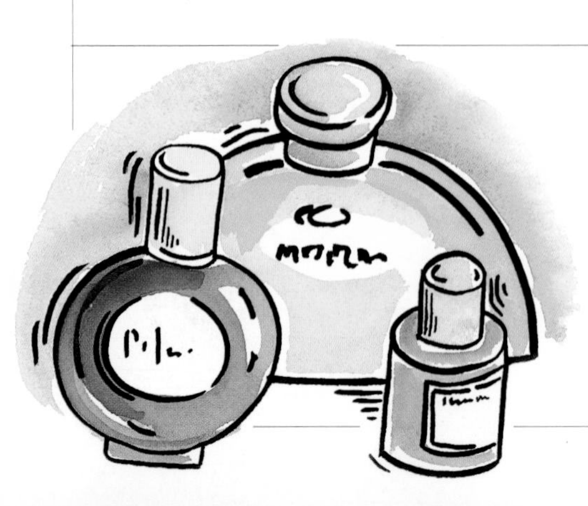

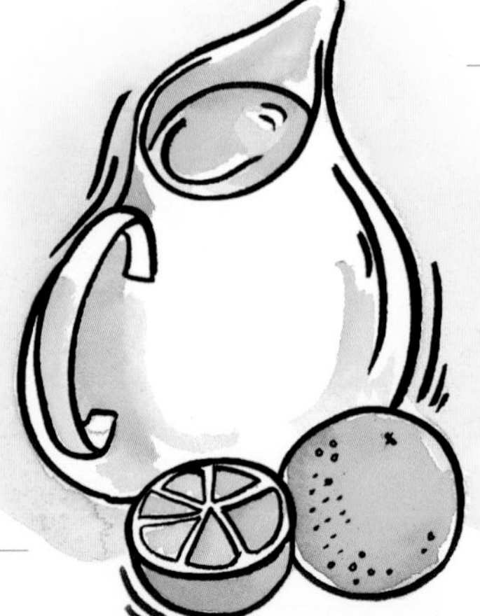

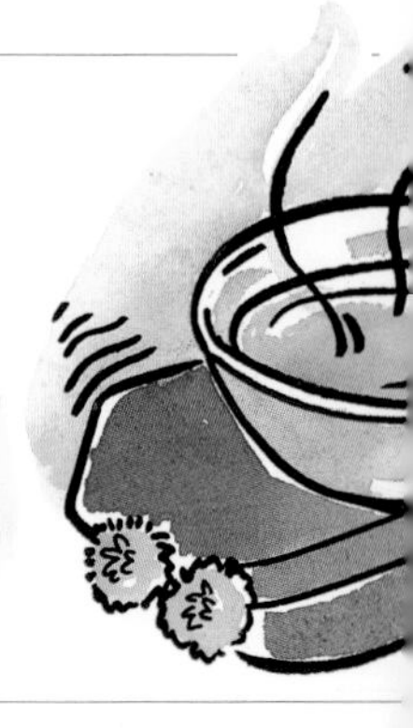

coughs, bronchitis, pleurisy, emphysema, asthma, angina, poor circulation, stomachache, constipation, diverticulitis, fibromyalgia, bursitis, carpal tunnel syndrome, feet and ankle pain, gout, arthritis, osteoporosis, ankylosing spondylitis, eczema/dermatitis, pregnancy, childbirth, cancer

Aromatherapy
Headaches, migraines, depression, earache, neck strain, backache, coughs, bronchitis, asthma, pleurisy, emphysema, palpitations, angina, stomachache, gallstones, constipation, irritable bowel syndrome, fibromyalgia, bursitis, gout, arthritis, osteoporosis, ankylosing spondylitis, heat rash, boils, blisters, tinea/ringworm, eczema/dermatitis, vaginismus and sore vagina, childbirth, cancer

Chiropractic
Headaches, neck and back strain, poor posture, sciatica, asthma

Osteopathy
Headaches, sinusitis, jaw strain, poor posture, fibromyalgia, repetitive strain injury, sciatica, neck and back strain, rheumatoid arthritis, joint sprains, breathing difficulties, asthma, digestive problems, infection, childbirth

Cranial osteopathy
Headaches, concussion after-effects, sinusitis, jaw problems, tinnitus, meningitis, recurring infections, neck and back strain, postnatal strain, and, in infants, colic, glue ear, hyperactivity, and disturbed sleep

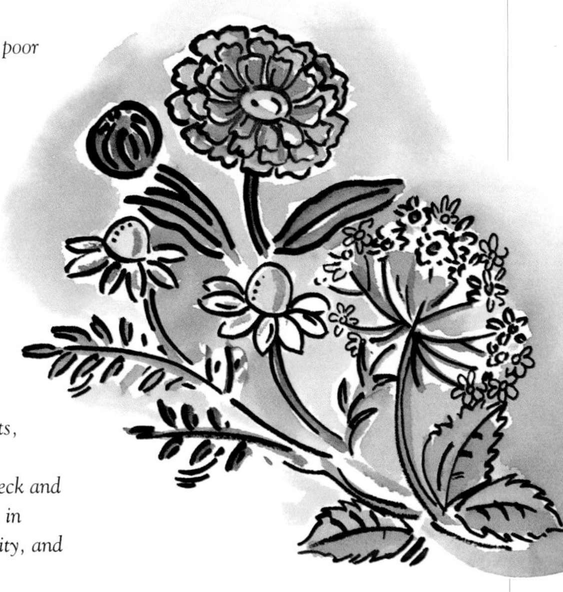

pressure, stomachache, irritable bowel syndrome, nerve pain, eczema, psoriasis, sexual problems, cancer

Creative arts therapies
Headaches, migraines, depression, obsessions, phobias, addictions, eating and digestive disorders

Acupuncture
Headaches, migraines, depression, addictions, tinnitus, sinusitis, neck and back strain, slipped disk, breathing problems, asthma, palpitations, poor circulation, stomachache, nausea, ulcers, gallstones, constipation, diarrhea, irritable bowel syndrome, diverticulitis, appendicitis, colitis, cystitis, kidney stones, nerve inflammation, fibromyalgia, bursitis, carpal tunnel syndrome, restless legs and leg pain, rheumatism and arthritis, ankylosing spondylitis, eczema, psoriasis, hernia, impotence, vaginismus, premenstrual syndrome, painful periods, childbirth pain, postnatal pain, cancer

fibromyalgia, bursitis, arthritis, ankylosing spondylitis, eczema, psoriasis, bruising

Healing
All, especially headaches, migraines, asthma, back pain, infections, cancer

Flower remedies
Psychological pain

Hypnotherapy
Mental and emotional pain: depression, phobias, addictions, obsessions; physical pain: headaches, neck and back ache, digestive and breathing problems

Counseling and psychotherapy
Mental and emotional pain: depression, phobias, addictions, obsessions; physical pain: headaches, neck and back ache, digestive and breathing problems

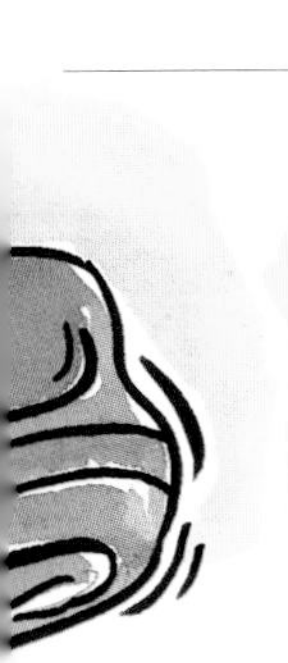

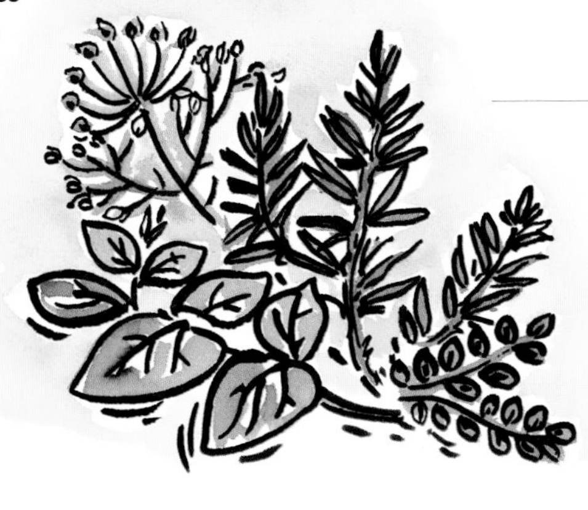

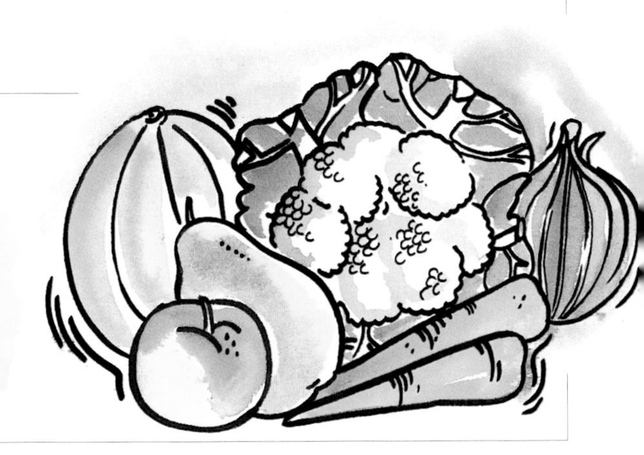

PHYSICAL THERAPIES

Therapies that work in a directly and obviously physical way by processes known and recognized by conventional medicine and science.

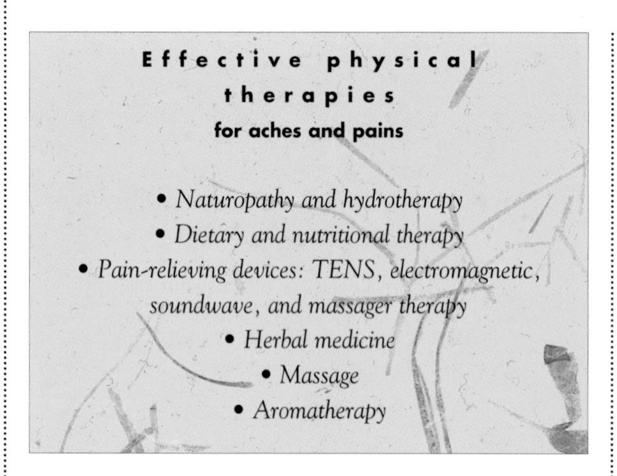

Effective physical therapies for aches and pains

- *Naturopathy and hydrotherapy*
- *Dietary and nutritional therapy*
- *Pain-relieving devices: TENS, electromagnetic, soundwave, and massager therapy*
- *Herbal medicine*
- *Massage*
- *Aromatherapy*

NATUROPATHY AND HYDROTHERAPY

Naturopathy means "natural treatment," and so naturopathy is the umbrella term now used in most western countries to cover a range of therapies that come under the heading of "natural medicine." In particular, as far as the effective natural treatment of pain is concerned, it includes hydrotherapy.

Developed from approaches to health and healing articulated over 2400 years ago by ancient Greek pioneers such as Hippocrates, the "father of medicine," naturopathy is based on the belief that the body will cure itself of anything as long as it takes in only pure air and water, is kept clean, indulges in healthy activity, and eats the right food.

This philosophy was all but forgotten in Europe during the Dark Ages but was revived and further developed in the 18th and 19th centuries, particularly in central Europe, by a new generation of pioneers, such as Preissnitz, Kneipp, Semmelweiss, Lindlahr, and Lust, who all believed that illness seldom occurs if the body is looked after in the way that nature intended. Modern naturopathy began in the United States, when Lindlahr and Lust arrived as emigrants there at the start of the 20th century (the term "naturopathy" was coined by Lust at that time).

Modern naturopaths follow much of the basic philosophy of their forebears, with some additions. For example, they believe that getting sick is a completely natural occurrence, and that methods of cure should follow the same natural principles. So, rather than being suppressed, symptoms of illness should be encouraged to "come out," and the body helped to fight back and find its proper balance again.

Naturopaths routinely prescribe brief fasting to get over infections, such as flu, and pay a great deal of attention to the health of the intestines (or bowels) where nutrients are absorbed into the bloodstream. The theory is that toxins in the bowels may have a part to play in the cause of many illnesses. Naturopaths encourage special diets to clear the gut and eliminate the overgrowth of hostile yeasts and bacteria that can

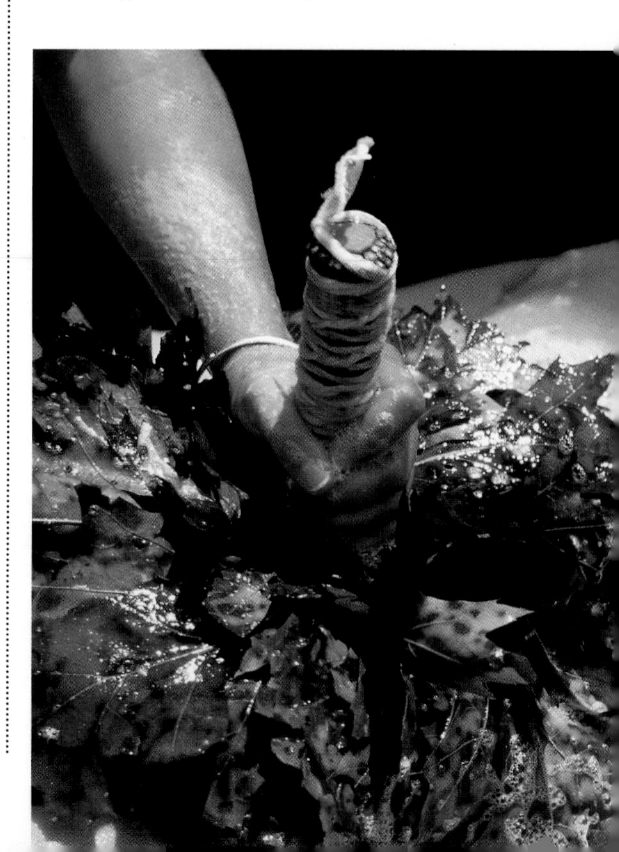

colonize the intestines and, they believe, contribute to toxicity, allergy, and poor immunity.

Known as "nature cure" or "natural hygiene," this "pure" approach survives among a few naturopathy practitioners, who think it wrong even to prescribe extra nutrients in the form of vitamin and mineral supplements, but it is no longer the usual approach of what is generally meant by natural medicine today. Modern naturopathy has widely extended its repertoire to include most of the therapies we now know as "natural," and its practitioners are generally trained at specialist colleges in a range of skills that include acupuncture, herbalism, homeopathy, manipulation, massage, hypnotherapy, nutritional and dietary therapy, and hydrotherapy.

This wide-ranging approach has become the standard training worldwide for those interested in practicing natural medicine in its broadest sense. Countries such as the United States, Canada, Australia, Germany, Israel, New Zealand, and South Africa run full three- and four-year courses leading to a recognized degree of doctor of naturopathy. (Britain, where the trend is proving slow to be accepted by those who run the natural therapies, is one of the few exceptions to this development.)

Birch twigs bunched together and used as a skin scrubber is one of a wide range of therapeutic techniques traditionally used in hydrotherapy. The woman in this picture is being treated at a Turkish bath.

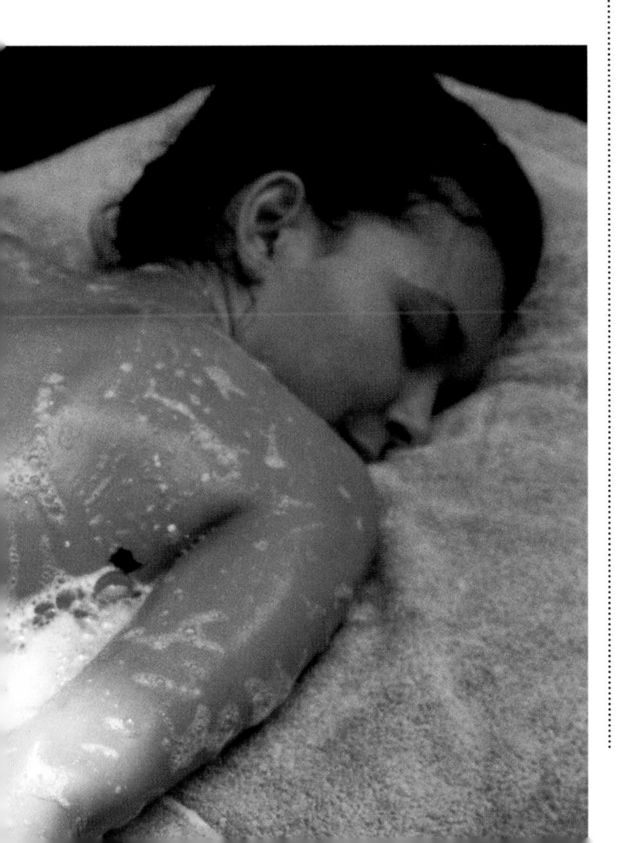

Special note

Most naturopaths would not regard many of the therapies coming under their umbrella as suitable for self-help, on the grounds that they can be dangerous if used without the proper training. In particular, acupuncture, herbalism, chiropractic and osteopathy, hypnotherapy, nutritional therapy with high doses of supplements, and even homeopathy, they will insist, should only be carried out by or under the supervision of a qualified practitioner.

This advice is sound and sensible when it comes to considering high-dose remedies for unusual or serious conditions—and therapies such as acupuncture, chiropractic, osteopathy, and hypnotherapy should never be carried out by nonspecialists. But for most everyday complaints, self-prescription and treatment by herbal and homeopathic remedies and nutritional supplements, in particular, is acceptable, and can be effective, as long as the remedies are bought from reputable suppliers and the instructions printed on the labels followed.

NATUROPATHY *as a general description of natural therapy is effective for aches and pains due to all causes, but for its benefits as a method of self-help, see under individual therapy headings.*

HYDROTHERAPY

Fortunately, one of the most effective naturopathic treatments for pain—hydrotherapy—is extremely suitable for self-help. Hydrotherapy treatment, which is increasingly in use in mainstream physical (or physio-) therapy, involves the therapeutic use of swimming, hot and cold compresses, douches, jet sprays, and hot and cold baths and showers. Steam ("Turkish") baths and saunas are both examples of hydrotherapy that is effective for pain relief.

Hydrotherapy is effective for all aches and pains due to headaches, migraines, eyestrain, earache, sinusitis, tooth and jaw ache, sore throats, neck strain, low back pain, coughs, bronchitis, asthma, pleurisy, circulation problems, stomachache, constipation, diarrhea, cystitis, hemorrhoids, nerve pain, fibromyalgia, bursitis, carpal tunnel syndrome, arthritis, heat rash, eczema, psoriasis, chlamydia, vaginitis, pregnancy, childbirth, and cancer.

DIETARY AND NUTRITIONAL THERAPY

Dietary and nutritional therapies share a similar outlook, but the two are not the same. Dietary therapy emphasizes correct eating and drinking to make and keep people healthy, while nutritional therapy is more concerned with the use of nutritional or food "supplements" to treat health problems. So dietary therapists (or dieticians) advise on what you should or should not eat, while nutritional therapists specialize in the recommendation of specific doses of vitamins and minerals for healing purposes.

There is a growing overlap between the two therapies, and it is possible that they may become a single discipline one day, but for the moment important differences remain. Few dieticians accept the need for extra nutrients if a healthy, balanced diet is followed. By contrast, few nutritional therapists, even though they support the idea of healthy eating, believe that the average western diet contains all the nutrients the body needs. This is mainly because they claim that modern methods of food production make most foods low in nutrients. Nutritional therapists often recommend high doses of vitamins and minerals for treatment purposes, whereas dieticians generally do not.

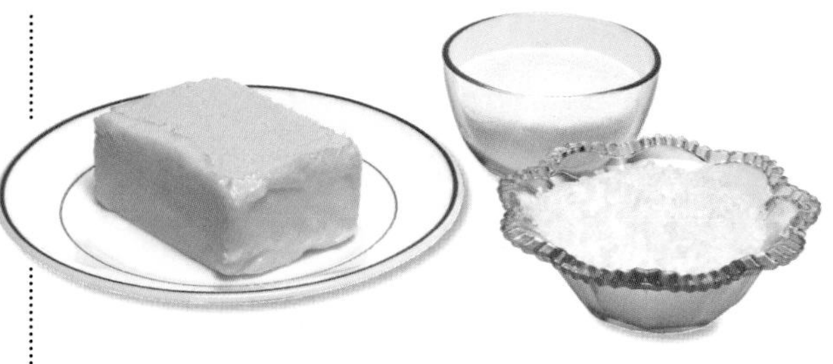

Items such as refined sugar, salt, and saturated fat should be avoided.

DIETARY THERAPY

The basis of dietary therapy is to maximize health by making sure people eat a regular amount (as much as needed, but no more) of wholesome food, with a good proportion of raw fruit, vegetables, and fiber, and as little as possible of saturated fat, salt, and sugar. So a dietary therapist may, for example, draw up a dietary plan for someone based on an analysis of what they have been eating and what they should be eating to improve their overall health.

Treatment by diet also involves knowing when not to eat—in other words, when to fast. Though not all doctors agree, a fast of no more than 24 hours, if carried out under proper supervision, is a perfectly safe and highly effective way of helping the body fight, for example, an infection. Fasting helps clear out toxins

The food combining diet

A diet known as the food combining diet, or Hay diet (after its creator, the American Dr. William Hay), is said to be particularly beneficial for the treatment of arthritic conditions and digestive problems. It entails not eating starch (e.g. pasta, bread, potatoes) at the same time as carbohydrates (e.g. fruit and vegetables), and not eating refined or processed food at all.

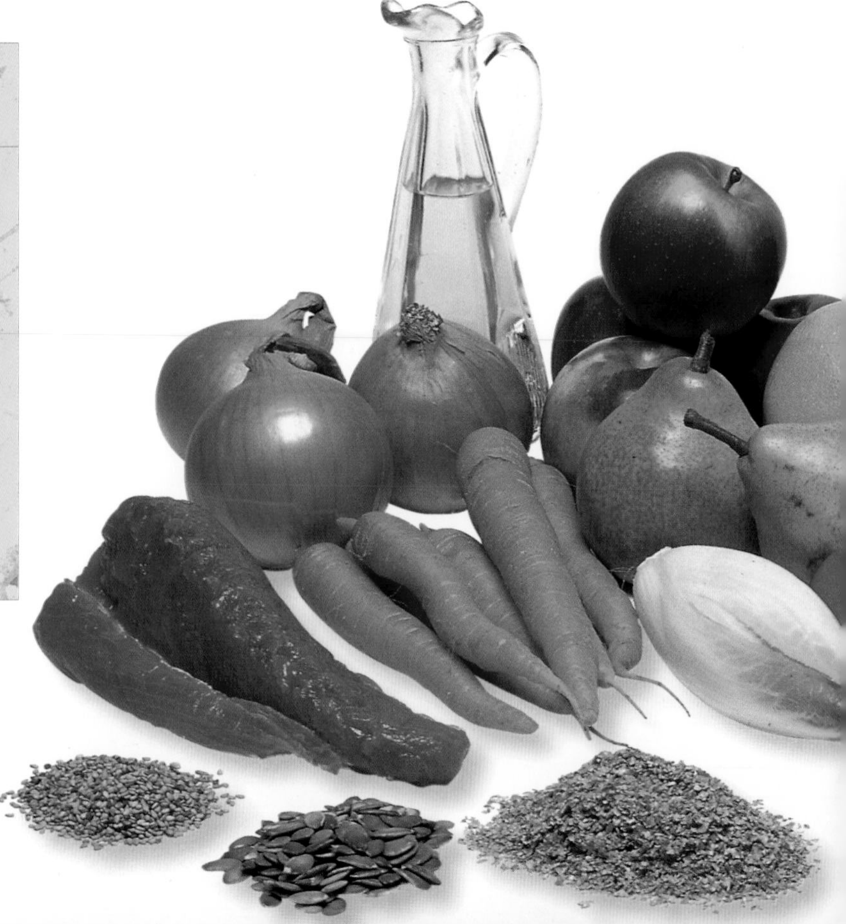

Guide to eating and drinking for a healthy heart

FOODS	EAT REGULARLY	EAT IN MODERATION	AVOID ALTOGETHER
Cakes, biscuits, and desserts	*Homemade cakes and biscuits made using low-fat recipes*	*Cakes and biscuits made with polyunsaturated margarine/oil (two or three times a week), ice-cream, skimmed milk puddings*	*Store-bought cakes and biscuits, cream cakes, dairy cream ice-cream, full-fat milk puddings*
Cereals and breads	*Wholemeal bread, porridge oats, rice, pasta, breakfast cereals*	*White flour, white bread*	*Fancy bread and pastries*
Dairy food and eggs	*Skimmed milk, cottage cheese, egg white, low-fat yogurt*	*Semi-skimmed milk, medium-fat cheese (three times a week), egg yokes (four a week)*	*Full-cream milk, cream cheese, blue cheeses, full-fat yogurt, coffee creamers*
Drinks and soups	*Water, fruit juice, clear soups*	*Alcohol, coffee, tea, low-fat drinking chocolate*	*Cream soups, full-fat milk drinks, cream-based drinks*
Fats and oils	*Olive oil (though all fats need to be limited)*	*Polyunsaturated margarines and oils, low-fat spreads*	*Butter, ghee, margarines not labeled high in polyunsaturates*
Fish	*Sardines, tuna, trout, salmon, white fish (not fried)*	*Shellfish*	*Fried fish, fish roe, fish pâté*
Fruit, vegetables, and pulses	*Most kinds of fresh fruit and vegetables, tofu, soya products*	*French fries and roast potatoes cooked in oil marked high in polyunsaturates or olive oil (once a fortnight), avocadoes*	*Chips/crisps, French fries cooked in oil not marked high in polyunsaturates or olive oil*
Meat	*Chicken, turkey (both without skin), lean ham*	*Lean beef, pork, lamb, bacon (unsmoked), liver, kidney*	*Visible fat on meat, sausages, pâté, duck, salami, meat pies*
Nuts and seeds	*Most kinds, except coconut and salted nuts*	*Salted nuts*	*Coconut*
Other	*Herbs, spices, mustard, cider vinegar, low-fat salad dressing*	*Low-fat salad cream and mayonnaise*	*Salad cream, mayonnaise, creamy dressings*
Preserves and sweets	*None*	*Jellies and jams, marmalade, honey, peanut butter*	*Chocolate spread, sugar, all sweets and confectionery*

Dietary therapy involves advising on what food to eat for optimum health and what to avoid. The foods displayed here are encouraged.

from the system and leaves the immune system free to concentrate on the healing process. Another aspect of dietary therapy is knowing what foods work best with one another—the concept known as "food combining" (see also page 118). The aim is to help the body "cleanse" on the one hand, and achieve "optimum nutrition" on the other. In this respect, at least, dietary therapy conforms to the ideals of naturopathy.

NUTRITIONAL THERAPY

Nutritional therapy as a discipline in its own right grew up in the second half of the 20th century. The idea of using concentrated nutrients in supplement form to treat illness began in the United States, where the first nutrient (or, more correctly, micronutrient) discovered—vitamin A—was identified by Elmer McCollum in 1913. Most influential researchers in this field continue to come from the US.

The therapy is based on the belief that the body can be helped by taking the right micronutrients in the right dose for a particular condition. So a consultation with a nutritional therapist is likely to lead to suggestions not only for a change in diet but also for the use of therapeutic doses of nutritional supplements.

Supplements come in tablet or capsule form, though they can also be powders and liquids. In this sense, they are no different from taking pills prescribed by your doctor, and this has led to some confusion and argument—particularly because, used therapeutically to heal rather than just to keep healthy, the doses recommended can sometimes be extremely high. For example, doses of 20 grams (20,000 milligrams) or more of vitamin C may be recommended to fight disease when the amount recommended by authorities in both the United States and Europe for normal daily consumption is just 60 milligrams.

Megavitamin therapy, as the use of high-dose nutrients is known, is not recommended except under the advice of a qualified practitioner. A few nutrients, notably vitamins A, D, and E, can be toxic if too much is taken, and most nutritionists will prescribe from their own special stocks anyway. Low-dose supplements, on the other hand, are readily available everywhere these days, and taking supplements bought from your local drugstore or health food store, in the doses recommended on the labels, is perfectly safe.

Dietary and nutritional therapies are effective for aches and pains due to migraines, depression, angina, circulation problems, hayfever, cold sores, asthma, pneumonia, tuberculosis, stomachache, indigestion/heartburn, nausea, ulcers, gallstones, constipation, diarrhea, irritable bowel syndrome, diverticulitis, appendicitis, inflammatory bowel disorder, hemorrhoids, gallstones, urinary tract infection, cystitis, kidney stones, nerve inflammation, fibromyalgia, carpal tunnel syndrome, gout, arthritis, osteoporosis, ankylosing spondylitis, eczema/dermatitis, psoriasis, pelvic inflammatory disorder, premenstrual syndrome, painful periods, and thrush.

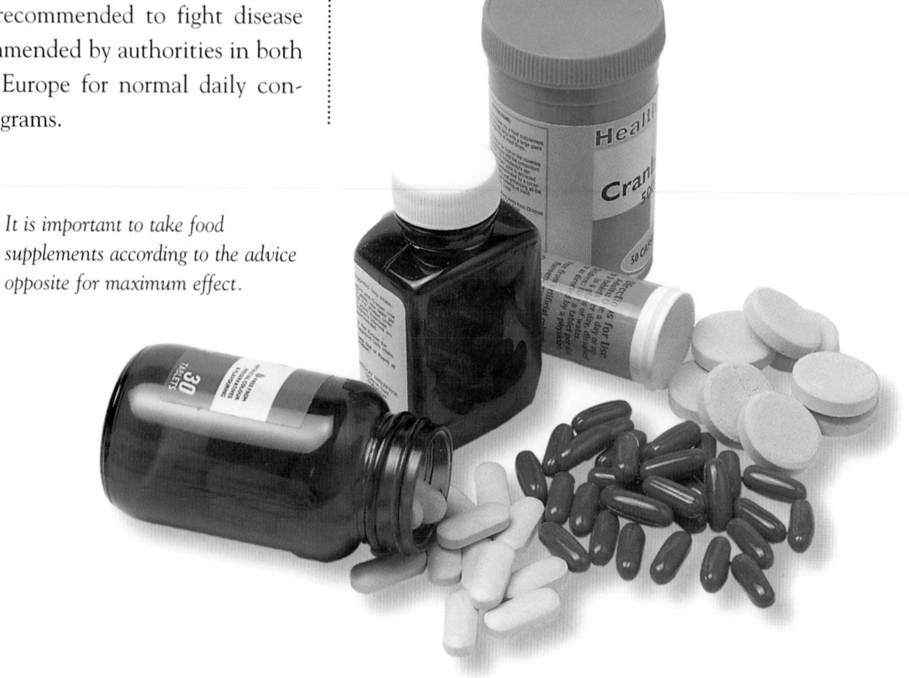

It is important to take food supplements according to the advice opposite for maximum effect.

Recommended daily intakes for vitamins and minerals

USA

Vitamins	Men (25–50)	Women (25–50)	Pregnancy	Lactation
Vitamin A	1000 μg	800 μg	800 μg	1300 μg
Vitamin B6	2 mg	1.6 mg	2.2 mg	2.1 mg
Vitamin B12	2 μg	2 μg	2.2 μg	2.6 μg
Vitamin C	60 mg	60 mg	70 mg	95 mg
Vitamin D	5 μg	5 μg	10 μg	10 μg
Vitamin E	10 mg	8 mg	10 mg	12 mg
Vitamin K	80 μg	65 μg	65 μg	65 μg
Folate	200 μg	180 μg	400 μg	280 μg
Niacin (B3)**	19 mg	15 mg	17 mg	20 mg
Riboflavin (B2)	1.7 mg	1.3 mg	1.6 mg	1.8 mg
Thiamin (B1)	1.5 mg	1.1 mg	1.5 mg	1.6 mg
Minerals				
Calcium	800 mg	800 mg	1200 mg	1200 mg
Iodine	150 μg	150 μg	200 μg	200 μg
Iron	10 mg	15 mg	15 mg	15 mg
Magnesium	350 mg	280 mg	355 mg	340 mg
Phosphorus	800 mg	800 mg	1200 mg	1200 mg
Selenium	70 μg	55 μg	75 μg	75 μg
Zinc	15 mg	12 mg	19 mg	16 mg

EUROPE

Vitamins	RDA	USL*	Minerals	RDA	USL*
Vitamin A	800 μg	2300 μg	Calcium	800 mg	1500 mg
Vitamin B6	2 mg	200 mg	Iodine	150 μg	500 μg
Vitamin B12	1 μg	500 μg	Iron	14 mg	15 mg
Vitamin C	60 mg	2000 mg	Magnesium	300 mg	350 mg
Vitamin D	5 μg	10 μg	Phosphorus	800 mg	1500 mg
Vitamin E	10 mg	800 mg	Zinc	15 mg	15 mg
Biotin	150 μg	500 μg			
Folic acid	200 μg	400 μg	Copper	—	5 mg
Niacin (B3)**	18 mg	150 mg	Chromium	—	200 mg
Pantothenic acid	6 mg	500 mg	Manganese	—	15 mg
Riboflavin (B2)	1.6 mg	200 mg	Molybdenum	—	200 μg
Thiamin (B1)	1.4 mg	100 mg	Selenium	—	200 μg

NOTE *Some nutrients have not yet been allocated recommended daily levels. This is because experts either do not consider them essential (they believe most people get enough of what they need in their daily diet), or they disagree on what the levels should be.*

**USL = upper safe level for daily self-supplementation (as recommended by the UK Council for Responsible Nutrition and the European Federation of Health Product Manufacturers Associations, 1997).*

***Niacin (B3) can be available as nicotinamide or nicotinic acid; take only one of these. USL for nicotinic acid is 150 mg daily; for nicotinamide 450 mg daily.*

KEY *mg = milligram (one thousandth of a gram); μg = microgram (one millionth of a gram).*

How to take supplements

- *Always take supplements with food, or as soon afterward as possible. The only exception is amino acids, which are best taken on an empty stomach.*

- *If you have decided on a course of supplements, take them regularly. Taking them irregularly is no use.*

- *Many vitamins and minerals work synergistically—that is, they work best together. Good examples are the B vitamins, and vitamin C and zinc. There are 12 or more known B vitamins (more are being identified all the time), and they operate by complementing one another. So as a general rule, it is best to take B vitamins as a "B-complex." Equally, vitamin C needs zinc to work properly. So vitamin C on its own is not as effective as when taken with zinc. Other vitamins and minerals have a similar relationship, and that is why taking a good-quality multinutrient supplement (a range of vitamins, minerals, and other nutrients in one tablet or capsule) is the best option for most people. For optimum results, though, it is a good idea to seek the advice of a qualified nutritional therapist before selecting a course of supplements.*

- *If taking a number of supplements, divide them equally between meals—for example, half at breakfast, and half at lunch; or a third at breakfast, a third at lunch, and a third at dinner. Make sure you spread the combination evenly throughout the day: do not take all of the vitamin C in the morning and all of the B-complex in the evening.*

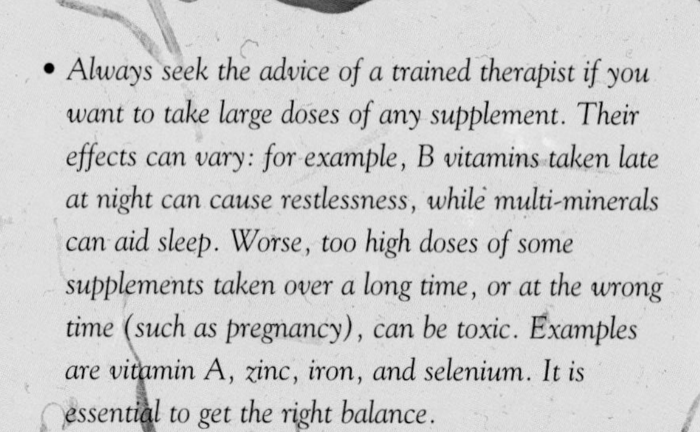

- *Always seek the advice of a trained therapist if you want to take large doses of any supplement. Their effects can vary: for example, B vitamins taken late at night can cause restlessness, while multi-minerals can aid sleep. Worse, too high doses of some supplements taken over a long time, or at the wrong time (such as pregnancy), can be toxic. Examples are vitamin A, zinc, iron, and selenium. It is essential to get the right balance.*

- *Do not expect overnight miracles, but do expect to feel benefits within the first three months. If you are not noticing positive changes then see a nutritional therapist for advice. Consult a therapist as soon as possible if you begin to feel unwell or are worried about side-effects or unusual symptoms.*

Regular intake of selected vitamins and minerals can help prevent illness as well as fight pain.

ELECTRONIC DEVICES

A number of devices for pain relief are now widely advertised, costing from a few dollars or pounds to several hundred. Though they appear to be very different, they all work by stimulating increased blood flow to the affected area, and interfering with pain messages getting to the brain. In effect they do mechanically exactly what we do when we ease the pain of banging ourselves by rubbing the spot. Rubbing not only increases blood flow, which accelerates the healing process, but "distracts" the nervous system, so that pain signals do not get through. Hand-held vibrating massagers, infrared toners, and soundwave devices do this with varying degrees of success, often depending as much on how comfortable the user feels with them as on any direct therapeutic effect.

More subtle devices that make use of the invisible waves of the electromagnetic spectrum, notably electricity and magnetism, have an established, and growing, record of helping with the symptoms of both acute and chronic pain. The best known method, now utilized in many conventional pain clinics throughout the world, is transcutaneous electrical nerve stimulation, or TENS. A new generation of devices that use magnetic frequencies below 25 Hz for pain relief is increasingly popular, and appears to be having some good success. Such devices are less readily available than the toners and massagers as a means of self-help, however, because of the need, in most cases, to consult a practitioner before starting and for supervision.

Electromagnetic therapy

Electromagnetic fields not only encourage the healing process, accelerating the rate at which both tissue and bones repair after accidents or surgery, but can also reduce levels of pain. Small magnets sewn into or attached to adhesive and other bandages are widely promoted as a self-help remedy for a number of conditions, including pain relief, but claims have been contradictory, and evidence so far inconclusive.

Some claim they work as an alternative to acupuncture, by stimulating chi ("subtle energy") at the energy "points" in the same way as needles, and others that the effect is similar to TENS. Better results have been recorded with Empulse, a device that claims to work by correcting deficiencies in brain waves using electromagnetic impulses.

TENS DEVICES

Transcutaneous electrical nerve stimulation (TENS) is the use of a device that sends electrical impulses from a battery or batteries to the nerves from electrodes attached to the surface of the skin at specific places on the body, usually on or near the site of the ache or pain. It works on the principle of the gate control theory (see page 11). The electrical impulses effectively fool the body into not feeling pain by "blocking out" the pain sensations trying to get through the pain "gate."

Since its development in the early 1970s, TENS has proved one of the most effective pain-relieving therapies now available, for both acute (immediate) and chronic (long-lasting) pain. It is especially useful for acute pain, providing up to 80 percent relief for all types of pain, and 50 percent for chronic pain. Recent developments in manufacturing mean that TENS devices are now available for home use by anyone with minimal training and at relatively little cost.

GigaTENS is a more sophisticated version that originated in Ukraine and is now being developed in the United States. It claims much more dramatic results by pulsing just a billionth of a watt at 52–78 GigaHertz (GHz), or a billion cycles per second. However, it remains controversial.

SOUNDWAVE THERAPY

The use of low-level soundwaves for pain relief is not new, even though it sounds as if it should be. The therapy, now usually called "intasound," was first developed in the 1920s in Sweden. But it is only in recent years that a hand-held device, developed in Denmark, has been in wide use as a quick and easy method of self-help. The device directs low-level soundwaves through tissues to stimulate blood flow at a deep level, promoting the repair of inflamed or damaged tissue at basic cellular level. Results are variable, but some people claim to have been helped dramatically.

TENS and soundwave therapy is effective for aches and pains due to migraines, sinusitis, arthritis, low back pain, slipped disk, sciatica, fibromyalgia, bursitis, cramp, post-herpes infection, sports injuries, breaks and sprains, and cancer.

HERBAL MEDICINE

Herbalism (the use of herbs or plants to heal) is probably the oldest form of medicine. It was almost the only type of effective treatment in the western world until the 18th century—and in many countries it is still the dominant method of healing.

Medical herbalism is enjoying a revival in the West as a result of public disenchantment with the unpleasant side-effects of so many pharmaceutical drugs, and the arrival of a growing number of practitioners trained in the rich oriental tradition. This is introducing a range of previously unknown and apparently effective remedies for many conditions, including pain. Oriental herbs are being incorporated into the repertory of western herbalists, who have been successfully drawing on the best of both European and North American traditions for some time.

Modern pharmaceutical medicine is largely based on herbal medicine, and it has been estimated that around 60 percent of all modern medicines are plant-based. But traditional herbalists object even to plant-based modern drugs, because they claim that the process of isolating and extracting specific compounds from plants—which pharmaceutical companies need to do to patent and commercialize a drug—concentrates the chemicals too much and removes the natural balancing effect of other substances in the plant. They also maintain that the body reacts against synthetic chemicals precisely because they are not natural.

To distinguish what they offer from both native herbal remedies and commercial synthetic drugs, modern herbalists in the West now tend to use terms such as "phytotherapy" and "botanical medicine" rather than herbal medicine to describe their work. Practitioners will still prepare their remedies individually from the raw ingredients, and offer them in the

Preparing herbal remedies

It is recommended that you consult a qualified herbalist before preparing homemade herbal remedies.

Infusions

An infusion is a kind of tea that can be drunk hot, cold, or iced. It is suitable for leaves and flowers. Add two cupfuls of boiling water to two teaspoonfuls of the herb. Leave to infuse for 10 minutes, stirring occasionally. Strain and sweeten with honey if you wish.

Decoctions

A decoction is used for the hard parts of the plant, such as roots, bark, and seeds, which must be boiled or simmered to release their essences. Add 1oz (30g) of the herbal mixture to each 16oz (500ml) of water in a pan. Do not use an aluminum pan, which will leach toxic traces into the mixture. Bring to a boil and simmer for about 10 minutes. Cool and strain, squeezing the herbs in order to extract all the juices.

Tinctures

A tincture is a way of preserving herbs for a period of up to two years. This is usually done in alcohol, which is also a good solvent for most of the active substances in the herb. Ready-made tinctures from a herb supplier tend to be stronger and last longer, but tinctures can be homemade by adding powdered herb to a 50 percent alcohol solution. Leave the herb to steep for two weeks, shaking daily, then strain and bottle. Add a tablespoonful to water or tea.

Poultices

A poultice, or plaster, can be used to apply herbs externally to an affected area. Mix the crushed herbs into a warm paste of flour or cornmeal and water, or bread and milk, apply to the skin and cover with a cloth. Keep moist by the addition of warm water at intervals. The herbs can also be mixed with a little warm water and placed between layers of gauze or cheesecloth before application to the skin.

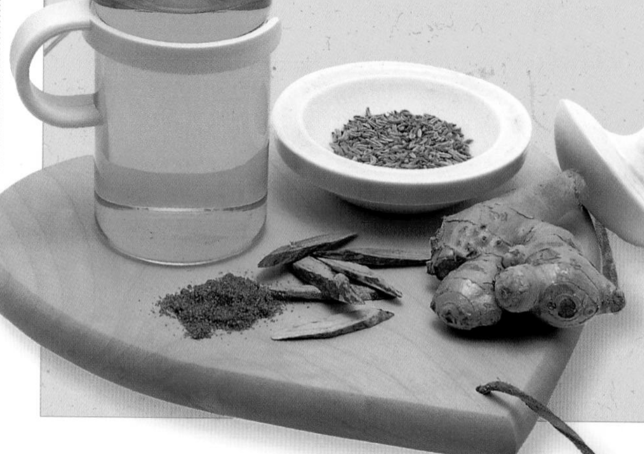

Ginger, licorice, saw palmetto, and celery seed decoction.

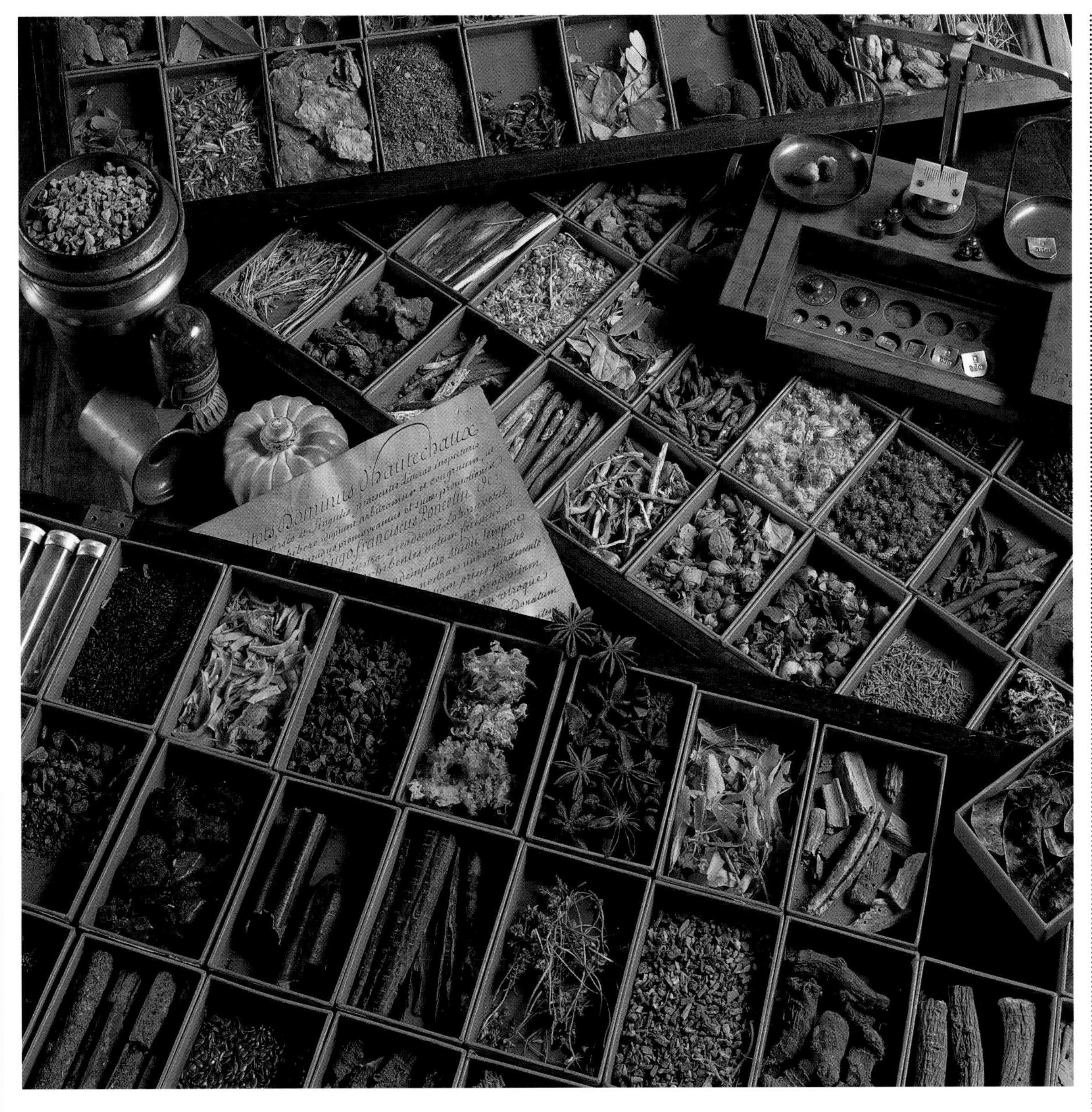

Western herbalists rarely display their herbs as in this picture any more, but in China, where more than 4000 herbs are still in wide use, the sight is a common one in most market places.

form of liquids, as dried herbs you can make into "teas," or as parts of the plant (root or leaves, for example) to take internally or apply externally.

Herbal remedies for the self-treatment of routine problems are increasingly available from drugstores and health food stores in tablet or capsule form. But individual treatment for more serious conditions, using raw herbs, is only recommended from a qualified herbalist. Herbs are powerful drugs, and some are dangerous in untrained hands. To make sure you use the right herb in the right dose for the right symptoms, without the risk of side-effects, go only to herbalists who are properly trained.

Herbal medicines are effective for aches and pains due to headaches, migraines, depression, eyestrain, earache, tinnitus, sinusitis, toothache and sore gums, mouth ulcers, sore throat, neckache, coughs, colds and flu, bronchitis, asthma, pleurisy, pneumonia, tuberculosis, angina, circulation problems, stomachache, indigestion/heartburn, nausea, ulcers, gallstones, constipation, diarrhea, irritable bowel syndrome, diverticulitis, appendicitis, inflammatory bowel disorder, hemorrhoids, urinary tract infection, cystitis, kidney stones, fibromyalgia, bursitis, gout, arthritis, ankylosing spondylitis, heat rash, boils, blisters, tinea/ringworm, eczema/dermatitis, psoriasis, prostatitis, herpes, prolapse, premenstrual syndrome, painful periods, vaginitis, cancer.

A brief guide to herbal remedies

Agrimony
tinea, diarrhea

Aloe vera
bruises, scalds, sunburn, blisters, shingles, mouth and stomach ulcers, vaginitis

Angelica (archangelica)
cough

Arnica
bruises, chilblains, whiplash, backache

Balmony
gallstones

Bilberry
stomach ulcers

Blackberry
eczema

Black cohosh
tinnitus, arthritis, prolapse, premenstrual syndrome

Black horehound
nausea, vomiting

Black willow
joint pain

Bogbean
nerve pain, arthritis

Boldo
gallstones

Boneset
colds, flu, fever

Borage
premenstrual syndrome, depression, anxiety

Bromelain
backache, angina

Broom
circulation pain

Buchu
cystitis, urethritis

Burdock
psoriasis, gout

Butterbur
asthma

Calendula
cuts, stings, scalds, sunburn, chilblains, heat rash, eczema, tooth abcess, hemorrhoids, vaginitis, chlamydia, cystitis, gingivitis, mouth ulcers

Cape aloe
constipation

Catmint
sore throat

Centaury
gallstones

Chamomile
hangover, hives, eczema, headache, earache, asthma, nerve pain, stomachache, nausea, indigestion, constipation, inflammatory bowel disease, cystitis, urethritis, thrush, morning sickness, premenstrual syndrome, insomnia

Chaste-tree
prolapse, premenstrual syndrome

Chickweed
hives, eczema

Cinammon
toothache, indigestion

Cleavers
boils, premenstrual syndrome

Clove
toothache

Comfrey
bruises, emphysema, nerve pain, gout, stomachache, hemorrhoids

Cornsilk
urethritis

Couch grass
cystitis, urethritis, prostatitis

Crampbark
cramp, backache

Cumin
cystitis

Dandelion
psoriasis, gallstones, constipation, circulation pain, prostatitis, premenstrual syndrome

Devil's claw
arthritis, joint pain

Echinacea
boils, psoriasis, colds, flu, earache, sinusitis, sore throat, bronchitis, pleurisy, pneumonia, tuberculosis, cystitis, prostatitis, chlamydia

echinacea

Elderflower
colds, flu, hayfever, sore throat, cough, pneumonia

Elecampane
cough, bronchitis, asthma, pleurisy, tuberculosis

Ephedra
hayfever, asthma

Euphorbia (pilulifera)
asthma

Euphrasia
eyestrain, hayfever

Fennel
bronchitis, indigestion, constipation, cystitis, premenstrual syndrome

Fenugreek
bronchitis

Feverfew
migraine, arthritis

Friar's balsam
frostbite

Fringetree
gallstones

Garlic
psoriasis, colds, flu, sinusitis, sore throat, bronchitis, pneumonia, sciatica, angina, circulation pain

Gentian
gallstones

Geranium (cranesbill)
diarrhea

Ginger
nausea, vomiting, headache, colds, flu, bronchitis, backache, indigestion, circulation pain, menstrual cramps, morning sickness

Ginko (ginkgo) biloba
cramp, tinnitus

Ginseng
asthma, nerve pain, premenstrual syndrome

Golden rod
sinusitis

Golden seal
nerve pain, gallstones, diarrhea, thrush, chlamydia, tinea, eczema, conjunctivitis, sinusitis, hayfever

Gravel root
kidney stones

Hawthorn
palpitations, angina, varicose veins

Hops
nerve pain, constipation

Horse chestnut
varicose veins, hemorrhoids

Horseradish
sinusitis, backache

Horsetail
prostatitis

Hypericum
bruises, cuts, burns, pneumonia, depression, anxiety, earache, backache, nerve pain, gastritis, cystitis, hemorrhoids, vaginitis

Hyssop
earache

Jamaican dogwood
backache, nerve pain

Juniper
pneumonia, gout

Kelp
cramp, premenstrual syndrome

Lavender
heat rash, headache

Lemon balm
depression, anxiety, insomnia, stomachache, indigestion, stomach ulcers, inflammatory bowel disease, palpitations, premenstrual syndrome

Licorice
hayfever, cough, tuberculosis, stomach ulcers, cold sores, sore throat, bronchitis, emphysema, premenstrual syndrome

Lily of the valley
angina, circulation pain

Lime
heat rash, palpitations, angina

Lobelia
earache, pneumonia, backache

Loganberry
eczema

Marshmallow
nerve pain, stomach ulcers, gallstones, heartburn, sinusitis, sore throat, asthma, stomachache

Meadowsweet
headache, toothache, backache, indigestion, phlebitis, heartburn, premenstrual syndrome

Mexican yam
premenstrual syndrome

Motherwort
palpitations, angina

Mullein
earache, cough, asthma, pleurisy, tuberculosis

Myrrh
frostbite, gingivitis, mouth ulcers, thrush

Nettle
hangover, eczema, psoriasis, gout, kidney stones

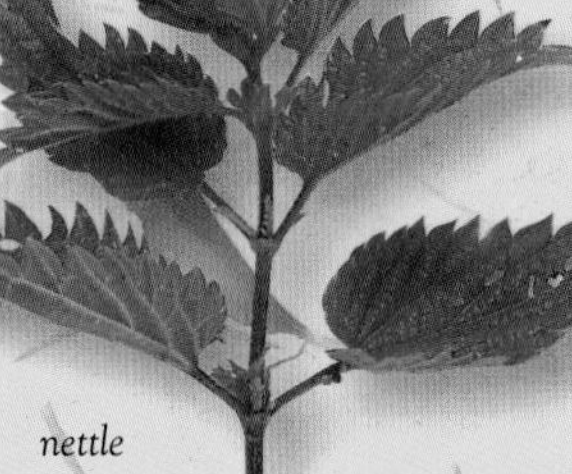

nettle

Parsley
gout, indigestion, kidney stones

Pasque flower
nerve pain

Passionflower
asthma, nerve pain, palpitations, headache

Pennywort (navelwort)
earache

Peony
hemorrhoids

Peppermint
hangover, heat rash, colds, flu, toothache, stomachache, nausea, indigestion, diarrhea, morning sickness

Pilewort
hemorrhoids

Plantain
sore throat, diarrhea

Primula
nerve pain

Propolis
tinea, sore throat

Pulsatilla
prostatitis

Pygeum
prostatitis, impotence

Raspberry
eczema, indigestion, menstrual cramps

Red clover
tinea, psoriasis

Roman chamomile
nausea, vomiting

Rosemary
depression, anxiety, headache, gallstones

Sage
tinea, tonsillitis

Saw palmetto
prostatitis, impotence

Slippery elm
boils, sore throat, asthma, nerve pain, stomachache, indigestion, constipation, inflammatory bowel disease

Spilanthas
sore throat

Staphysagria
prostatitis

Stone root
gallstones, kidney stones

Thyme
mouth ulcers, sore throat, asthma, pneumonia

Valerian
depression, insomnia, headache, anxiety, backache, nerve pain, palpitations

White willow
toothache

Willow
nerve pain, gout, headache, backache, hemorrhoids, premenstrual syndrome

Wintergreen
gout

Witchhazel
insect stings, burns, scalds, hemorrhoids, genital herpes

Yarrow
hangover, colds, flu, earache, cough, pneumonia, cystitis, urethritis, angina, hemorrhoids, fever

Yellow dock
boils, psoriasis

CAUTION *Research into the effects of herbs is an ongoing process. As a result of the findings of such research, some herbs are "scheduled"—that is, they can only be prescribed by a qualified herbalist. The list of scheduled herbs regularly changes, and to make matters more complicated, different countries often have different recommendations. We therefore recommend that you use ready-made preparations that can be purchased from reliable health food and drugstores. If you want to make your own herbal remedies, we strongly recommend that you first consult a qualified herbalist or an appropriate organization for advice. A list of useful addresses is given on page 155.*

MASSAGE

Massage is one of the old and highly effective "touching" treatments widely ignored in the West until recently. Whether utilized as a method of relaxation, or as a more complex "detoxifying" therapy, its benefit for a wide range of conditions, including pain relief, is now so well recognized that it is in growing use in hospitals and nursing clinics everywhere.

The effectiveness of massage lies in stimulating blood flow, relaxing nerves and muscles, and in the psychological benefits of feeling "cared for." The variations available are enormous, from the relatively strong techniques used in Swedish massage to methods so gentle that they hardly seem like massage at all, and have more in common with the "soft-tissue" manipulation used by some osteopaths or "hands-on" healers. Massage can cover all of the body or just a small area, such as the neck and shoulders. The most effective massage is that applied to the entire back. The photographs below show the main ways of giving an effective and satisfying massage, using techniques taught at all leading massage and bodywork schools. They can be applied perfectly safely to any age group of either sex, including children and babies.

The person being massaged should lie horizontal on a comfortable but firm surface in a warm room. It is a good idea to have a couple of large towels at hand also to keep the person warm. The massager should use a neutral oil, so that the hands slide easily over the skin (a number of oils are available in most good health stores and drugstores).

Massage is effective for aches and pains due to headaches, migraines, depression, eyestrain, sinusitis, neck strain, backache, coughs, bronchitis, pleurisy, emphysema, asthma, angina, poor circulation, stomachache, constipation, diverticulitis, fibromyalgia, bursitis, carpal tunnel syndrome, feet and ankle pain, gout, arthritis, osteoporosis, ankylosing spondylitis, eczema/dermatitis, pregnancy, childbirth, and cancer.

Some basic massage techniques

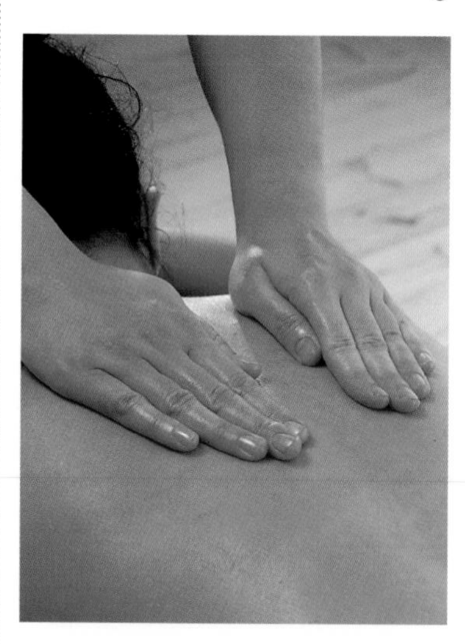

Palm effleurage *(French for "light touching") should be performed at the beginning and end of every massage session. After applying oil, place the palms of the hands side by side on the area to be massaged, and stroke slowly and rhythmically, applying very light pressure. Gradually increase the pressure with each stroke, particularly when stroking in the direction of the heart. Keep fingers close together and turn the fingertips slightly up so that they do not dig into the flesh.*

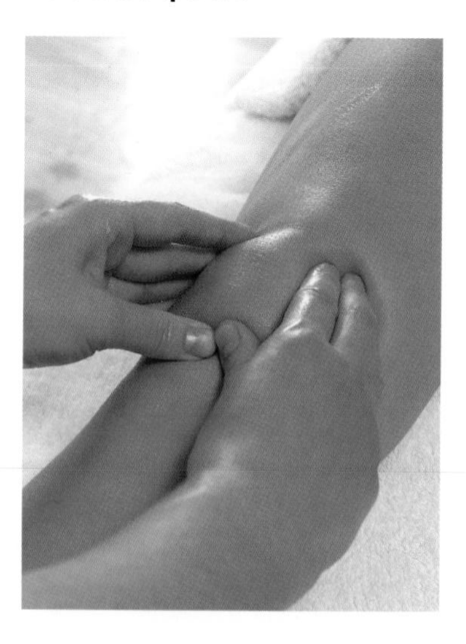

Thumb effleurage *is used to relax tight and tense muscles in areas where the bone is close to the surface. Using the thumbs of both hands, apply a very short, circular movement, concentrating on a small area of muscle at a time. Alternate between one thumb and the other until a softening of the tissue is felt. Move along the skin in this way, trapping the skin with each movement rather than sliding over it. You should apply slightly more pressure than with palm effleurage.*

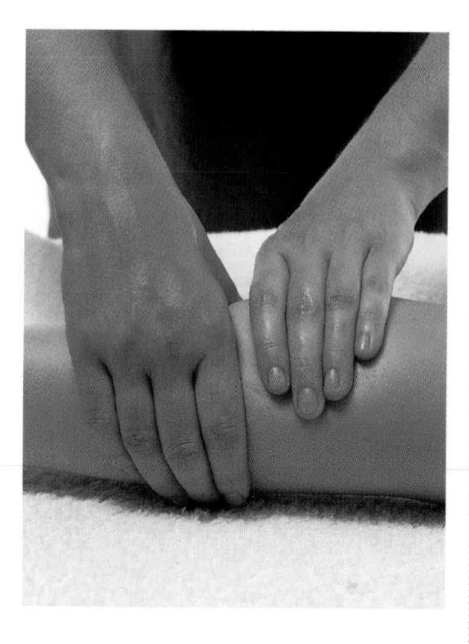

Petrissage *is a French word for kneading. It is a type of wringing movement used to loosen bunches of knotted muscle fibers. Pick up the muscle and apply pressure between the fingers of one hand and the thumb of the other in order to compress and lift the muscle. Having squeezed and twisted the muscle tissue, release it, then lift up again for a repeat compression. Do not slide the fingers along the skin or dig into the tissues.*

Lymph drainage massage

Lymph drainage massage (or lymphatic massage) is a special technique offered by some natural therapists to clear toxins from the lymphatic system, a vital part of the body's immune system. The therapist begins with the glands (or, more correctly, nodes) in the neck and tries gently to move the lymph fluid by massaging the nodes until any swelling is reduced. It is a safe, simple, and sometimes dramatically effective treatment, especially for painful swelling caused by infection.

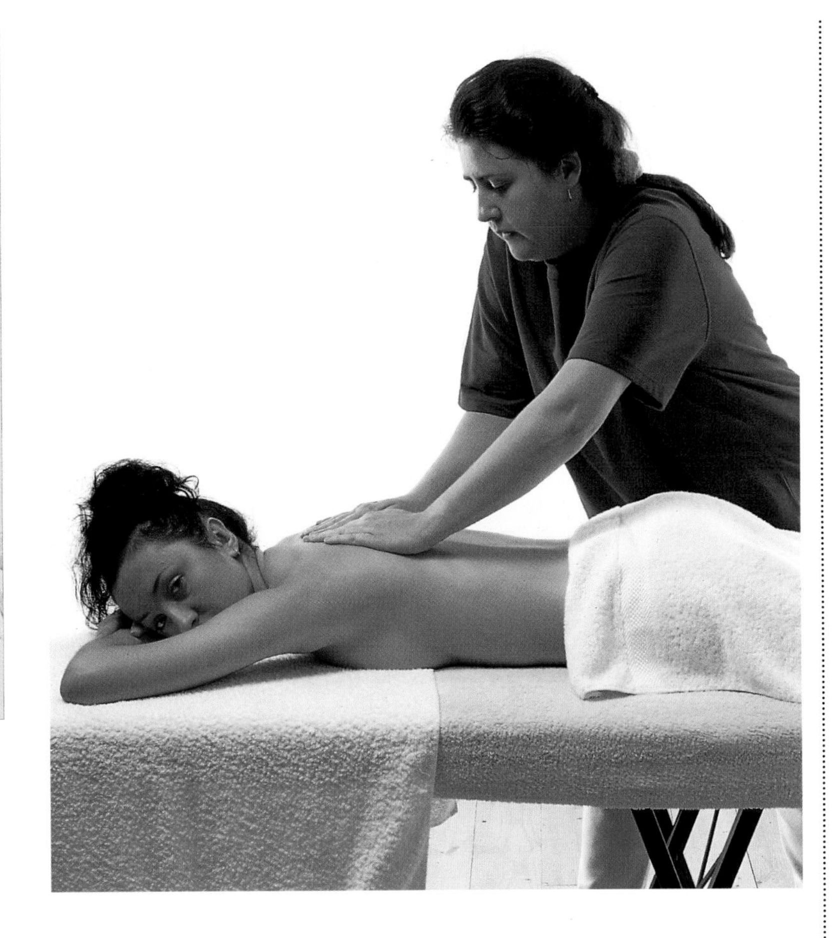

Massage can be both relaxing and invigorating. Self-massage is possible but it is better if you can find someone to do it to you.

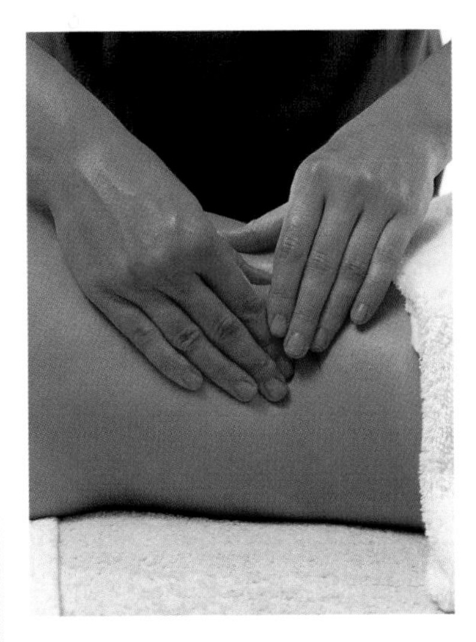

Kneading *itself is used for large areas of flesh where there is no bone immediately below the soft tissue, for example, the waist area and thighs. Pick up the flesh in one hand and pass it over to the other hand, then grasp another handful, and repeat the process in a regular, smooth rhythm. The action is rather like kneading bread. Try to keep the fingers straight and together, and avoid allowing the fingertips to dig into the flesh. This technique is both relaxing and invigorating.*

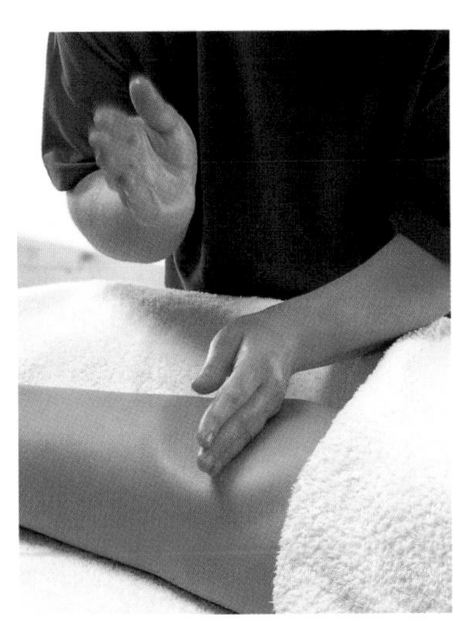

Hacking *is a percussive stroke that increases circulation in the skin and stimulates the nerve endings. It is excellent for toning muscles. Holding your fingers together, apply a light percussive strike with the little finger edges of each hand in turn. Keep the wrists loose as you bring each hand up and down quickly in a smooth chopping motion. Carry out the movement in a controlled and steady manner for a couple of minutes. Do not apply too much pressure.*

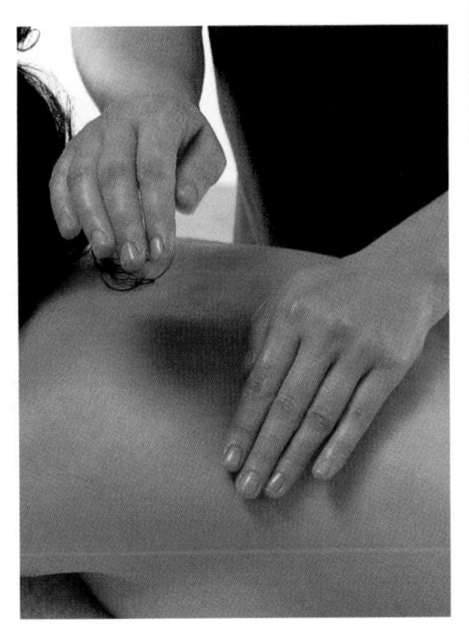

Cupping *is another percussive stroke. Bend the hands where the fingers join the palms as if you were holding a small ball. Tap each cupped hand in turn on the skin, keeping the wrist almost straight and moving the entire forearm up and down. Try to keep the fingers and thumbs close together so that a mini-vacuum is created (this will produce a sound like trotting hooves). The vacuum draws blood to the surface of the skin and is extremely invigorating. Stop after a few minutes.*

AROMATHERAPY

Aromatherapy treats the body with oils distilled from plants considered to have healing properties. Most of the plants used are well-known and often powerful medicinal herbs. The concentrated oils are known as "essential oils," and are notable for their strong and characteristically pleasant odor.

The word aromatherapy means "smell therapy," and so includes treatment by inhaling and vaporizing the oils. But these days aromatherapy is generally taken to mean massaging with aromatic oils, and claims to be the continuation of a tradition practiced widely in the ancient world, particularly Egypt.

Research in France, where the therapy was revived in the 1920s by chemist René-Maurice Gattefosse, has shown that massaged essential oils penetrate the skin, moving into the bloodstream and the lymphatic system within four hours—much as medicinal herbs or drugs do. But therapists believe that the smells given off also have therapeutic value through the olfactory nerves in the nose. Others claim psychological effects for the oils similar to those made for flower remedies.

It is now well established that massaging essential oils can help with a wide range of pain problems, from angina and arthritis to migraine and backache. In addition to working like any herb, they also tone and relax, so helping to ease tension and improve mobility. Most people find the overall effect so pleasurable that it is not surprising that the therapy is also said to benefit depression and fatigue.

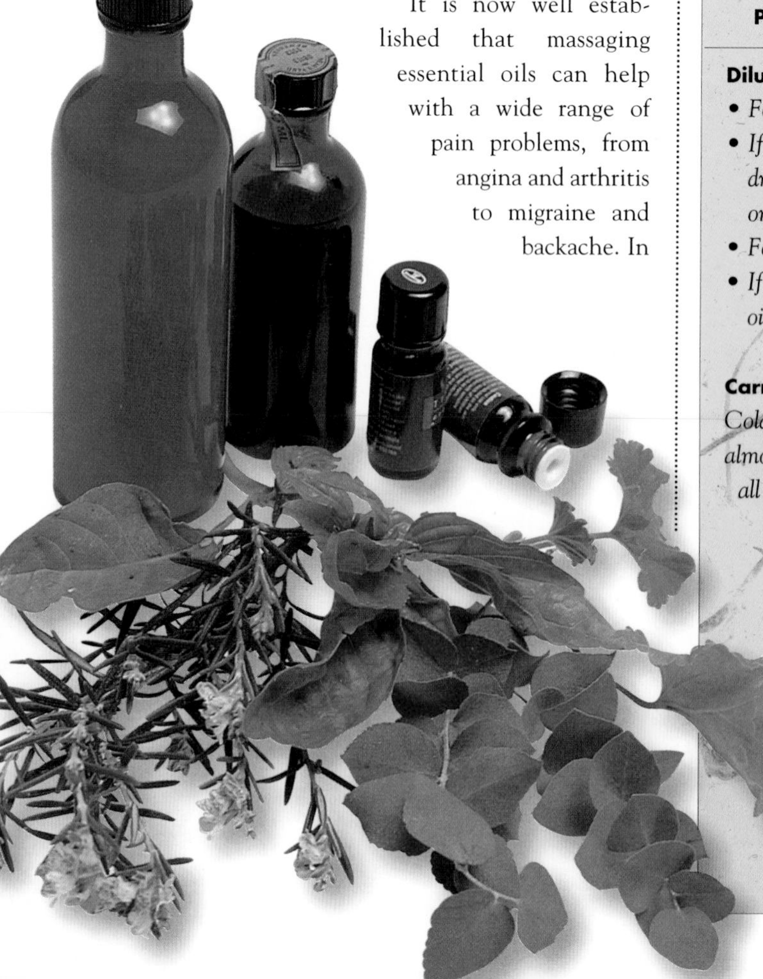

CAUTION The oils contain plant compounds and some are dangerous if taken internally, or used by very young children and pregnant women. Always consult a properly qualified aromatherapist about what oils not to take as much as those that are recommended.

Aromatherapy is effective for aches and pains due to headaches, migraines, depression, earache, neck strain, backache, coughs, bronchitis, asthma, pleurisy, emphysema, palpitations, angina, stomachache, gallstones, constipation, irritable bowel syndrome, fibromyalgia, bursitis, gout, arthritis, osteoporosis, ankylosing spondylitis, heat rash, boils, blisters, tinea/ringworm, eczema/dermatitis, vaginismus and sore vagina, childbirth, and cancer.

Preparing essential oils

Dilutions

- *For bathing, put five drops directly into the water.*
- *If using oils directly on the body, put around 20 drops into 2oz (50ml) of carrier oil. For the face, only use 10 drops in the same amount of carrier oil.*
- *For children, reduce the quantity to 5–10 drops.*
- *If vaporizing the oils, put around five drops into the oil holder and fill up with water.*

Carrier oils

Cold-pressed vegetable oils such as peach, sweet almond, grapeseed, sunflower, and safflower oils are all very good. Coconut oil is particularly appropriate for floral-based essential oils.

Storage

Store in a dark, airtight glass bottle and keep in a cool, dry place out of the reach of sunlight, such as the refrigerator. Both carrier oils and essences will oxidize with time. Adding a little wheatgerm oil will slow down the process but will not prevent it, so do not mix too large a quantity.

A brief guide to essential oils

Angelica
pleurisy

Arachis
eczema

Basil
emphysema, nerve pain, fatigue, joint pain

Bergamot
psoriasis, cough, asthma, cystitis, thrush, depression

Birch
backache

Cajuput
headache, emphysema

Calendula
blisters, tinea, eczema

Camphor
asthma, pneumonia

Capsicum
arthritis

Cedarwood
bronchitis, emphysema

Chamomile
eczema, cough, backache, gout, arthritis, morning sickness

Clary sage
backache, stress, depression

Clove
toothache, mouth ulcers, nerve pain

Cypress
cough, tuberculosis, gout, backache, arthritis, stress, varicose veins, prostatitis, pelvic inflammatory disease

Eucalyptus
headache, migraine, cough, sinusitis, bronchitis, asthma, pneumonia, emphysema, tuberculosis, backache, nerve pain, gout, arthritis

Fennel
eczema

Frankincense
cough, asthma, depression

Geranium
eczema, shingles, cold sores, fatigue, gout, diarrhea, depression, insomnia

Ginger
tuberculosis, backache

Hyssop
eczema, cough, bronchitis, asthma, emphysema

Jasmine
stress, depression

Jojoba
impotence, vaginitis

Juniper
eczema, asthma, headache, migraine, tuberculosis, backache, nerve pain, diarrhea, cystitis, stress

Lavender
sunburn, blisters, eczema, psoriasis, sinusitis, cold sores, asthma, pneumonia, backache, nerve pain, gout, arthritis, joint pain, cystitis, prostatitis, vaginitis, thrush, pelvic inflammatory disease

Lemon
pneumonia, stress, varicose veins, morning sickness

Lemon grass
premenstrual syndrome

Lime
varicose veins

Marjoram
headache, tuberculosis, neckache, backache, fatigue, constipation

Melissa
headache, depression

Myrrh
cough, pleurisy, nerve pain

Neroli
tuberculosis, depression, insomnia, anxiety

Nutmeg
fatigue

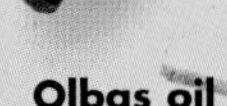

calendula (marigold)

Olbas oil
headache, migraine, colds, flu, bronchitis, nerve pain (Olbas oil contains juniper berry, eucalyptus, menthol, clove, wintergreen, cajuput, and mint oils)

Orange
stress reduction

Patchouli
impotence, depression

Peppermint
nausea, vomiting, headache, migraine, sinusitis, asthma, emphysema, tuberculosis, nerve pain, gout, diarrhea, morning sickness

Pine
pleurisy, pneumonia, emphysema, nerve pain

Rose
impotence, thrush, anxiety, depression, insomnia

Rosemary
sprains, headache, migraine, neckache, asthma, pleurisy, tuberculosis, backache, nerve pain, fatigue, gout, arthritis, joint pain, constipation, stress

Sage
shingles, pleurisy

Sandalwood
psoriasis, cough, bronchitis, nerve pain, diarrhea, cystitis, varicose veins, impotence, depression

Scots pine
gallstones

Sweet marjoram
sprains

Tea tree
bites, boils, blisters, mouth ulcers, cold sores, pleurisy, pneumonia, tuberculosis, diarrhea, vaginitis, thrush

Thyme
shingles, cold sores, cough, emphysema, fatigue, nerve pain, prostatitis

Tiger balm
arthritis

Vetiver
depression

Wintergreen
headache, migraine, asthma, nerve pain

Ylang ylang
impotence, depression, insomnia

CAUTION
The following oils should never be used during pregnancy: angelica, cinnamon bark, clary sage, hyssop, juniper berry, lovage, myrrh, origanum, penny-royal, rosemary, sage, savory, sweet fennel, sweet marjoram, thyme.

MOVEMENT THERAPIES

Therapies based on physical movement that work both physically and psychologically by processes increasingly accepted by conventional medicine and science.

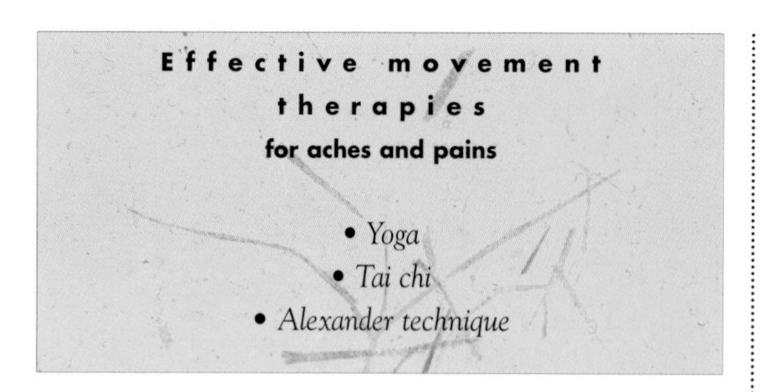

Effective movement therapies
for aches and pains

- *Yoga*
- *Tai chi*
- *Alexander technique*

Therapies that owe their benefit to movement are mostly oriental in origin, and hundreds of years old. In reality, activities such as yoga and tai chi are not so much therapies as arts: that is, they were devised not to cure disease but to promote spiritual enlightenment and physical enrichment. Both yoga and tai chi owe their effectiveness, when done properly, to a combination of physical movement linked to the cultivation of mental concentration and emotional harmony. In the sense of being neither simply physical nor just psychological but both at once, they are unique—and doubly effective. Like all oriental movement arts, they aim to promote unity of body, mind, and emotions—thereby achieving the perfect balance that experts believe equates with good health. Health, in effect, is the bonus rather than the aim.

Western movement therapies share little of this philosophy, though some place the same importance on the interaction between body and mind and have an equally good record in the treatment of pain, particularly chronic pain. The best known is the Alexander technique, but others with success (if less easy to find outside the United States) are Hellerwork and the Trager approach.

Beginner's salute to the sun

one

In this simplified version of the traditional yoga sequence, start by raising your arms straight above your head, in line with your ears. Lean forward slightly and bend your knees.

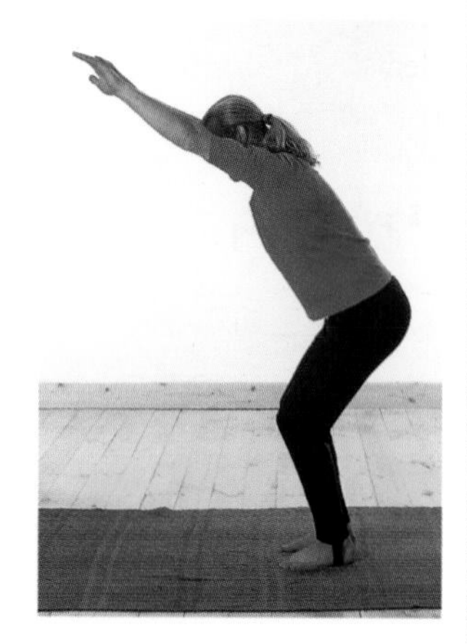

two

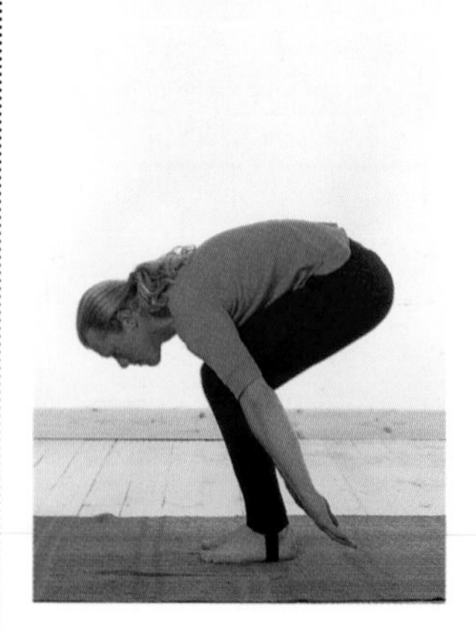

Bend your body forward in a smooth, flowing motion until your torso touches your thighs. Keep your knees bent. Drop your arms behind your calves and hold your head in line with your body.

three

Return to position 1, then continue smoothly upward, arching the back slightly and keeping the arms above the head. Your knees should still be bent. Repeat the sequence several times.

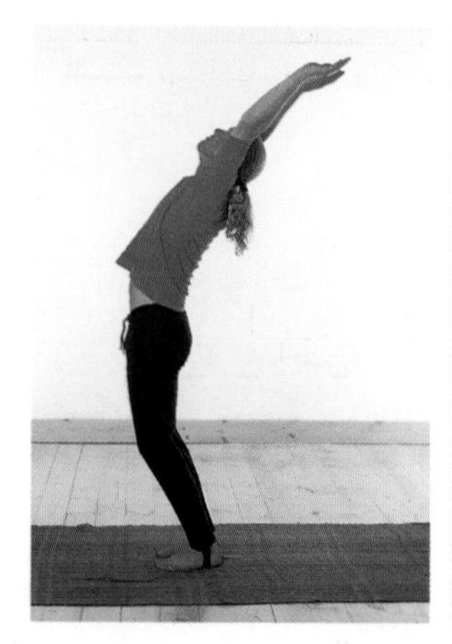

YOGA

Believed to have originated in India some 5000 years ago, yoga is one of the most effective movement therapies for many types of pain, particularly pain as a result of restricted mobility from accident, injury, or inflammation of muscles, nerves, and joints as a result of back conditions, arthritis, or multiple sclerosis. Yoga promotes not only physical mobility but a positive mental and emotional approach that can have profound psychological benefits. So it is effective also for controlling circulation problems, stress, and stress-related conditions, depression, chronic breathing problems, and digestive disorders.

Even though yoga exercises have been proved to benefit every part of the body, down to the smallest facial muscles, experts stress that yoga is very much a "whole person" approach to health and so generally do not recommend physical exercises (*asanas*) in isolation from a program of correct breathing (*pranayama*), or mental and emotional exercises.

There are various forms of yoga—including specialized types, such as kundalini yoga and tantra yoga—but the kinds most usually taught, and which incorporate the above elements, are hatha yoga, raja yoga, and ashtanga yoga. Because of such differences, yoga is best learned from a good instructor rather than from a book or video, at least initially. These days, yoga is so widespread that it should be easy to find classes.

Spinal twist

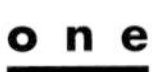

one

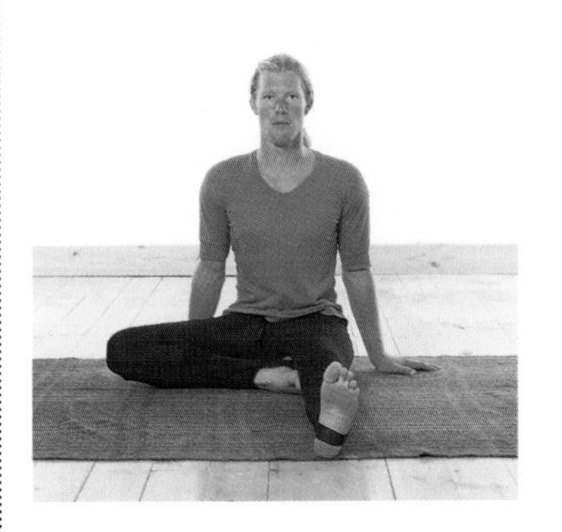

You should perform this posture first in one direction, then in the other. Sit on the floor with your legs stretched out in front of you. Keep your back straight and use your hands for support. Bend your right knee out to the side and bring the sole of your foot in toward your groin until it touches the thigh of your left leg.

Yoga is effective for aches and pains due to headaches, migraines, depression, neck and back pain, asthma, angina, high blood pressure, constipation, irritable bowel syndrome, nerve pain, arthritis, ankylosing spondylitis, osteoporosis, sexual problems, pregnancy, and childbirth.

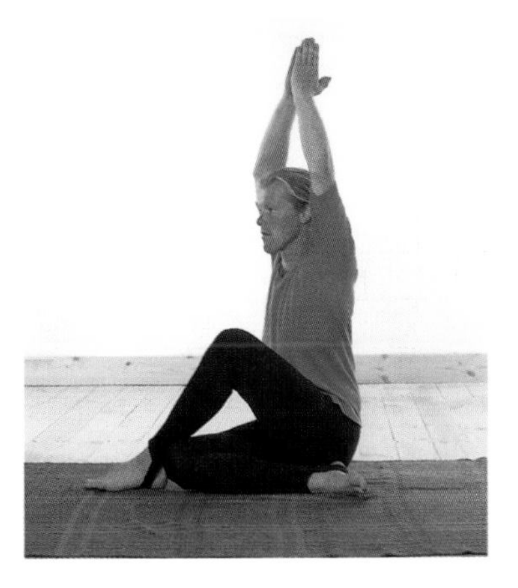

two

Bring your left leg over your right knee. Use your arms for support and balance but do not lean on them. Slowly raise your hands over your head, palms together.

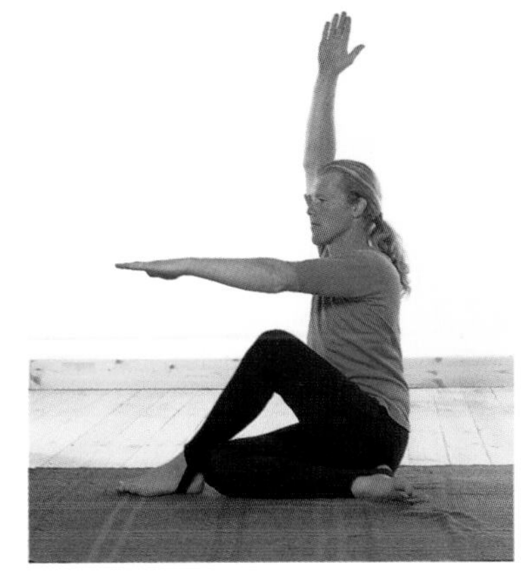

three

Hold that position for several seconds, then slowly bring your left arm down until it is straight in front of you at shoulder height. Keep the palm face downward.

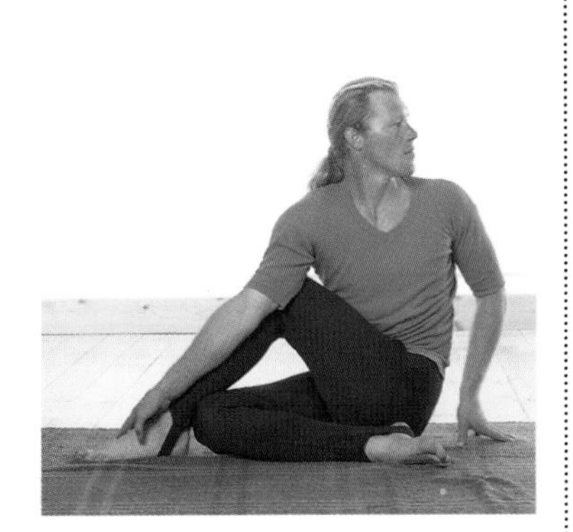

four

Bring your right arm down on the outside of your left leg and hold your foot for balance. Twist your body around and use your left arm for support. Hold for 30 seconds.

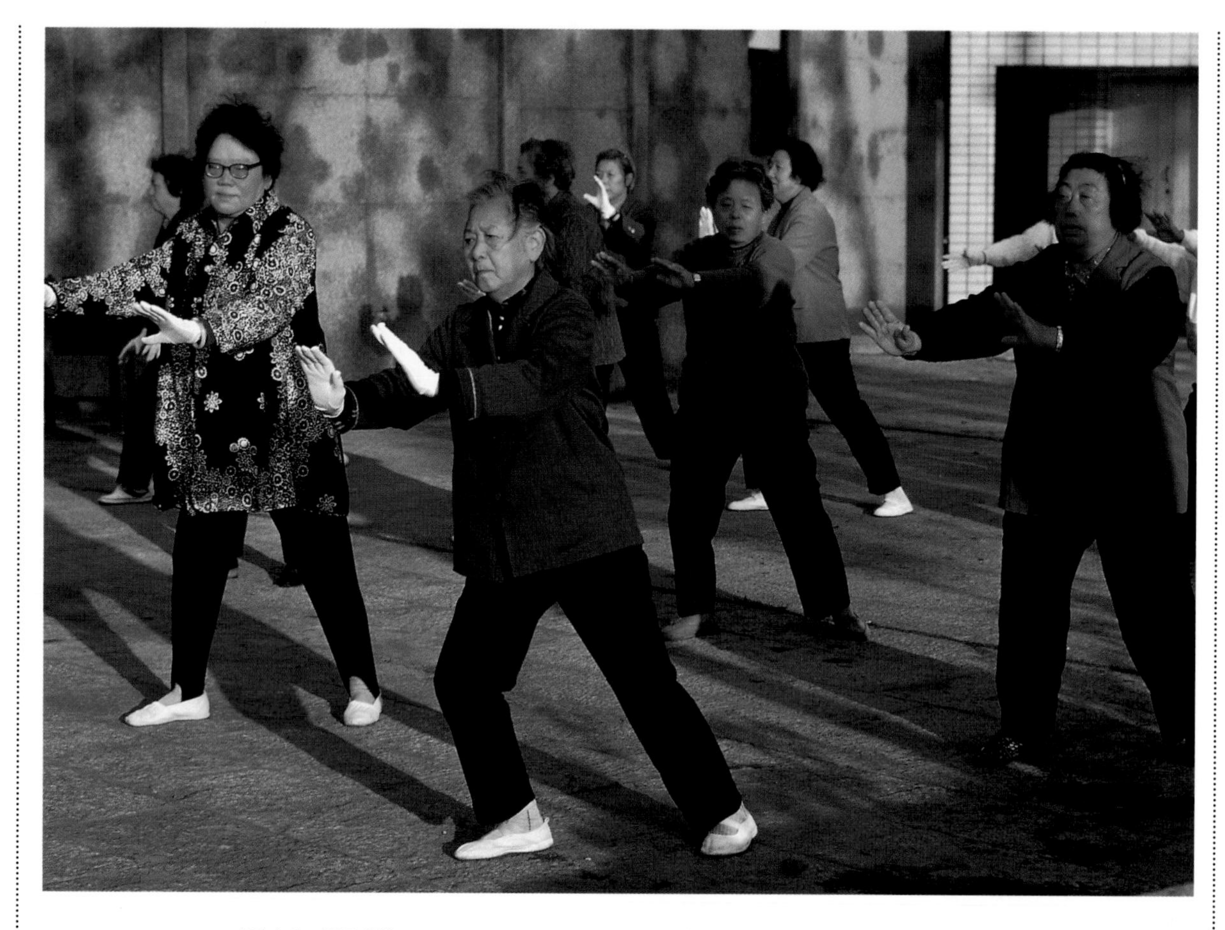

Tai chi being practiced in public parks and places is a common sight in China. The exercises are usually done in the morning.

TAI CHI

Tai chi—or t'ai chi ch'uan in full—is a form of movement originating in China, where it is still so popular that it is common every morning in most major parks and public places to see dozens, and even hundreds, of people going through their daily routines. Like yoga, tai chi is now favored in the West and widely practiced.

The essence of tai chi, which grew out of an even earlier Chinese system known as *chi kung* (or *qi gong*), is the slow and graceful style of its movements, which have led to its being described as "meditation in motion." The aim is to develop *chi* ("subtle energy," or "life force") in the body as an antidote to aging, and to encourage the growth of spiritual enlightenment, as in yoga. Like yoga, it can be used to promote healing and maintain health.

Tai chi is less physically demanding in some respects than yoga, and experts claim that with regular practice it is possible to build up huge reserves of mental and emotional strength. Because of its special combination of physical and psychological benefits, tai chi is especially effective for aches and pains where physical discomfort has resulted from psychological problems, and vice versa.

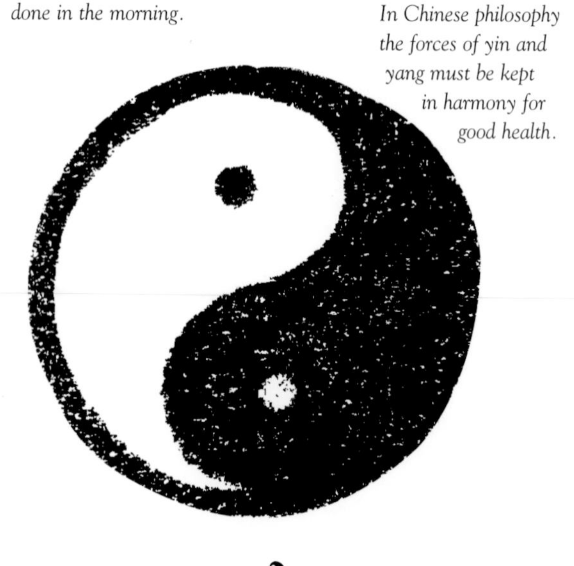

In Chinese philosophy the forces of yin and yang must be kept in harmony for good health.

Tai chi is effective for aches and pains due to headaches, migraines, depression, neck and back pain, asthma, angina, high blood pressure, constipation, irritable bowel syndrome, nerve pain, arthritis, osteoporosis, sexual problems, pregnancy, and childbirth.

ALEXANDER TECHNIQUE

The Alexander technique was developed early in the 20th century by an Australian actor called F. Matthias Alexander, who solved a recurring problem with his breathing and voice when he found that his posture was to blame. The success of the technique in the years since led to its popularity with performers of many kinds the world over.

What Alexander established was that use affects functioning: in other words, bad postural habits that we develop over the years affect the body's ability to function properly. His technique is a way of learning how to use the body as it is designed to work—and how, in most of us, it started out working.

The techniques must be learned from teachers in the first place (practitioners prefer the word teacher to therapist), but once learned are easy enough to do yourself at home. Generally between four and six lessons are needed to correct—or "unlearn"—poor postural habits, though some people need more. The lessons are based around everyday activities and movements, such as sitting, standing, and walking, and basically help you to use your body without being so badly affected by the stresses and tension of living.

Hellerwork and the Trager approach

Originating in the United States this century, these therapies aim to re-educate the body to function correctly by encouraging the unconscious mind to adjust "misalignments" in the musculo-skeletal system. This is done by a trained practitioner through a combination of manipulation and movement.

Hellerwork is a bodywork therapy aimed at promoting health through "realignment." The Trager approach includes a system of mind exercises called "mentastics" that can be practiced at home and is said to be particularly effective for pain control.

Hellerwork and the Trager approach are effective for aches and pains due to headaches, migraines, stress, asthma, musculo-skeletal problems, and nerve pain.

The Alexander technique is effective for aches and pains due to poor posture, especially headaches, migraines, neck and back problems, fibromyalgia, and circulation and breathing problems, including asthma.

Posture-correcting exercise: how to stand up

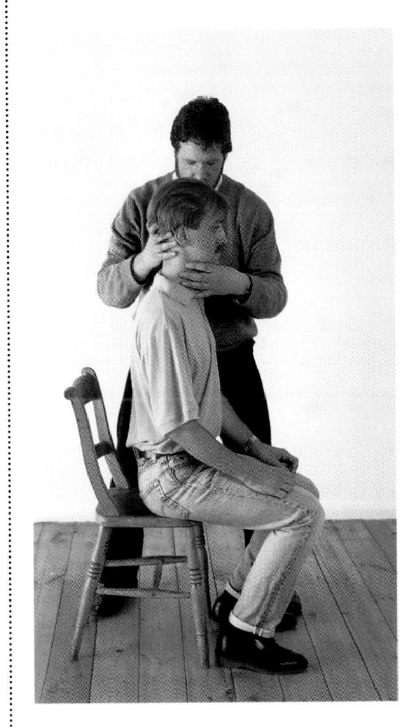

Before the model begins to stand, the teacher corrects the alignment of his head, neck, and back by supporting the chin and base of the skull in the correct positions.

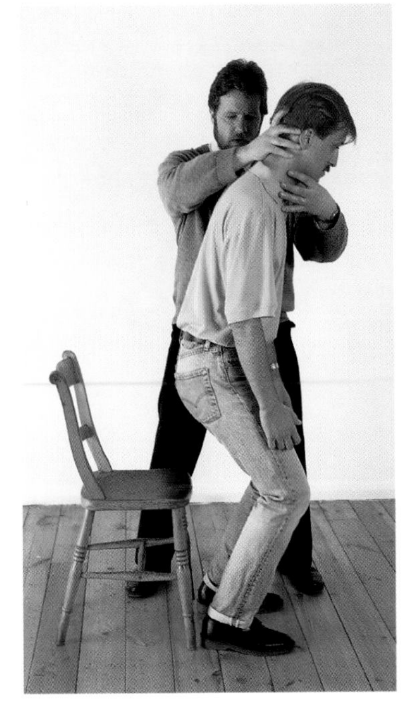

As the model stands up, the teacher keeps his head in line with his back, making sure the head does not become retracted and that the back is straight, not hunched.

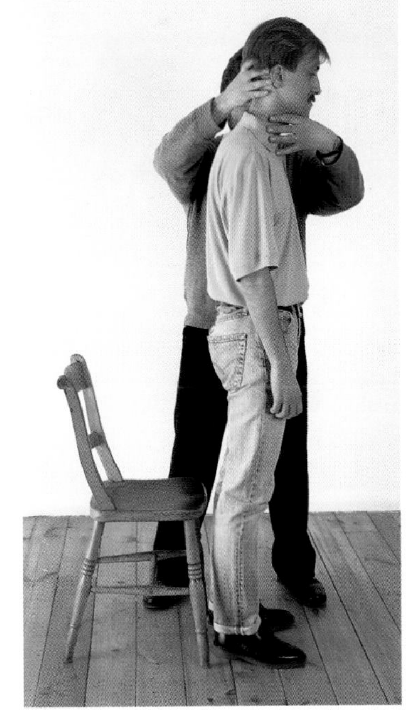

As the model arrives in the standing position, the teacher continues to support the head, helping him to achieve a more lengthened and balanced standing posture.

PSYCHOLOGICAL THERAPIES

Therapies based on mental and emotional exercises that produce physical effects by processes increasingly understood and accepted by conventional medicine and science.

Effective psychological therapies
for aches and pains

- *Self-hypnosis*
- *Relaxation therapies: visualization, meditation, autogenic training, biofeedback*
- *Creative arts therapies: art therapy, sand play therapy, dance therapy, music therapy, drama therapy*

Self-hypnosis affirmations

Try the following affirmations in front of a mirror:

- *I am calm and confident.*
- *I love and approve of myself.*
- *I am a wonderful human being.*
- *I am the authority in my life and no one else is.*
- *I am strong and my mind/heart is healing itself.*
- *I am filled with healing power.*

SELF-HYPNOSIS

Self-hypnosis is more accurately described as autosuggestion. Put simply, autosuggestion is thinking yourself well, and is the process of using the power of the mind to heal the body. In self-help it can involve repeating a word or phrase over and over, and this is more usually known today as an "affirmation."

Perhaps the most famous affirmation is that coined by the French chemist and hypnotist Emile Coué, who developed autosuggestion (or Couéism) more than a century ago: "Every day in every way, I am getting better and better." Repeated 15 to 20 times twice a day, morning and night, it has helped some seemingly hopeless problems, including chronic pain, addictions, and phobias.

The best-known affirmations today are those of the American therapist Louise Hay. By identifying a number of negative thought-patterns and beliefs, and teaching how to understand the detrimental effect these have on the body, she claims to have helped many people. Affirmations are best performed on a daily basis looking into a mirror.

Self-hypnosis can be a means of entering the inner world of imagery, with powerful therapeutic results. It can be learned from a qualified teacher, then practiced at home indefinitely. It is effective for most aches and pains, from physical and mental conditions.

RELAXATION THERAPIES

Learning how to relax has been shown to have a powerful healing effect on both the body and mind. This is true not just of illnesses as a result of psychological tension and stress but physical problems also. Physical pain of all kinds, acute and chronic, can be helped by discovering the relaxation therapy that works best for you individually.

One of the best ways of relaxing body and mind is physical exercise, particularly strenuous exercise. Pain sufferers cannot always manage exercise—although a warm bath, or just stretching and breathing deeply, as you do when yawning and sighing, can be

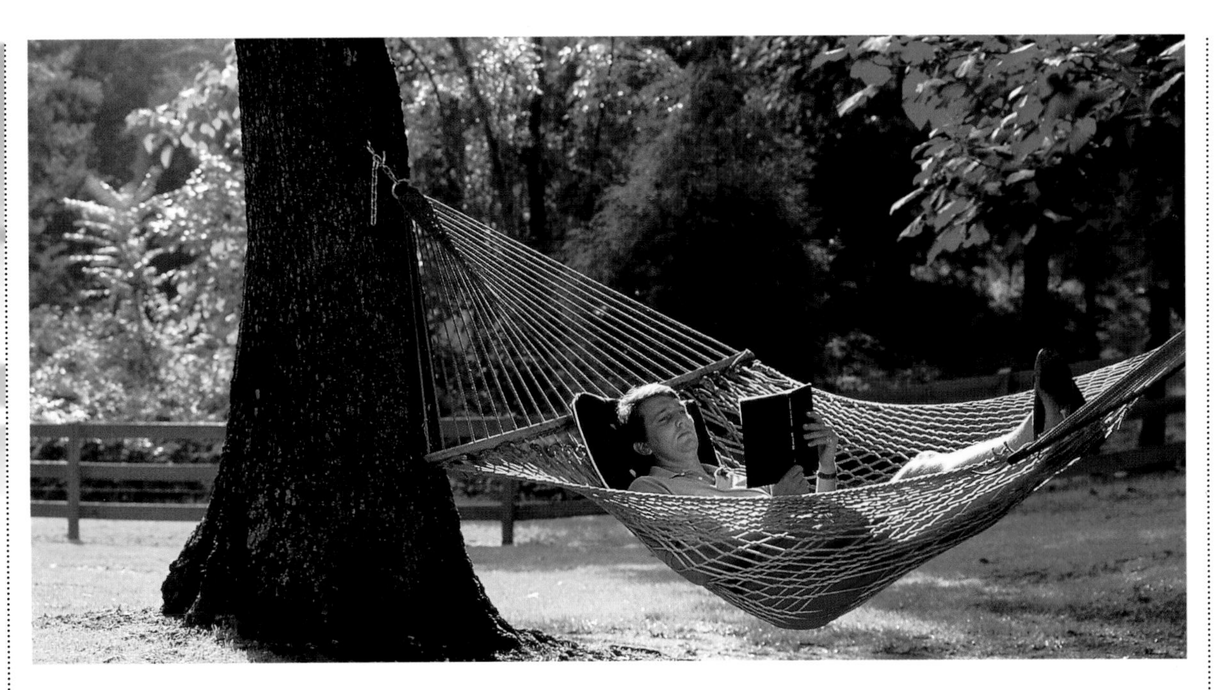

very relaxing—but there are alternatives. The most effective relaxation therapies that do not involve physical effort are visualization, meditation, and biofeedback. All three involve relaxing the body totally by making a conscious mental effort. They can be done quite quickly with the right instruction and practice.

VISUALIZATION

Visualization is the technique of using the power of the mind—specifically the imagination—to help the body. It has been used effectively in the treatment of illnesses as mild as a cough and as serious as cancer. Against cancer, for example, sufferers have been encouraged to imagine an army of healthy cells destroying all the cancer cells and replacing them with undamaged cells.

Although results are variable —depending very much, it seems, on the personality of the person doing the visualizing—positive results have been recorded. Visualization seems to be particularly useful for people who are able to allow their imaginations to express themselves freely. Perhaps for this reason, children and young people tend to have more success. But adults can achieve good results also if they let themselves.

As an example, try imagining yourself in a place you know, where you feel content. Gradually become part of the scene. See yourself fit and well, with a cheerful outlook and without pain. Over a period of time, notice if there is any change in your symptoms.

No one is quite sure how visualization actually works—the process seems to be similar to the self-hypnosis of affirmations—but the power of the mind to influence the body, for better or worse, is clearly at the root of the process.

Relaxation techniques may help to relieve pain in times of ill health, but it is important to relax regularly at all times in order to maintain good health.

Relaxation therapies are effective for aches and pains due to headaches, migraines, depression, back strain, breathing problems, asthma, angina, circulation problems, high blood pressure, stomachache, irritable bowel syndrome, nerve pain, eczema, psoriasis, sexual problems, and cancer.

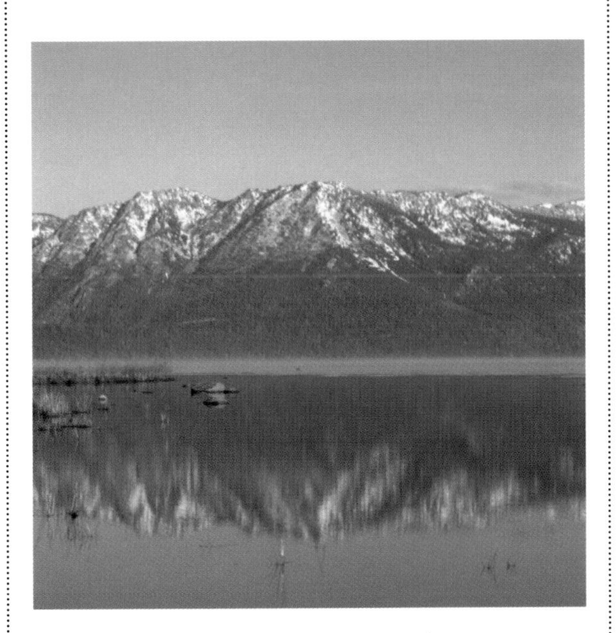

The benefits of relaxation in the management of pain are immense, and picturing a pleasing image in your mind is a useful way to achive a calm and positive outlook.

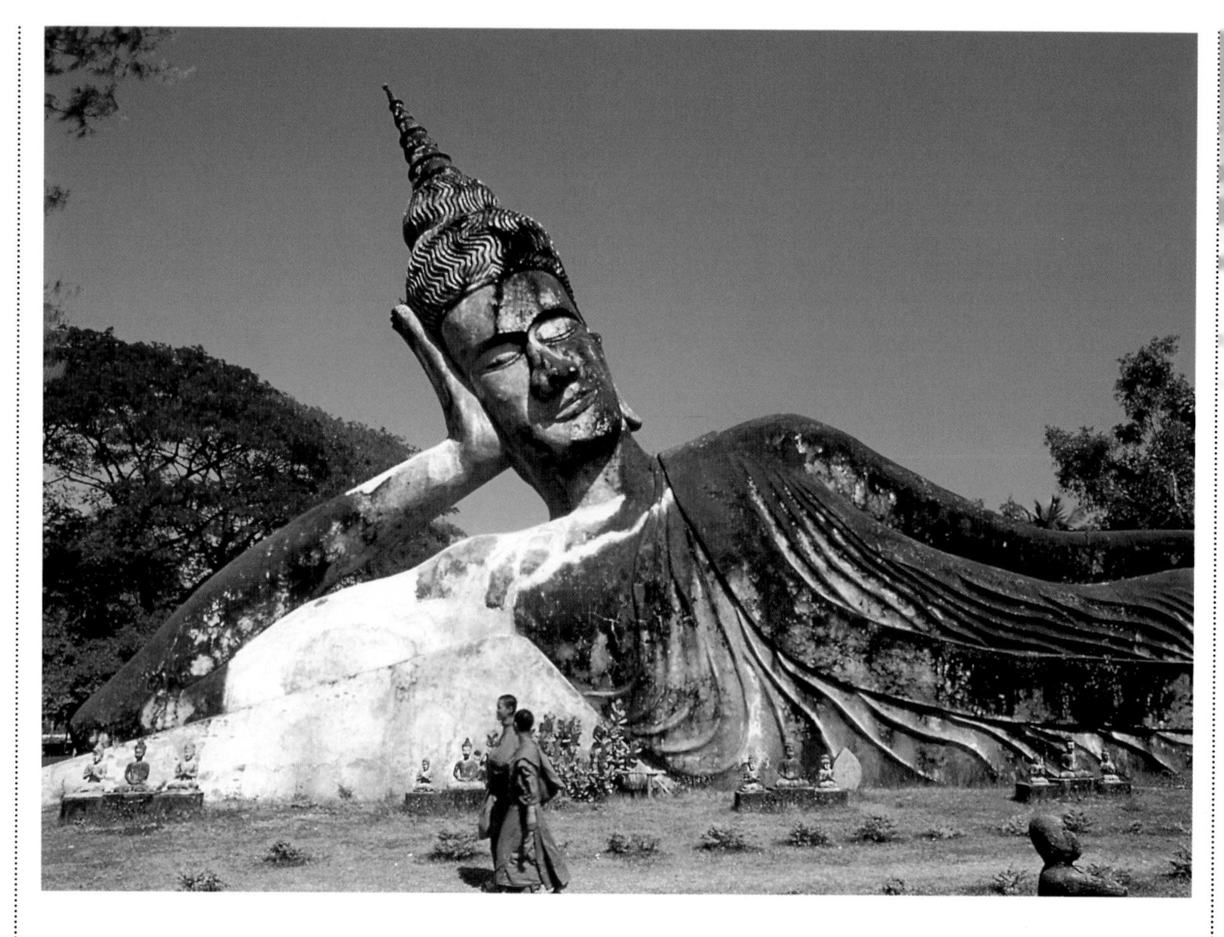

Meditation has been a fine art for centuries in the Orient, and is widely depicted in Buddhist statues—and not always in the classic "lotus" position.

MEDITATION

When the mind is at rest, it has, like the body, a much greater capacity for healing itself. Meditation is a way of resting your mind beyond simply thinking nothing or daydreaming. It has been best described as "passive concentration" or "active attention."

There is a wide variety of meditative techniques, some of which are promoted by religious organizations. The most famous of such techniques is probably transcendental meditation (TM). But there is, or should be, nothing mystical or mysterious about meditation. It is not a religion, and you do not have to sit in the famous "lotus" position, with your eyes closed and your legs in a knot, to benefit. An example of an effective western version of meditation without ritual is autogenic training (see right).

The benefits of meditation are becoming increasingly known. There is good evidence, for example, that as well as supporting the body's immune system, meditation also lowers stress and induces a strong sense of peace and tranquillity that many find helpful regardless of its therapeutic value. In the Netherlands, health insurance became cheaper for people who practice transcendental meditation after it was shown to lower blood pressure and so protect against heart and circulation problems.

Anyone can meditate, but it takes a bit of practice to do it properly, which is why it is a good idea to be shown how to do it by someone experienced in the first place. The aim is to relax the body and then try to do the same with the mind. This can be a little difficult in the beginning, but it becomes easier with practice.

The Sanskrit symbol for the "sacred sound" OM, used widely in meditation to clear and focus the mind.

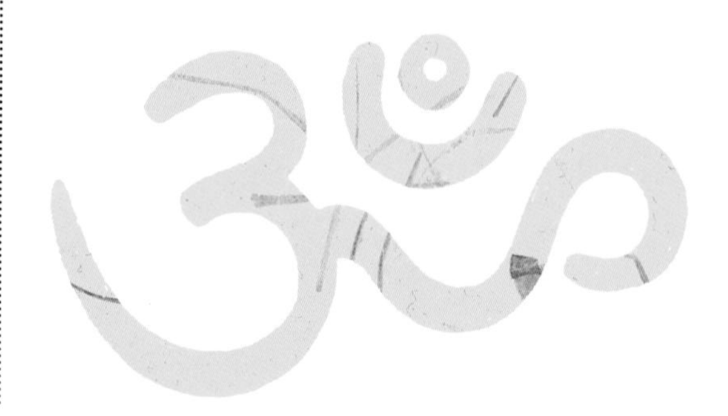

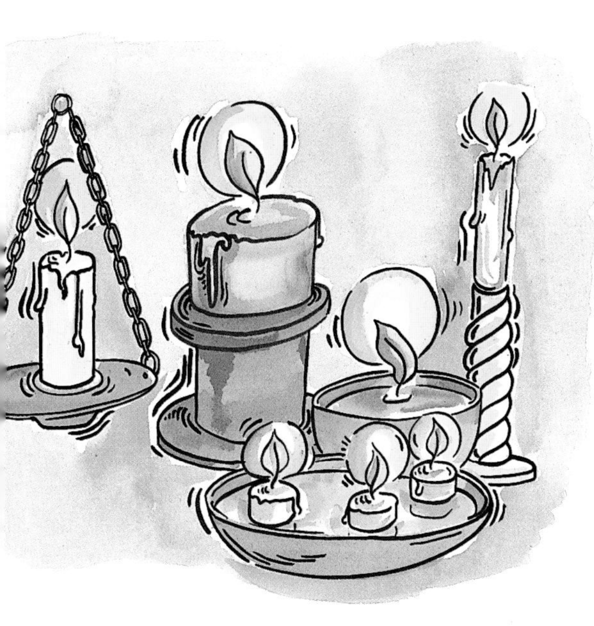

Focusing on a burning candle is a good way to help the concentration during meditation.

AUTOGENIC TRAINING

Autogenic training was developed more than 70 years ago by a German psychiatrist and hypnotist, Dr. Johannes Schultz, who wanted to discover an alternative method to equal the results of hypnotism. His system is related to meditation (it is often called "western meditation"), self-hypnosis, and yoga.

Autogenic training uses six standard exercises that involve directing your attention inward and focusing your mind on different parts of the body. You train yourself to be aware of:

- *sensations of heaviness in your body*
- *warmth in your arms and legs*
- *the calmness and regularity of your heartbeat*
- *your easy and natural breathing*
- *warmth in your abdomen*
- *coolness in your head.*

The exercises are normally taught by trained practitioners at weekly individual or small group sessions over an eight-week period. Students are usually taught how to do the exercises in one of three positions: lying, sitting in an armchair, sitting in an upright chair. The idea is that the exercises can be done anywhere at any time, but the recommended practice is three times a day after eating.

BIOFEEDBACK

Research over many years at the US space center NASA proved the benefits of biofeedback. Originally developed to control motion sickness in astronauts, it was found to have additional benefits as a method of overcoming the effects of stress. As a result, biofeedback therapy is now established as an extremely safe, gentle, and effective way of promoting relaxation.

Biofeedback uses a meter to help you recognize how your body is behaving at any given moment by means of fine electrodes held either in the hand or connected to a band tied around your head. For example, the meter will register one reading when you are tense and a different reading when you are relaxed. By using the meter to monitor the physical effects produced by specific feelings, you gradually learn, with the help of a trained therapist, how to influence your responses and so educate your body to do more of what helps you and less of what hurts.

From its introduction in the United States in the 1950s, biofeedback technology has developed considerably, and it now includes a wide range of devices, from simple hand-held battery-operated appliances that anyone can buy and use, to reclining armchairs linked to sophisticated computer monitors, which show heartbeat and blood-pressure patterns as well as brain waves and blood chemistry, that are generally only used by therapists at specialist centers.

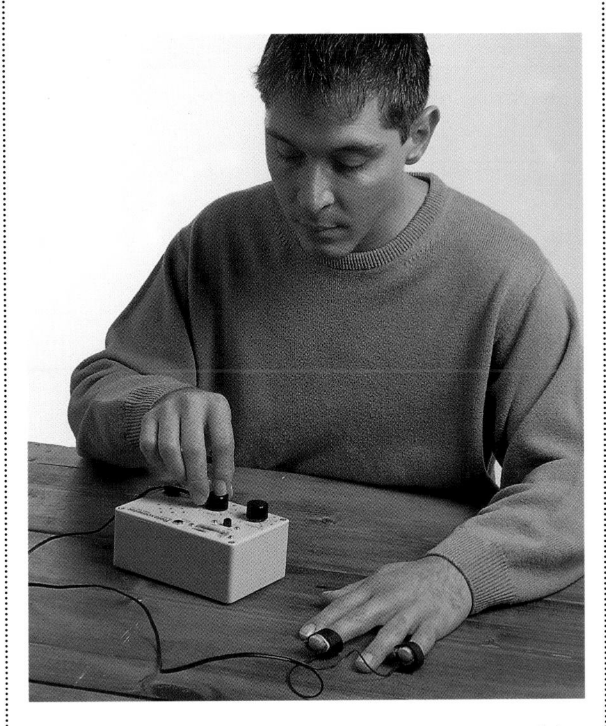

A simple biofeedback device can help train the mind to control the body. It allows you to see just how effective different relaxation techniques are by monitoring changes in blood pressure.

CREATIVE ARTS THERAPIES

As the name implies, creative arts therapies use dance, painting, music, drama, and other forms of creative activity to enable people to express themselves in purely nonverbal (but not silent) ways. Hence they are also often called "expression therapies." The nonverbal aspect is the significant part of this highly effective and growing form of psychotherapy. The method is in rapidly increasing use for people of all ages and abilities with psychological problems, including depression, who have difficulty in expressing themselves adequately in words. The arts have been shown to be a potent tool for communicating not only with others but with yourself—and there is no need to be good at any of the art forms involved to do it.

ART THERAPY

Art therapy usually means the use of paint to express yourself, but can also include modeling or sculpting with clay. In all cases, the standard of the works created is less important than the opportunity to express inner feelings freely. Painting can be used either as a physical form of visualization or as a way of venting inner feelings (of anger, joy, grief, and so on). In the case of visualization, some people find it easier or more satisfying to paint scenes of serenity and happiness than imagine them. The painting is more likely to be abstract or surreal than realistic, but the free expression put into it is what matters, with generous use of color and shape.

Sculpting or modeling can be used in much the same way to release strong feelings. It is the physical act—of splashing on paint or throwing and molding clay with your hands—that offers the release. By watching carefully how a person works and exploring the process together, a trained therapist can help people toward insights into their problems, and healing. Art therapy is also an effective way of relieving tension without supervision.

SAND PLAY THERAPY

Sand play therapy uses a sand tray and miniature models to represent anything the user chooses. By placing items in the "world" of the tray, people can represent the past, present, or future, and work therapeutically on their problems with the help of a trained therapist. This medium is best known for helping children, but adults also find it beneficial.

Clay modeling or sculpting is a way that helps people express feelings without having to talk about them.

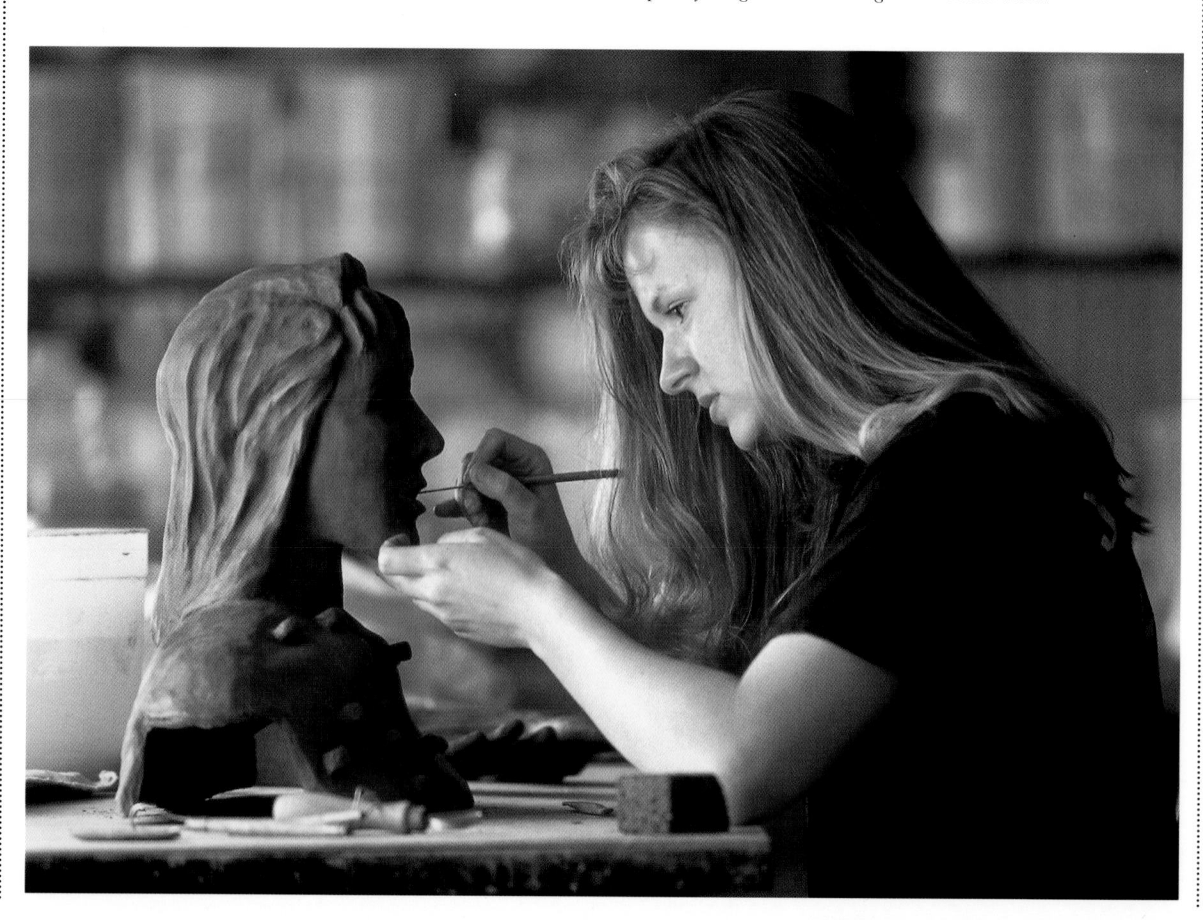

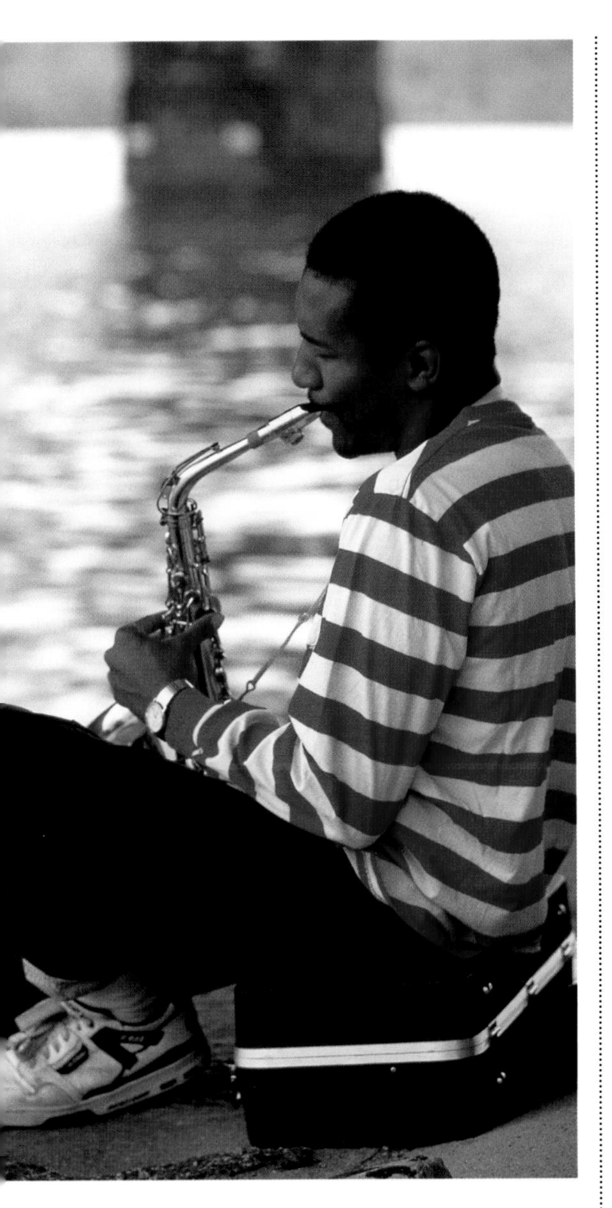

Playing a musical instrument can help people express inner feelings through music rather than words.

DANCE THERAPY

Dance (or dance movement) therapy uses physical movement to "draw out" or express inner feelings that a person may not be able to talk about. Based on the work of the 1920s pioneer Rudolf von Laban, dance therapy is most effective when done in groups under the guidance of a trained therapist, so it is not an ideal form of self-help. But dancing freely to music (see "Music therapy," below) is, on the other hand, an excellent way to release inhibitions and relieve stress.

MUSIC THERAPY

Music therapy uses the combination of sound and the playing of musical instruments to allow free expression of emotions that might not otherwise find an outlet. So, for example, beating a drum or singing (even shouting) whatever you want, how you want, is part of the therapy. But it could mean simply listening to music that moves you, and perhaps dancing to it (see also "Dance therapy," above). As with the other creative arts therapies, working with a trained therapist is more usual and effective, but music therapy is also an excellent method of self-help.

DRAMA THERAPY

Drama therapy is allied to psychodrama. It may involve, for example, discovering hidden, suppressed, or repressed feelings through acting out imaginary situations in a group. Pretending to be someone or something else can open up insights into problems and allow ways of experimenting with solutions. Formulated in the 1920s by Jacob Moreno—first in Europe, and then in the United States—this is another effective therapy that is now well-established everywhere.

Creative arts therapies are effective for aches and pains due to a very wide range of psychological problems, from the everyday, such as headaches, migraines, eating, and digestive disorders, to deep-seated psychological trauma, including manic depression, obsessions, phobias, and addictions.

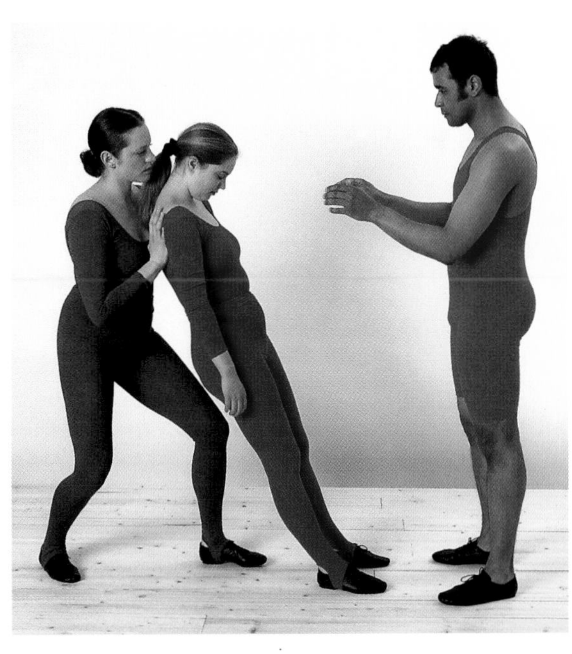

Drama therapy helps people express inner feelings though acting out imaginary situations in the company of others.

SUBTLE ENERGY THERAPIES

Therapies that work by processes that are only partly physical and are not yet fully understood or accepted by conventional medicine and science.

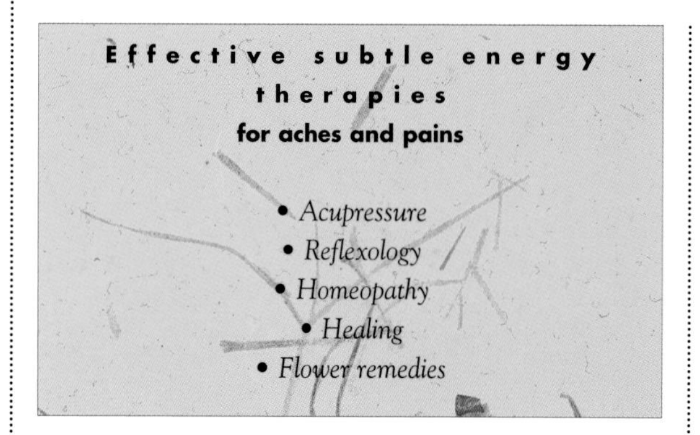

Effective subtle energy therapies for aches and pains

- *Acupressure*
- *Reflexology*
- *Homeopathy*
- *Healing*
- *Flower remedies*

A number of therapies encourage the body to heal itself by stimulating not just physical energy—the kind of energy you can get from eating the right foods, for example—but what is known as "subtle energy." Subtle energy is energy said to exist at a subtle or invisible level. That is, it is non-physical, or "psychic." Other terms commonly used instead of subtle energy are "life energy" or "life force." Leading examples of subtle energy or life force therapies effective in the treatment of pain are acupuncture, acupressure, reflexology, homeopathy, and healing.

Because life force has not so far been scientifically measured, evidence of its existence remains inconclusive and controversial: some people swear by it, while others declare it to be imaginary. Despite this, therapies such as acupuncture, homeopathy, and healing have a long history of success and scientific studies to back them up, and are used regularly by a growing number of doctors.

Examples of other subtle energy therapies sometimes said to help pain are crystal therapy, gem therapy, and radionics. Though there is as yet no proper research to support any of them, crystals and gems certainly look good, and if they work—and some clearly do for some people—they are a form of healing. There is no evidence that they are harmful, and at worst they are simply ineffective.

CAUTION Practice of many of the subtle energy therapies, particularly healing and radionics, is illegal in some countries, including a certain number of American states—even by qualified medical practitioners. The reason appears to be traditional hostility to the idea of healing by what are perceived by many to be "supernatural" means.

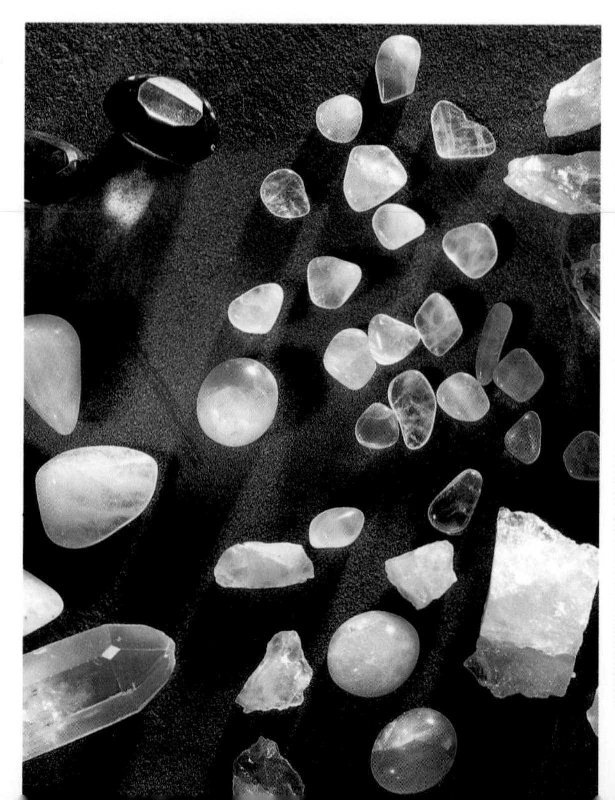

Despite lack of scientific evidence, many therapists use gems and crystals to help healing. The theory is that crystals such as rose quartz work by reattuning a person's hidden "vibrations."

ACUPRESSURE

Often referred to as "acupuncture without needles," acupressure is a widely used and highly effective form of therapy in which finger or hand pressure (and sometimes elbow, knee, or heel pressure) is applied to the same points of the body as in acupuncture. Some people believe it may have been an earlier form of acupuncture, or a variation developed for those who did not have or did not like needles. The principles of acupressure are the same as those of acupuncture—but most modern forms were developed in Japan rather than China. The best-known variation is *Shiatsu* (meaning "finger pressure" in Japanese), but other names you are likely to come across are *Do-In*, *Jin Shen* (or *Shin*), and *Shen Tao*.

Since the use of needles is not really possible—or even allowed in some countries—as a method of self-help, acupressure is the best way to achieve the well documented pain-relieving benefits of acupuncture, without the needles. Pain caused by musculo-skeletal and nerve problems are said to respond particularly well to acupressure.

The "body maps" below show some of the many acupressure points that can be useful in the treatment of pain.

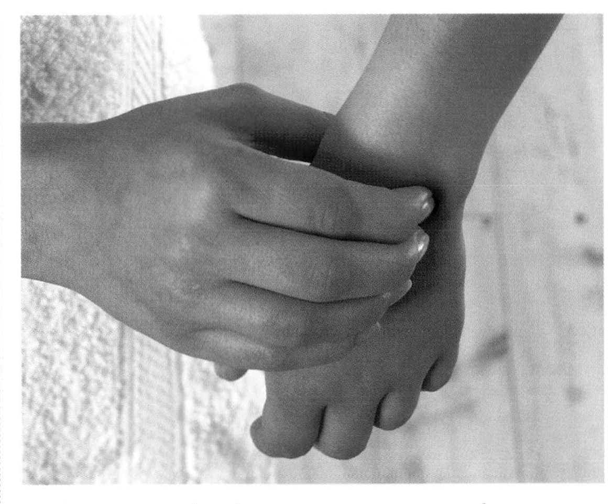

Apply pressure to the relevant acupressure points with your thumb or fingers—pressure should be firm and steady.

Acupressure is effective for aches and pains due to headaches, migraines, sinusitis, hayfever, back pain, coughs, asthma, angina, palpitations, circulation problems, stomachache, nausea, gallstones, diarrhea, irritable bowel syndrome, urinary tract infection, cystitis, kidney stones, nerve pain, fibromyalgia, bursitis, carpal tunnel syndrome, feet and ankle problems, gout, arthritis, pelvic inflammatory disease, premenstrual syndrome, painful periods, childbirth, and cancer.

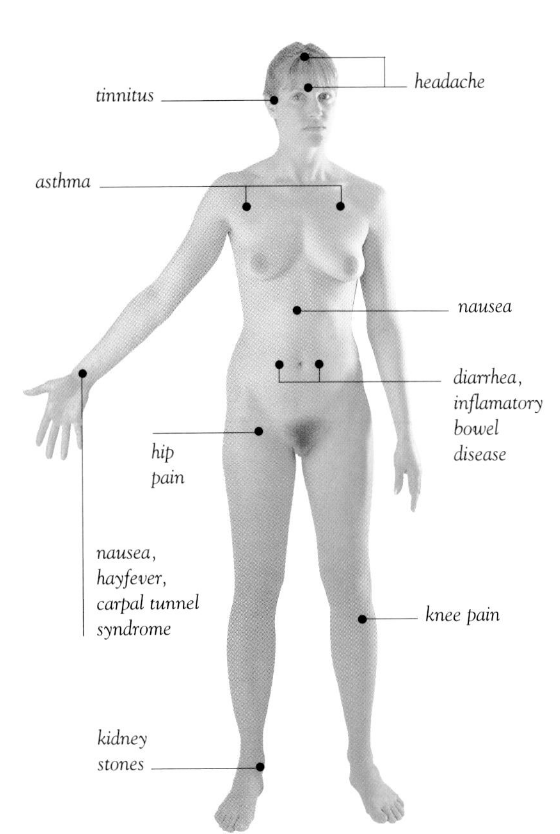

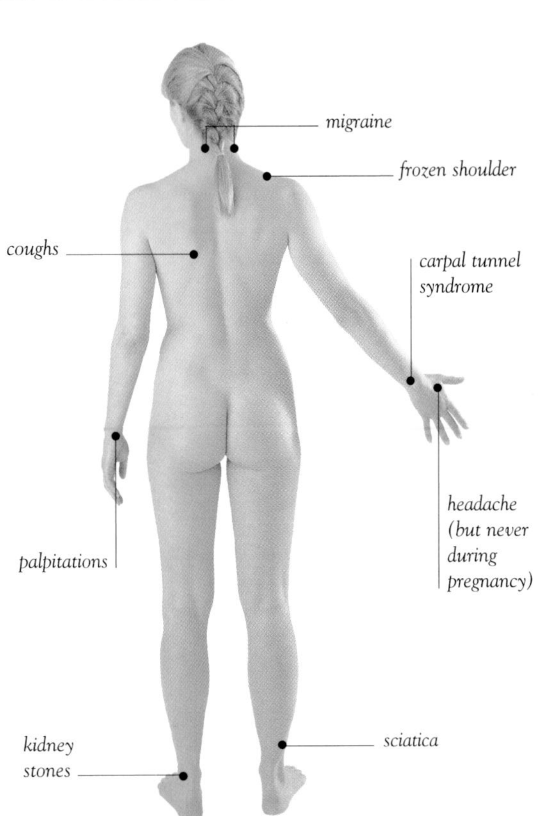

REFLEXOLOGY

Reflexology (or reflex therapy) could be simply described as foot massage, but most therapists insist it is much more than this. Said to be a revival of a healing method widely practiced in the ancient world, reflexology probably has links with acupressure and acupuncture, and so is, strictly speaking, an energy therapy rather than a physical one. But this categorization is challenged by many reflexologists, who see their work as broadly in line with other physical therapies. In Britain, reflexology has been officially recognized by the Chartered Society of Physiotherapists, the national body for physical therapists, since 1993.

Nevertheless, reflexology is based on the idea that lines of energy run through the body and these lines link all the major organs to specific "reflex" points in the feet. According to reflexologists, the bottom of each foot can be mapped with areas, or "zones," which correspond to these various organs, and the organs can be affected by putting the reflex points under pressure.

Pressure is usually applied using the thumb and fingers. No pain means no problem—but any discomfort is said to indicate a difficulty in the corresponding area of the body, and pressure is applied to the painful point. Sometimes this is distinctly uncomfortable, but working on the point for a few moments usually causes the pain to ease, and a response is felt in the affected organ. So, for example, a headache might be relieved by having pressure applied to the base of the big toe (which corresponds to the base of the neck), and congested lungs by pressing the ball of the foot. Reflex therapy is a variation using much gentler pressure.

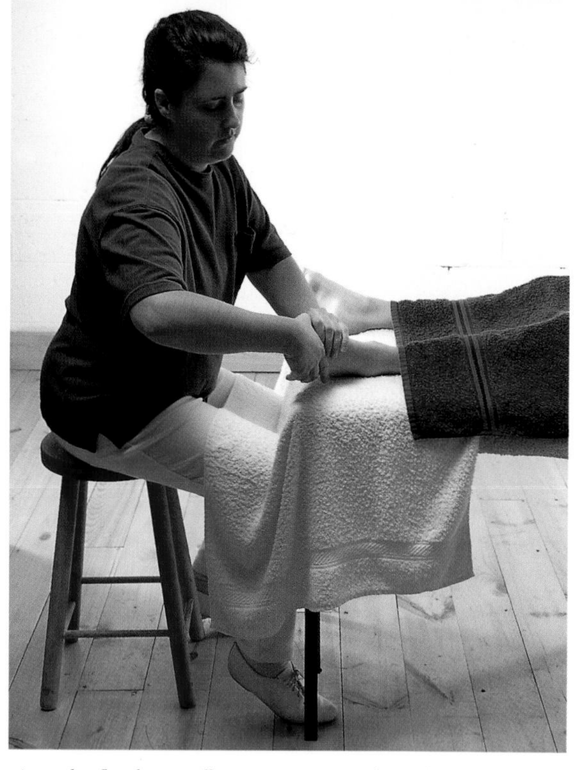

A good reflexologist will attempt to attune themselves to the person they are treating as well as manipulate the feet.

Reflexology does not claim to be able to remove inflammation or infection, but therapists believe treatment can speed recovery and help maintain it. Most patients say it has a strongly relaxing effect, and this will improve circulation and benefit most bodily functions. Some evidence of its relaxing qualities is the fact that many people feel like sleeping after a treatment.

Some basic reflexology techniques

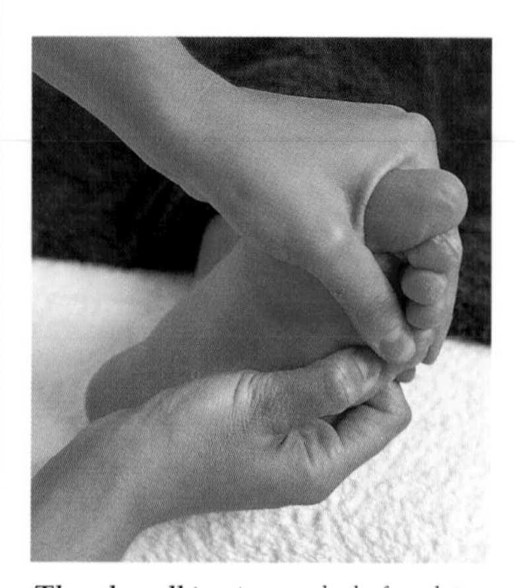

Thumb-walking *is a method of applying pressure to a line of reflex points. Bend the joint nearest the nail but keep the lower one comfortably straight. Each time the thumb bends, take a tiny sliding step forward. Talc on the skin will help.*

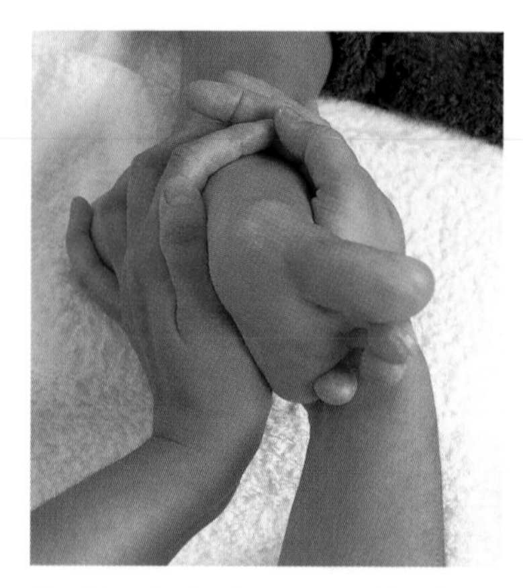

Stroking *the feet between working the various reflex points is extremely relaxing. Cup the foot between the palms of both hands and slide the hands slowly from toes to ankle and back again in a smooth, circular motion.*

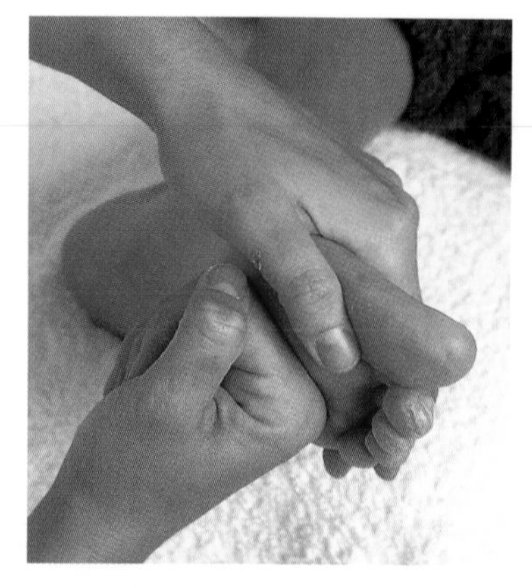

Caress *the foot by making a fist with one hand and pressing the backs of the fingers into the ball of the foot—do not use the knuckles. Rotate the fist slowly in a circular motion. This technique can also be performed with the heel of the hand.*

A modern, high-tech version of reflexology, known as Vacuflex, has recently been introduced from Denmark and South Africa, which claims to achieve better results more quickly by using special felt boots and a system of suction pads. Air is drawn out of the boots by a pump, and the feet are given an allover squeeze from the vacuum that results. The suction pads are then used in much the same way as "cupping" (see "Acupuncture," pages 150–151) to stimulate various reflex points on the feet, legs, arms, and hands.

Reflexology is effective for aches and pains due to headaches, migraines, depression, pneumonia, emphysema, stomachache, indigestion/heartburn, nausea, constipation, irritable bowel syndrome, nerve pain, feet and ankle pain, and cancer.

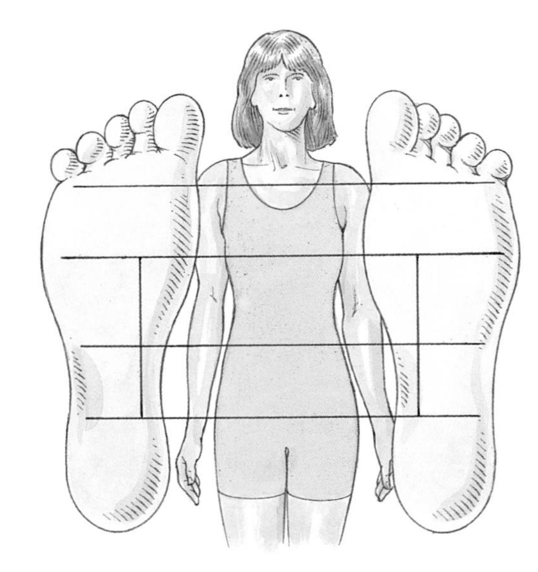

Reflexologists believe that areas of the feet correspond to parts and organs of the body, with the toes aligning with the head and shoulders, the ball of the foot with the chest and lung area, the arch of the foot the internal organs, and the heel the pelvic region.

This "foot map" shows some of the many reflex points. There are some variations between different schools of reflexology, but the majority would follow most of the points shown here.

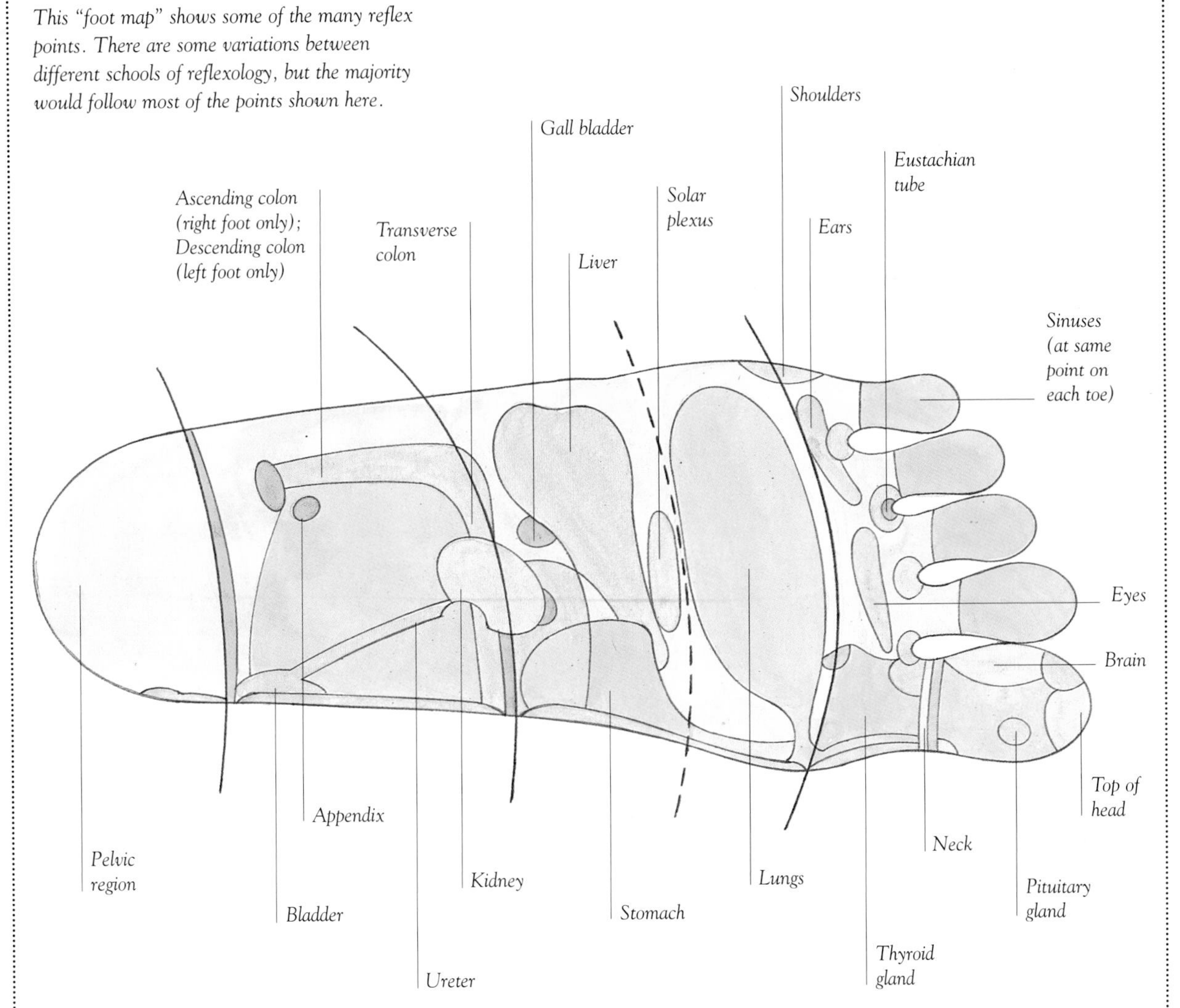

HOMEOPATHY

Homeopathy is a "complete," or self-contained, system of medicine developed some 200 years ago by a German doctor called Samuel Hahnemann. Basing his ideas on early Greek principles of medicine, Hahnemann discovered by treating himself that a very small amount of what causes a disease also cures it. This gave rise to his principle of "like cures like," which remains the basis of homeopathy.

Homeopathic remedies are used by taking only the smallest amounts of a specific substance, usually from plants or minerals, diluting them in water with a little alcohol, and shaking them vigorously. This vigorous shaking, known as "succussion," is central to how homeopathy is said to work. The process of diluting and shaking is done several times. Unlike most conventional doctors, who believe that the higher the concentration of something the stronger it is, homeopaths believe the remedy gets more potent each time it is diluted and shaken—hence the term "potentization" to describe the process. Homeopathic remedies are usually given as small white tablets onto which the potentized mixture was dripped.

Homeopaths, like most natural therapists, usually see physical symptoms of disease as as indication of something deeper, and they will always want to see a patient personally and take a detailed history to get to the bottom of what they think is wrong before prescribing. That is why self-prescribing is not recommended by most homeopaths, even though homeopathic remedies are available in drugstores and health food stores.

There has been no explanation acceptable to scientists of why and how homeopathy works. But several clinical trials appear to show that it does work—and a growing number of doctors are now specializing in it. A few studies have shown positive results with animals, and this has led to more veterinarians also turning to homeopathy.

Homeopathy is widely available in most countries, but may be restricted to registered practitioners; ask your national Homeopathic Association for information. In Britain it is the natural therapy that has been available longest under the state health service. A derivative of homeopathy is flower remedies.

peony and cornflower

Homeopathy is effective for aches and pains due to almost any physical condition resulting from "buried" psychological problems, such as shock, bereavement, and depression, but it is effective also for eyestrain and infections, migraines, sore throat, hayfever, coughs, asthma, stomachache, indigestion/heartburn, colitis, Crohn's disease, flatulence, urinary tract infection, cystitis, kidney stones, fibromyalgia, bursitis, arthritis, ankylosing spondylitis, eczema/dermatitis, psoriasis, and bruising.

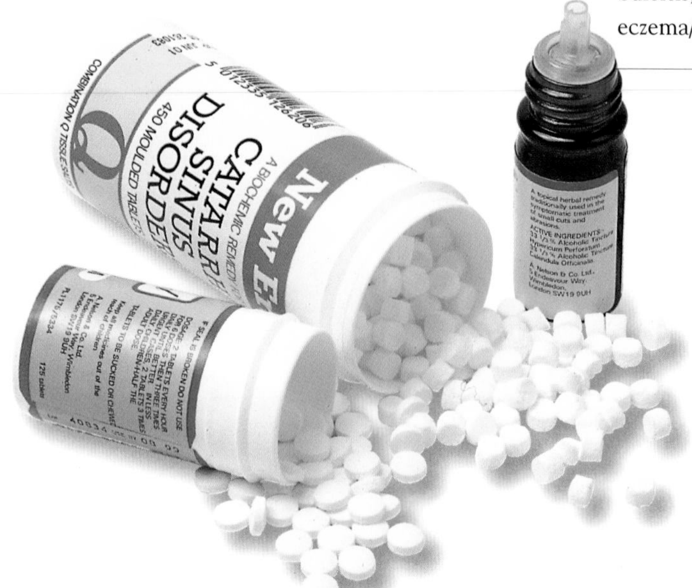

Homeopathic remedies are usually taken as small pills, though some practitioners also give them as a liquid or powder. Homeopaths normally advise not handling the remedies but dropping them into the mouth and allowing them to dissolve slowly.

A brief guide to homeopathic remedies

Aconite
burns, scalds, toothache, conjunctivitis, earache, cough, bronchitis, nerve pain, palpitations

Agaricus
frostbite, chilblains

Allium cepa
hayfever

Apis
bee stings, jellyfish stings, bites, frostbite, conjunctivitis, hives, shingles, sore throat, nerve pain

Arnica
bruises, sprains, eyestrain, headache, whiplash, backache, slipped disk, nerve pain, gout, arthritis, joint pain

Arsenicum album
motion sickness, cough, stomachache, vomiting, diarrhea, conjunctivitis, sore throat, hayfever, bronchitis

Belladonna
sunstroke, conjunctivitis, earache, tooth abcess, sore throat, tonsillitis, headache, nerve pain, gout

Bellis per
bruises

Berberis
kidney stones

Borax
nausea, vomiting, anxiety

Bryonia
cough, bronchitis, nerve pain, arthritis, joint pain, stomachache

Calcarea phos
toothache, kidney stones

Calendula
stings

Cantharis
cystitis

Carbo veg
chilblains

Causticum
diarrhea

Chamomila
earache, toothache

Cinchona off
tinnitus

Cocculus
nausea, vomiting

Cuprum
sunstroke, cramps

Euphrasia
conjunctivitis

Ferrum phos
earache, conjunctivitis

Gelsemium
headache

Glonoin
sunstroke, dizziness

Graphites
eczema, psoriasis

Hepar sulf
boils, earache, tooth abcess, cold sores, sore throat

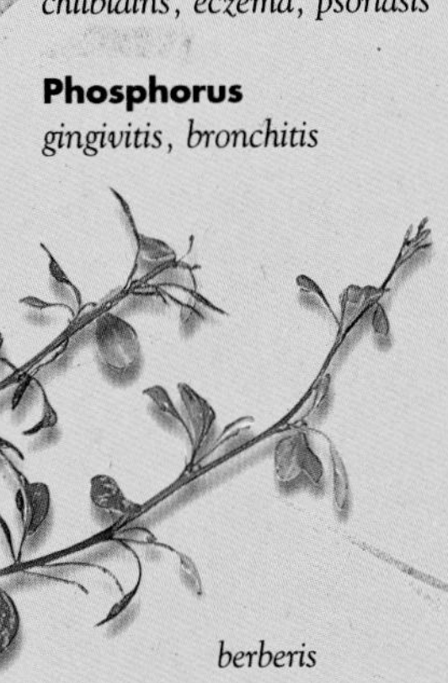

berberis

Hypericum
bites, tooth abcess, whiplash, nerve pain

Ignatia
headache

Ipecacuanha
motion sickness, vomiting, morning sickness

Lachesis
bruises, sore throat

Ledum
insect stings, jellyfish stings

Lycopodium
migraine, sore throat

Magnesia phos
kidney stones

Mercurius corrosivus
conjunctivitis

Mercurius solubilis
sore throat, tonsillitis

Mezereum
shingles

Natrum mur
migraine, cold sores, eyestrain

Nux vomica
nausea, vomiting, migraine, stomachache, morning sickness, headache

Petroleum
chilblains, eczema, psoriasis

Phosphorus
gingivitis, bronchitis

Phytolacca
sore throat

Pulsatilla
frostbite, nausea, vomiting, motion sickness, headache, toothache, conjunctivitis, cough, bronchitis, vomiting, diarrhea, morning sickness

Pyrethrum
insect stings

Rhus tox
blisters, hives, eczema, shingles, cold sores, backache, nerve pain, arthritis, joint pain

Rumex
cough

Ruta
bruises, sprains, eyestrain, backache, arthritis

Sabadilla
hayfever

Salicylic acid
tinnitus

Sarsaparilla
kidney stones

Sepia
nausea

Silicea
boils, migraine, earache, tooth abcess

Spigelia
migraine

Staphysagria
bites, cystitis

Sulfur
eczema, psoriasis, bronchitis

Symphytum
bruises

Tabacum
nausea, vomiting, dizziness

Tamus ointment
chilblains

Urtica urens
hives

HEALING

Healing—better known by most people as faith healing or spiritual healing—is probably the simplest, safest, and most natural of all therapies in that it involves nothing but the touch, or sometimes only the thoughts, of the healer. According to American researcher Daniel Benor, who published two volumes of research into the subject in 1993, there is more evidence in favor of the therapeutic effects of "hands-on" healing than of any other form of natural therapy except hypnotherapy. The powers some healers seem to have of alleviating pain and curing disease, even at a distance, is consequently acquiring its own scientific definition. It is now called "non-local medicine."

Whether the healing is caused by the healer, by some mysterious force that is channeled through him or her (some call it "universal energy" or "God power"), or by the stimulation and reinforcement of the body's own healing powers is an open debate at the moment. But whatever the truth of the matter, healing has apparently worked for many people, and is not to be ignored.

THERAPEUTIC TOUCH

Therapeutic touch (TT) is a modern version of healing by the laying-on of hands. The term is used particularly in the United States, where healing by what are claimed to be supernatural means is illegal in some states. Started in the 1970s by Dolores Krieger, an American professor of nursing, TT is based on a belief in the actual transfer of energy from the toucher to the person being touched, and is in increasing use.

REIKI

Reiki healing is another variation that has become popular in recent years. Created by a Japanese priest, Dr. Mikao Usui, in the early part of the 20th century, *reiki* (pronounced "ray-kee," and meaning "universal life force") is claimed to be a rediscovery of an ancient Tibetan Buddhist technique of healing involving the transfer of restorative energies from one person to another. Reiki therapists have set up centers in North and South America, Europe, and Australasia as well as Japan, with over 250,000 practitioners worldwide.

Healing can be effective for aches and pains due to almost every condition—but especially for headaches, migraines, asthma, back pain, infections, and cancer.

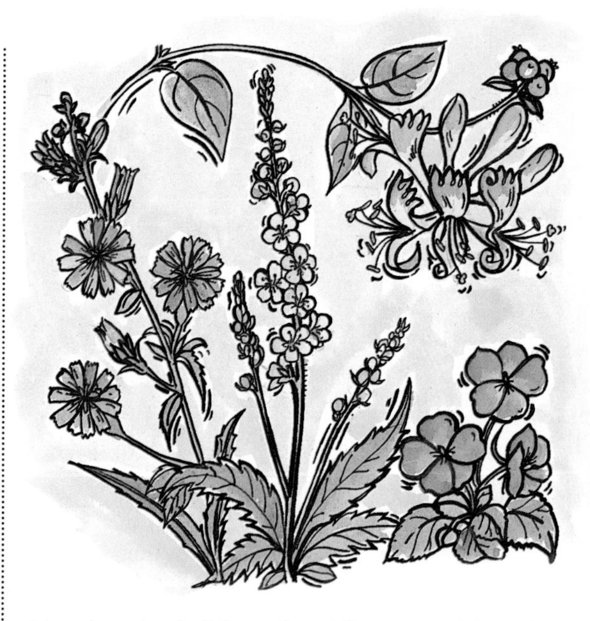

More than a hundred flowers from different parts of the world are now used in an ever-growing range of these popular remedies.

FLOWER REMEDIES

Flower remedies treat physical conditions by treating the psychological problems that are believed to lie behind them. The most famous are the Bach remedies, named after British homeopath Dr. Edward Bach, who originated them in the 1920s and 1930s. Dr. Bach, who was convinced that a negative outlook affects both the body and the events in our lives (as well as the way we face up to them), developed a set of 38 remedies for every type of human emotion, from anger to vulnerability. Each remedy is intended to treat the individual rather than the illness he or she is suffering from.

Flower remedies use the "essences" of flowers and trees, but though plant-based, they are more homeopathic than herbal in the way they are said to work. In other words, they act psychologically and psychically rather than chemically. Today there are some two dozen companies producing over 100 essences in more than 50 countries. The main problem with flower remedies is that no one has so far explained scientifically how they might work. Despite this, flower remedies are used throughout the world by many thousands of people who swear by their benefit.

Flower remedies are said to be effective for a wide range of conditions due to underlying psychological problems that can result in aches and pains.

A brief guide to the Bach flower remedies

Agrimony
Encourages those who hide their worries behind a cheerful exterior to express their inner pain

Aspen
Allays fears that are vague or unconscious in origin, including fear of death

Beech
Encougages tolerance in those who are arrogant or overcritical of others

Centaury
Helps those who feel unassertive, weak-willed, or imposed upon by others to achieve their goals

Cerato
Helps people who doubt their own judgment to have faith in themselves

Cherry plum
Provides reassurance for those who feel they may be on the verge of a breakdown

Chestnut bud
Helps people who find it hard to become wiser through experience, or who repeat old patterns, to learn by their mistakes

Chicory
Enables those who are overpossessive of loved ones to let go

Clematis
Aids concentration in those who are dreamy or vague

Crab apple
Known as "the cleanser," this helps those who feel shame about themselves to put everything in perspective (also useful for hayfever or rhinitis)

Elm
Restores confidence in those who take on more than they can deal with and become overwhelmed

Gentian
Restores faith in the process of life in those who are despondent or depressed through a known cause

Gorse
Restores hope for those who have given up and are in despair, particularly in cases of chronic pain

Heather
Helps those who are obsessed with themselves develop compassion for others

Holly
Dampens negative feelings of rage, jealousy, anger, or other negative emotion; paradoxically, it also helps you contact your true feelings when you feel cut off from life

Honeysuckle
Helps those nostalgic for the past to let go and embrace the present

Hornbeam
Restores energy in those who are temporarily unmotivated or procrastinate; often called the "Monday morning" remedy

Impatiens
Encourages patience and tolerance in those who find it hard to work in a team

Larch
Enhances self-confidence in those who are overcome with feelings of inferiority or fear of failure

Mimulus
Gives courage to those with phobias and fears of known or tangible things

Mustard
Helps reinstate optimism in those who experience sudden depression and despair without a known cause

Oak
Rebuilds strength and endurance in those who overachieve or set themselves impossibly high goals but can no longer cope

Olive
Regenerates peace and balance after long periods of overwork or emotional exhaustion

Pine
Helps those with an overdeveloped sense of guilt to forgive themselves

Red chestnut
Encourages those who are obsessive in their concern for others, to the point where they project all their own fears onto them, to put their fears into perspective

Rock rose
Reassures those who experience panic, terror, or sudden alarm

Rock water
Not actually a flower but derived from spring water in natural locations, this remedy helps those who keep themselves under rigid self-control or self-denial to become more lenient toward themselves

Schleranthus
Helps those who are indecisive to make decisions and allays uncertainty and mood swings

Star of Bethlehem
Reassures after shock or trauma, sudden loss, or accident

Sweet chestnut
Gives hope to those in a state of hopeless despair

Vervain
Restores balance to those who are are overenthusiastic and fanatical

Vine
Encouranges those who are ruthless or power-hungry to be more understanding of others

Walnut
Protects those who are experiencing periods of transition and also facilitates change

Water violet
Helps those who are withdrawn, reserved, or proud to open up to others

White chestnut
Dispels persistent unwanted throughts and restores peace of mind (also useful for insomnia)

Wild oat
Encourages decisiveness in those who are searching for their true direction, purpose, or career, and thus fulfilment

Wild rose
Recreates motivation in those who are apathetic or resigned

Willow
Encourages a positive frame of mind in those who feel bitter and blame others

Rescue Remedy
Calms and comforts in times of emergency and stress (contains Star of Bethlehem for shock, rock rose to deal with panic, impatiences for impatience and tension, cherry plum for fear of losing control, and clematis to help focus the mind and prevent fainting)

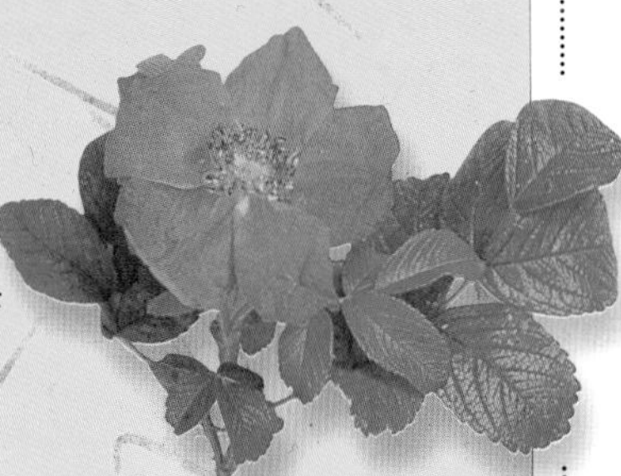

wild rose

OTHER EFFECTIVE THERAPIES

The following therapies, though known to be effective in the treatment of many aches and pains, are NOT suitable for self-help, and should only be performed by fully trained and qualified practitioners. They are included for information and brief reference only.

From a qualified practitioner only

- *Acupuncture*
- *Manipulation: chiropractic, osteopathy, cranial osteopathy*
- *Hypnotherapy*
- *Counseling and psychotherapy*

ACUPUNCTURE

Acupuncture—the use of very fine needles to treat illness—originated in China more than 4000 years ago, though the earliest books on the subject did not appear until 475 BC. In Chinese philosophy, disease is seen as often brought about by an over or under amount of "wind, cold, damp, or heat" in the "humors" or "elements" of the body. This sort of imagery has found little support among modern doctors, but the practical benefits of treatment have.

Among an estimated three million practitioners worldwide are a growing number of doctors as well as physical (or physio-) therapists who use acupuncture in the treatment of pain and addictions. Western hospitals have also started using acupuncture as an anesthetic where drugs are not appropriate or possible.

Acupuncture uses very fine gold, silver, or steel needles—so fine that most people do not feel them being inserted or removed—to stimulate the body's subtle energy (known as *qi* or *chi* in Chinese) at one or more of hundreds of points (different schools disagree about the exact number of points), situated along the 14 "meridians," or energy channels, said to run through the body. This process is believed to balance out the flow of subtle energy in the body and so help its natural self-healing tendency.

Most doctors do not accept this explanation, but because research has shown definite benefits they practice a more clinical form of the therapy known as "western acupuncture," often preferring to use a weak electric current attached to the needles for greater effect (a variation referred to as electro-acupuncture), especially those applied to points in the ear, a procedure known as auricular acupuncture, or auricular therapy.

The most usually accepted theory today of how and why acupuncture works is that it interferes with pain messages to the brain, either by "distracting" the brain in the same way as TENS and other electronic devices, or by promoting the release of the "pleasure hormones" (endorphins and enkephalins) that close the "pain gate" (see page 11).

More traditional variations are the techniques known as moxibustion and cupping. In moxibustion, a gentle heat is applied to an energy point, using *moxa*, a dried herb (usually common mugwort). This is either attached to the needle so that the heat transfers down the needle to the energy point, or it is rolled into small cones and slowly burnt over the point on top of a protective covering. Sometimes a few cones are used together. The belief is that this "draws" and heats the energy, making more energy available.

Cupping is the use of small cups or jars (usually made of glass) to stimulate and "draw" the body's energy points in much the same way as moxibustion. A lighted taper is held inside the jar and then quickly removed to create a vacuum so that the jar clamps itself to the body and "sucks" on the point. The cup is

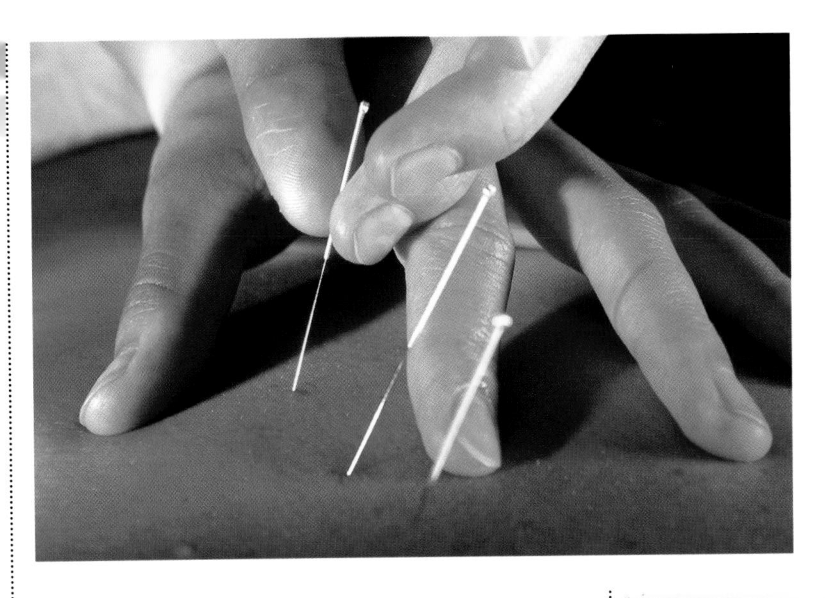

Very thin needles, usually of stainless steel or gold, are used in acupuncture to activate the body's chi or "life force." Practitioners insert them into the skin at very specific points in the hopes of clearing any blockages in the flow of chi.

left in place for perhaps 10 minutes for full effect. For local congestion and inflammation, cupping is often used with needles.

As the example of moxibustion shows, acupuncture is used closely with herbs in China and other parts of Asia, and belongs to a comprehensive system of diagnosing and treating disease known collectively as traditional Chinese medicine (TCM). The list of herbs used in Chinese medicine is vast, and many are extremely strong, so practitioners of TCM in the West tend to be Chinese, because few westerners have the necessary skill or experience to use them safely. Western practitioners of TCM seem to concentrate solely on the use of acupuncture and moxibustion—though, strictly speaking, that is not true TCM.

See also "Acupressure," page 143, "TENS devices," page 123, "Herbal medicine," pages 124–127, "Reflexology," pages 144–145.

Acupuncture is effective for aches and pains due to almost any problem, but particularly headaches, migraines, depression, addictions, tinnitus, sinusitis, neck and back strain, slipped disk, breathing problems, asthma, palpitations, poor circulation, stomachache, nausea, ulcers, gallstones, constipation, diarrhea, irritable bowel syndrome, diverticulitis, appendicitis, colitis, cystitis, kidney stones, nerve inflammation, fibromyalgia, bursitis, carpal tunnel syndrome, restless legs and leg pain, rheumatism and arthritis, ankylosing spondylitis, eczema, psoriasis, hernia, impotence, vaginismus, premenstrual syndrome, painful periods, childbirth pain, postnatal pain, and cancer.

This 19th-century Japanese acupuncture chart shows the meridians or "channels" along which "life force" or chi is believed to flow.

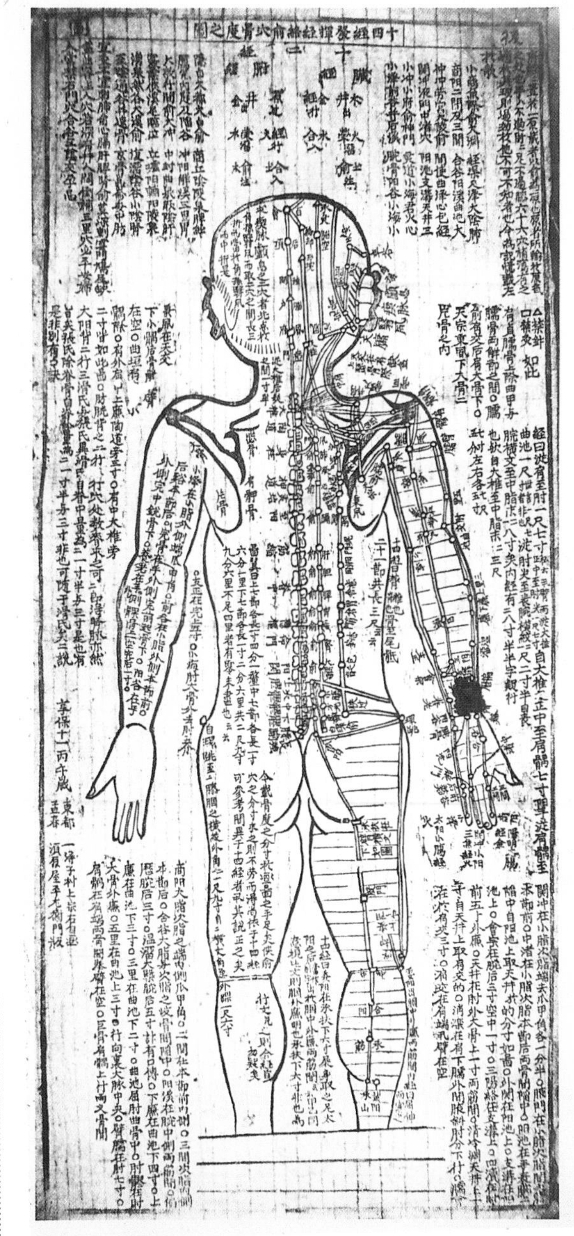

MANIPULATION

Expert manipulation of the body, and especially the bones, muscles, and tissues of the spine, has long been known to help a range of persistent long-term (or chronic) problems, including pain. Manipulative therapies most helpful for pain are chiropractic, cranial osteopathy (or cranio-sacral therapy), and osteopathy—though more recent versions such as Rolfing, myotherapy (or trigger point injection therapy), the Rosen technique, and the Bowen technique all claim to treat aches and pains from musculo-skeletal problems successfully. None is suitable for self-help, though. They can be dangerous if carried out by nonspecialists, and so must only be performed by fully trained and qualified practitioners.

CHIROPRACTIC

The word chiropractic comes from the Greek and means "manual practice." Like osteopathy, chiropractic aims to restore health and "balance" by manipulation of the bones, muscles, and tissues of the body, particularly the spine, so that everything is in its correct place and is working properly. Techniques vary, from the famous bone-cracking "high-velocity thrusts" used by some practitioners to the relatively gentle approach adopted by supporters of the McTimoney method and its derivative McTimoney-Corley therapy.

The main difference between osteopathy and chiropractic is that osteopaths consider the main effect of their treatment is on the blood supply, while chiropractors believe the nerves are the important element. Conventional chiropractic is also generally more vigorous than osteopathy, and its practitioners are somewhat more conventionally "medical" in approach, including the use of x-rays in diagnosis. (See also "Alexander technique," page 135, "Massage," pages 128–129.)

Chiropractic is effective for aches and pains due to headaches, neck and back strain, poor posture, sciatica, and asthma.

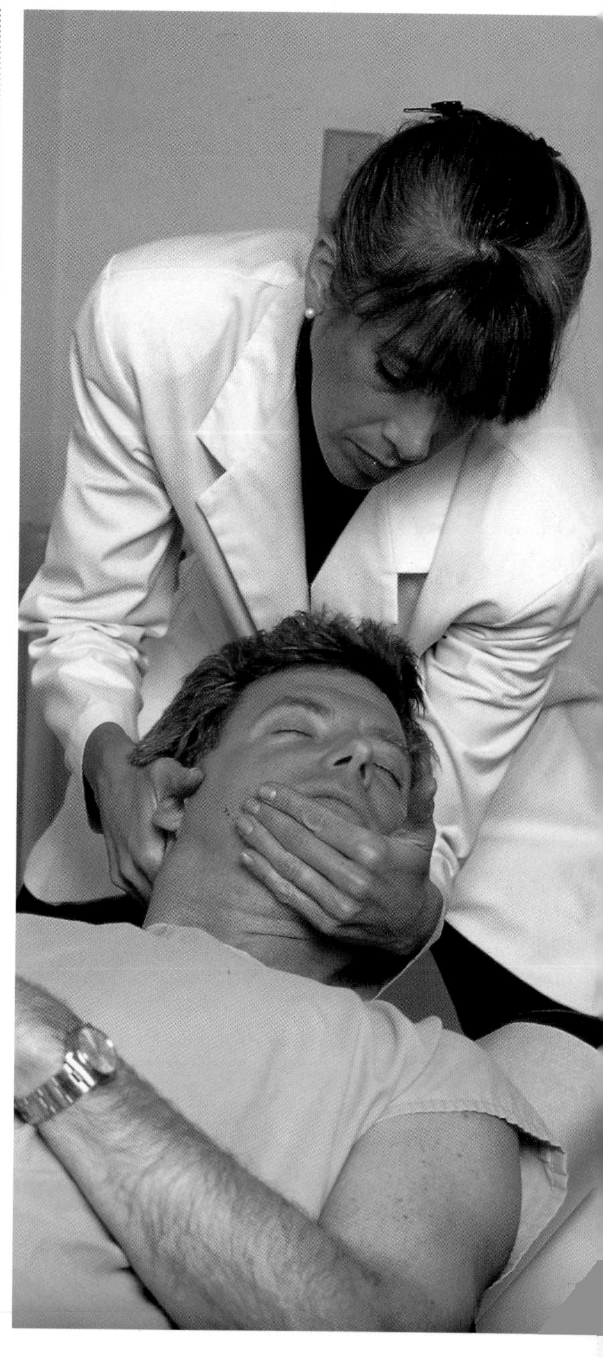

A chiropractor manipulates a patient's neck to help with a problem of the spine. Techniques such as this require lengthy training and great care and should never be attempted by anyone untrained.

OSTEOPATHY

Osteopathy—the word means "bone treatment"—is not just treatment for bones and bad backs, even though it is best known for that. Osteopathy works to improve the overall structure of the body, and its practitioners claim that it can benefit almost any disorder, including pain, by manipulation of the bones, muscles, and the so-called "soft tissues" of the body.

Like chiropractic, osteopathy began in the United States more than 100 years ago, and is today so established there that its practitioners are all conventional doctors with extra training in manipulation. Outside the US, osteopaths are generally not doctors, and train in special colleges. Though the better colleges teach many of the same things as medical schools, they put greater emphasis on naturopathic techniques, such as diet, nutrition, and allergy-testing—all of which can be useful in the treatment of pain (see also "Naturopathy," pages 116–117).

Osteopathy is effective for aches and pains due to headaches, sinusitis, jaw strain, poor posture, fibromyalgia, repetitive strain injury, sciatica, neck pain, back strain, rheumatoid arthritis, joint sprains, breathing difficulties, asthma, digestive problems, infection, and childbirth.

CRANIAL OSTEOPATHY

Cranial osteopathy, and its latest variation known as cranio-sacral therapy, is a method of "balancing" the body by the very gentlest manipulation of the bones—of the head especially, and also, to some extent, the spine. The bones of the head and spine are attached to the central nervous system and surrounded by a fluid (known as the cerebro-spinal fluid), and the belief is that if the passage of this fluid becomes blocked for any reason, physical or emotional "dis-ease" occurs. By placing the hands lightly on the patient's head, and using the softest pressure, the therapist aims gently to release these restrictions and restore balance and proper function to the body.

Cranial osteopathy originally developed in the United States and is said to be especially beneficial for children and babies, if performed by properly trained therapists. (See also "Alexander technique," page 135, "Massage," pages 128–129.)

Cranial osteopathy is effective for aches and pains due to headaches, concussion after-effects, sinusitis, jaw problems, tinnitus, meningitis, recurring infections, neck and back strain, postnatal strain, and, in infants, colic, glue ear, hyperactivity, and disturbed sleep.

HYPNOTHERAPY

Hypnotherapy (or hypnosis) is a unique approach to dealing with problems by helping people connect at a deeply unconscious or subconscious level with the mental or emotional states that may underlie them. This is normally done by a therapist inducing a state of deep relaxation to help a person "get in touch with" the cause or causes of the distress, or to imagine ways in which they could cope more easily. Once the cause or causes are known—a childhood trauma, for example—it may be easier to deal with it consciously through counseling or psychotherapy. That is why some hypnotherapists are also psychotherapists.

Hypnotherapy is also a way of learning to relax deeply. The many "subliminal" tapes and CDs now on the market use a form of hypnosis to aid relaxation—though some therapists have voiced concerns about the safety of such products.

Hypnosis is a very old therapy, known to native shamans in most cultures throughout the world, but its use in the West has been tarnished by the antics of stage hypnotists since the 19th century. Despite this, hypnotherapy is a genuinely helpful therapeutic technique that is now not only well researched but in increasing use by doctors everywhere.

CAUTION Hypnotherapy is a very powerful form of therapy, and clearly open to abuse, so it is important to check out a therapist thoroughly before agreeing to treatment. The best way is to verify that he or she is registered with a recognized professional organization.

Hypnotherapy is effective for aches and pains due to mental and emotional problems of all kinds, especially depression, phobias, addictions, and obsessions, along with the physical pain, such as headaches, neck and back ache, and digestive and breathing problems, they can sometimes bring.

COUNSELING AND PSYCHOTHERAPY

In simplest terms, psychotherapy and counseling are "talking" therapies. As the description implies, talking therapies generally encourage sitting quietly and talking about yourself and your problems to a trained and experienced listener, who will help you express your feelings, find insights, and see solutions for yourself. In most western countries it is increasingly common to find professional counselors and psychotherapists at health centers and clinics.

COUNSELING

Counseling has become such a well-organized, regulated, and widespread therapy that it is no longer considered unconventional, as it once was. Safe and gentle, counseling is an important and effective way of helping many people cope with major periods of stress and strain, including occasional consequences of extreme psychological as well as physical pain due, for example, to a failed relationship, redundancy, debt, or a sense of sexual inadequacy.

PSYCHOTHERAPY

Like regular counseling, psychotherapy is a method of allowing people to talk through emotional and mental problems, and receive support and guidance for them. Psychotherapy, though, goes much further, tackling the deeper, often hidden, underlying causes of illness by trying to get people to understand and face up to psychological problems within themselves. This can be done either on an individual basis or as part of a group.

Since its start at the beginning of the 20th century, with pioneers such as Freud, Jung, and Reich, psychotherapy has developed a wide spectrum of activity, covering almost every type and style of approach, from the complex (psychoanalysis) to the down-to-earth (laughter therapy). Examples you are likely to come across include co-counseling (or re-evaluation counseling), encounter therapy, Gestalt therapy, humanistic psychology, Jungian or analytical psychology, bioenergetics, psychoanalysis (Freudian psychotherapy), Rogerian therapy, psychosynthesis, transpersonal psychology, transactional analysis, and cognitive therapy.

Therapists—and they include growing numbers of doctors nowadays—who specialize in any of these methods tend to be familiar with most others, and so can guide someone to the right approach if they cannot help that person themselves. (See also "Relaxation therapies," pages 136–139, "Self-hypnosis," page 136, "Creative arts therapies," pages 140–141.)

Counseling and psychotherapy are effective for mental and emotional pain of all kinds, especially depression, phobias, addictions, and obsessions, in addition to the physical pain, such as headaches, neck and back ache, and digestive and breathing problems, they can sometimes cause.

A group psychotherapy session in progress. Psychotherapy does not have to be done in groups and therapy can be just as effective on a one-to-one basis.

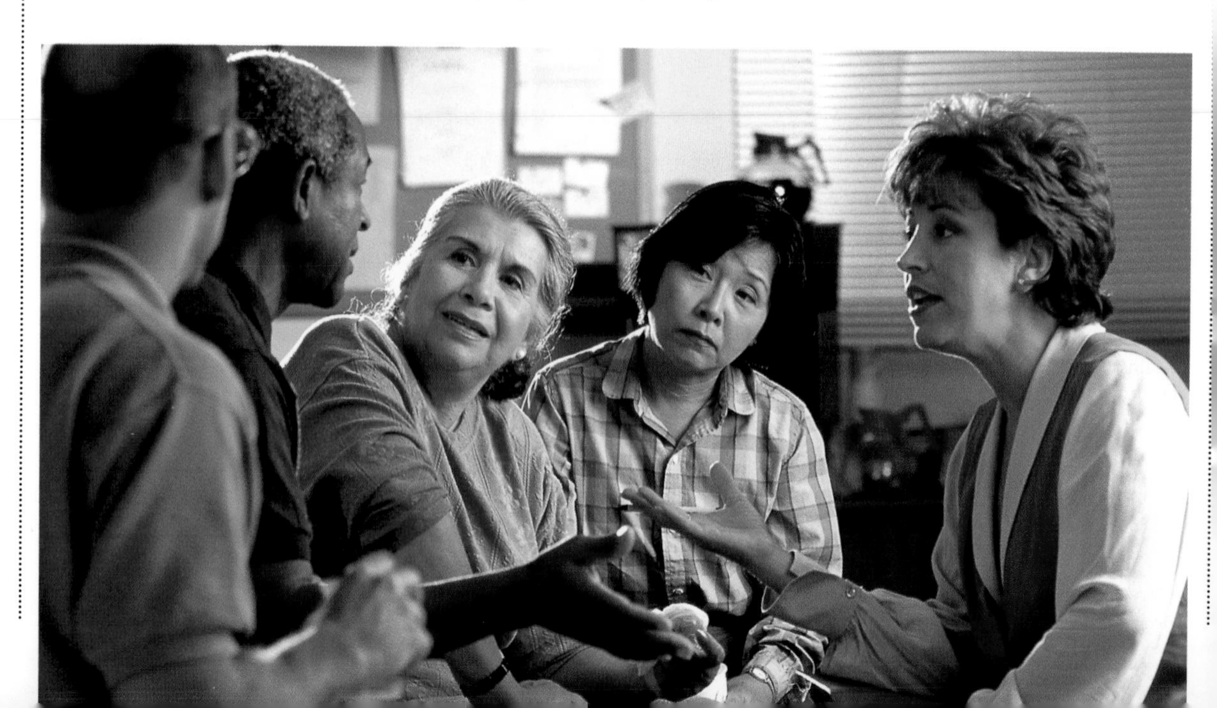

APPENDIX

Bibliography

Acupressure, Carola Beresford-Cooke (Macmillan, USA, 1996)

Alternative Medicine—The Definitive Guide, ed. Burton Goldberg (Future Medicine Publishing, USA, 1994)

Aromatherapy, Anna Selby (Macmillan, USA, 1996)

The Book of Pain Relief, Leon Chaitow (Thorsons, UK, 1993)

The Complete Family Guide to Alternative Medicine, ed. Richard Thomas (Element Books, USA, 1996)

The Complete Illustrated Guide to Reflexology, Inge Dougans (Element Books, UK, 1996)

The Complete Yoga Course, Howard Kent (Headline Press, UK, 1993)

Coping Successfully with Pain, Neville Shone (Sheldon Press, UK, 1995)

Dr. Amarnick's Pain Relief Program, Claude Amarnick (Garrett Publishing, USA, 1995)

Drug-free Pain Relief, George T. Lewith & Sandra Horn (Thorsons, UK, 1987)

Family Guide to Natural Medicine, ed. Patrick Pietroni (Reader's Digest, USA, 1993)

Herbal Remedies, Tamara Kircher & Penny Lowery (Macmillan, USA, 1996)

How to Conquer Pain, Vernon Coleman (European Medical Journal, UK, 1994)

Miracles Do Happen, C. Norman Shealy (Element Books, USA, 1995)

Natural Pain Relief, Jan Sadler (Element Books, UK, 1997)

The Natural Way series, ed. Richard Thomas (Element Books, UK, 1994–96)

The Nature Doctor, H.C.A. Vogel (Mainstream Publishing, UK, 1990)

The Pain Relief Handbook, Chris Wells & Graham Nown (Vermilion, UK, 1993)

The Radical Home Doctor, Lynne McTaggart (Wallace Press, UK, 1995)

Tai Chi, Paul Crompton (Macmillan, USA, 1996)

You Don't Have to Feel Unwell, Robin Needes (Gateway Books, UK, 1994)

Useful addresses

American Holistic Medical Association
6728 Old McLean Village Drive,
McLean VA 22101, United States

National Center for Homeopathy
801 N. Fairfax Street, No. 306,
Alexandria VA 22314, United States

Office of Alternative Medicine
9000 Rockville Pike, Building 31,
Room 5B–38, Bethesda MD 20892,
United States

Canadian College of Naturopathic Medicine
2300 Yonge Street, 18th floor,
PO Box 2431, Toronto M4P 1E4,
Canada

Canadian Holistic Medical Association
42 Redpath Avenue, Toronto,
Ontario M4S 2J6, Canada

Canadian Natural Health Association
439 Wellington Street, Toronto
Ontario M5V 2H7, Canada

Australian Medical Faculty of Homeopathy
49 Cecil Street, Denistone East,
NSW, Australia

Australian Traditional Medicine Society
27 Bank Street, Meadowbank,
NSW, Australia

National Herbalists Association
Suite 305, BST House, 3 Smail Street,
Broadway NSW 2007, Australia

British Homeopathic Association
27A Devonshire Street, London
W1N 1RJ, United Kingdom

Council for Complementary and Alternative Medicine
Suite D, Park House, 206–208 Latimer
Road, London W10, United Kingdom

Register of Complementary Practitioners
PO Box 194, London SE16 1QZ,
United Kingdom

Finding a therapist

The emphasis in this book is on self-help remedies. However, before embarking on a course of self-help, we strongly recommend that you first establish contact with a therapist or teacher who can explain and demonstrate the finer points of each particular therapy. After this, you can continue on your own.

To find a suitable therapist, the best answer is a personal recommendation from someone you can trust to give good advice. Or, you can seek advice from your doctor's office or local health center. If local effots fail, try contacting a national organization for advice (see left). Even if they cannot help you themselves, they may at least be able to point you in the right direction.

Courses

Nowadays, it is possible to study a wide range of natural therapies on courses that lead to nationally recognized qualifications. Below are a few examples of institutions where such courses are available.

National College of Naturopathic Medicine
11231 S.E. Market Street, Portland
OR 97216, United States

The Dominion Herbal College
7527 Kingsway, Burnaby, British
Columbia V3N 3C1, Canada

Australasian College of Natural Therapies
56 Foveaux St, PO Box K1356
Haymarket 1240, Surry Hills,
NSW 2012, Australia

Australian College of Natural Medicine
362 Water Street, Fortitude Valley
QLD 4007, Australia

Middlesex University
Queensway, Enfield, Middlesex
EN3 4SF, United Kingdom

INDEX